The Princeton Review®

Cracking the Nursing School Entrance Exams

Kristen Marie Haight, RN, MS, CPNP-PC
and the Staff of The Princeton Review

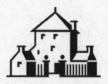

Random House, Inc. New York

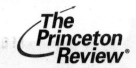

The Princeton Review, Inc.
111 Speen Street, Suite 550
Framingham, MA 01701
E-mail: editorialsupport@review.com
1-800-2-Review

NLN PAX-RN is produced by the National League for Nursing.
TEAS is produced by the Assessment Technologies Institute ™ LLC.
NET is produced by Educational Resources, Inc.

ISBN: 978-0-375-42742-8
ISSN: 2161-5462

Editor: Selena Coppock
Production Editor: Kathy G. Carter
Production Coordinator: Deborah A. Silvestrini

Printed in the United States of America on partially recycled paper.

10 9 8 7 6 5 4 3 2 1

2012 Edition

Editorial

Rob Franek, VP Test Prep Books, Publisher

Seamus Mullarkey, Editorial Director

Laura Braswell, Senior Editor

Selena Coppock, Editor

Random House Publishing Team

Tom Russell, Publisher

Nicole Benhabib, Publishing Manager

Ellen L. Reed, Production Manager

Alison Stoltzfus, Associate Managing Editor

ACKNOWLEDGEMENTS

I am honored to have worked with and written among the talented, the unseen and often hidden, mysterious persons behind the high ceilings and great big revolving glass doors welcoming the daunting Madison Avenue entrance of The Princeton Review. I am most grateful to Selena Coppock, my editor, comic relief, and friendly resource—without whose expertise and wit, this project could not have come to fruition. Many thanks to Calvin Cato for using words, *literally*, to express the mathematical certainty of geometric rules applied to circles, swimming pools, and sundecks. Thank you, Seamus Mullarkey and TPR staff, for welcoming me and coffee-visitation at any hour, any day, and for unconditional moral support behind the scenes. Kudos are in order for our off-site team members at Random House and Penn Foster.

Great big thanks to my parents, loving family, and friends. I would not have had the talent or innate tools if it were not for my gifted parents: teacher, writer, artist, and columnist, Louise D. Haight; and teacher, science guru extraordinaire, Rev. Peter RC Haight. Thank you, Daddy, for helping me remember what you taught years ago and for putting up with many questions and double-checking my work for *all* those hours, *all* those pages, *all* those evenings. Thank you family and friends for understanding where I had to be during the time-consuming production and completion of this book.

Special thanks to just some of the people who had given me inspiration and guidance during the earlier years of my nursing profession as well as the friendships, support, and counsel added, found abundantly through the present: Florence Nightingale; Dr. Dorothea Orem, RN; Martha Rogers RN, PhD; Dr. Felix Bocchino; Mrs. Mary Jane Reardon, RN; my grandparents: Alfred and Theresa Dellamarco, and grandmother: Gertrude E. Haight, LPN; Aunt Lizzie Donato, RN; Aunt Cathy Dellamarco, LPN; Mary Dwyer, RN; Cyndi Mallon, RN; Debbie Mitchell, RN; Ann Aurigemma, RN, CPNP; Nidia Ortiz, RN, CPNP; Sarla Santos RN, CNS; Cary Berwald, MD; Jessica Orbe, MD; Marguerite Aglialoro; Phyllis Marchitelli, RN; Manuel P. Santos, MD; and Monika Symms, MD.

I am grateful to the many patients and families who have been entrusted to my care over the years and those who have inspired me to continue and for the little *and not so little* angels who watch afar from clouds above. For obvious reasons, your names cannot be mentioned, but know you are and will always have a special place in my heart.

CONTENTS

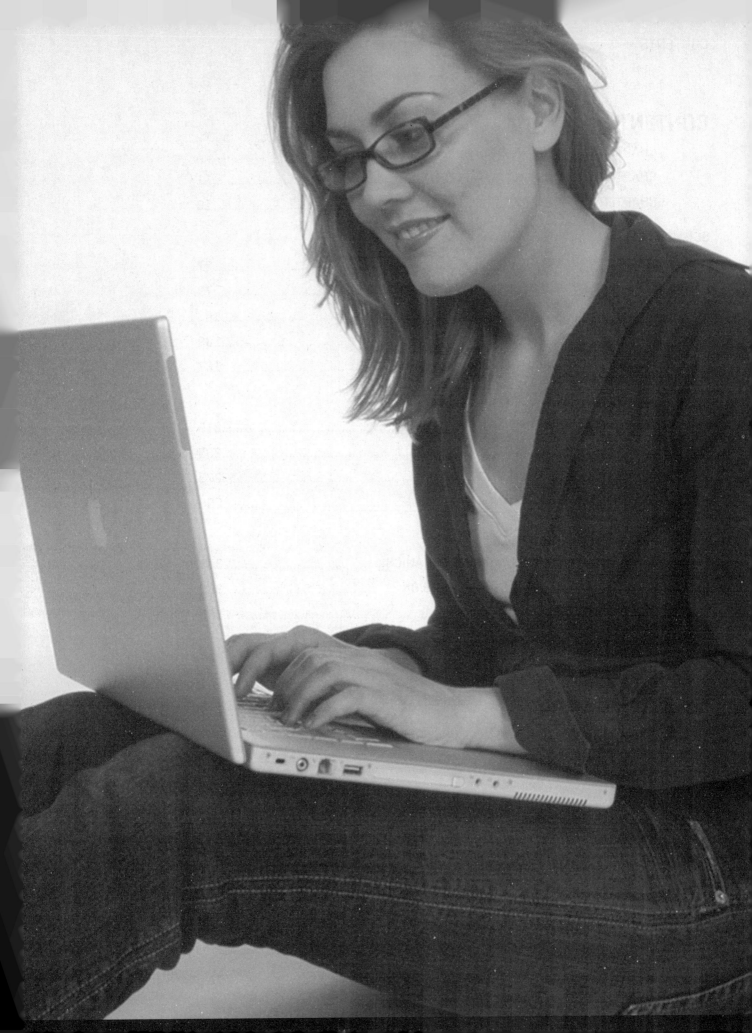

...So Much More Online!

More Practice...

- Practice your NLN PAX-RN, NET, TEAS test-taking skills.

- Access three full-length practice exams: one NLN PAX-RN, one NET, one TEAS

- Work through the chapters and Cracking drills in this book, focusing on the sections where you need specific review.

- Then take the practice test for your chosen exam.

- Go back and review any sections where you still need work.

- Then, prepare to tackle your nursing school entrance exam with skill and ease!

Register Your Book Now...

- Go to PrincetonReview.com/cracking

- You'll see a welcome page where you should use the ISBN to register your book. The ISBN for *Cracking the Nursing School Entrance Exams* is 9780375427428.

- You will then see a page where you can make an account with PrincetonReview. com so that future log-ins will be a breeze.

- Now you're good to go!

Look For These Icons Throughout The Book

 Go Online   More Great Books

Chapter 1
Getting Started

Congratulations on purchasing The Princeton Review's *Cracking the Nursing School Entrance Exams.* Preparing for this exam is an important step on the path to the career of nursing. We are here to help you prepare for that exam, be it the Nursing Entrance Test (NET), the National League for Nursing RN Pre-Admissions Exam (NLN PAX-RN), or the Test of Essential Academic Skills (TEAS). Different nursing schools require different exams and have unique scoring requirements, so each reader will have a specialized course and goal. We will introduce helpful test-taking strategies, lead you through a complete content review (covering science, math, and verbal skills), give you a list of the most important vocabulary you should know, and then conclude things with a few final pre-exam tips. Sounds like a lot to tackle, huh? So let's get moving!

WHAT IS THE PRINCETON REVIEW?

The Princeton Review is an international test-preparation company with branches in all major U.S. cities and several cities abroad. In 1981, John Katzman started teaching an SAT prep course in his parents' living room in New York City. Within five years, this course evolved into The Princeton Review, the largest SAT prep program in the country.

Our phenomenal success in improving students' scores on standardized tests is due to a simple, innovative, and radically effective philosophy: Study the exam, not just what the exam claims to test. This approach has lead to the development of techniques for taking standardized tests based on the principles the test writers themselves use to write the exams.

The Princeton Review has found that its methods work not just for cracking the SAT, but for any standardized test. We've already successfully applied our system to the GMAT, LSAT, MCAT, and GRE, to name a few. Obviously you need to be well versed in many subjects to do well on the NET, TEAS, or NLN PAX-RN, but you should remember that any standardized test is partly a measure of your ability to think like the people who write standardized tests. This book will help you prepare for the NET, TEAS, or NLN PAX-RN by using our detailed content review and applying test-taking strategies.

We offer books and online services that cover an enormous variety of education and career-related topics. If you're interested, check out our website at PrincetonReview.com.

THE NURSING ENTRANCE TEST (NET)

About the Test

The NET is a computer-based exam administered by Educational Resources, Inc. (www.eriworld.com). This exam has five sections: math, reading comprehension, stress level, social interaction, and learning style. The most important sections are the math and reading comprehension. Although the other three sections don't count toward your score, you must complete all five sections to receive a score.

The Breakdown

The math and reading sections are made up of multiple-choice questions, with four answer choices per question. You have 60 minutes to complete the math section, which is comprised of 60 questions. Educational Resources, Inc. says that the content is basic mathematics, which includes arithmetic and basic algebra. You have 30 minutes to complete the reading comprehension section, which is comprised of 25–35 multiple-choice questions. For the reading comprehension section, you will be given a passage of 100–200 words to read. The questions after the passage will ask you to identify the main idea of a passage, make inferences, tell the purpose of the passage, draw conclusions, and make predictions. Note that the NET doesn't have a science section. So if science is not your strong suit, this exam might be a good choice for you. (You should bone up on science during nursing school, though, as you will need it for the NCLEX-RN and your nursing career.) The three sections that don't count toward your score are stress level, social interaction, and learning style. The stress level section is a self-generated profile in which you explore the way you respond to stress in social settings and the workplace. The social interaction section includes questions about leadership style and social skills. In the learning style section, you must specify if you agree or disagree with the statements presented.

Here's a chart to give you a visual representation of the exam sections for which you can study and prepare:

Section of NET	Question Type	Number of Questions	Time	Content
Math	Multiple-choice, with four choices per question	60	60 minutes	• Arithmetic • Basic algebra
Reading Comprehension	Multiple-choice, with four choices per question	25–35	30 minutes	• Identifying the main ideas of a passage • Making inferences • Telling the purpose of a passage • Drawing conclusions from a passage • Making predictions

Scoring

The NET doesn't have a passing score—each nursing school decides the score range for admission to its institution. So do some research on your preferred school(s) to find what score you need to shoot for. You will receive separate scores for the reading comprehension and math sections. Statistics are used to compare you to other test takers to see where your score lands you on the range of scores.

Take a Look

Here are a few questions that are like those you might see on the NET.

Mary travels 50 miles on 2 gallons of gasoline. If she wants to travel 75 miles, how many gallons of gasoline will she need?

A. 1.5
B. 2
C. 3
D. 3.5

Here's How to Crack It

You can express this problem in the following proportion: $\frac{50}{2} = \frac{75}{x}$. Cross multiply to obtain $50x = 150$. Divide both sides by 50 to find the value of x. In this case, $x = 3$, so choice C is correct. To take another approach, you can think of it this way: If Mary travels 50 miles on 2 gallons of gas, she travels 25 miles on 1 gallon of gas. So 75 miles will take 3 gallons of gas, since 1 gallon of gas will take Mary 25 miles. Choices A and B are definitely wrong because she would need more gas to travel 75 miles than she would to travel 50 or fewer. Don't be fooled by choice D, which is close to the correct answer but not correct. Do your math carefully and you should have no problem.

Here's a passage and question like the ones you will see on the NET Reading Comprehension section.

Vegan diets or vegetarian diets include plant-based food for consumption. Vegans consume foods like vegetables, fruits, nuts, grains, seeds, and so on. In 1944, the term *vegan* was coined by Mr. Donald Watson, the co-founder of British Vegan Society in England. The American Dietetic Association claims that vegetarian diets may be more widespread among adolescents with eating disorders. But evidence suggests that the embracing of a vegetarian diet does not necessarily cause eating disorders, rather that "vegetarian diets may be selected to camouflage an existing eating disorder."

The risk factors associated with animal foods, detrimental impact of animal foods on health, religious adherences or beliefs, and the desire to safeguard animals are some of the factors leading to an upsurge in vegetarian diets. Vegan diets can be classified as follows:

- The vegan diet, which is only plant based, rejects meat and animal products.
- The lacto-vegetarian diet includes plant-based foods and dairy products such as cheese, yogurt, and so on.
- The lacto-ovo vegetarian diet includes plant-based foods, dairy products, and eggs.
- The flexitarian (semi-vegetarian) diet includes plant-based foods, with a moderate amount of fish and meat.

According to the passage, which of the following factors led to an upsurge in vegetarian diets around the world?

A. Celebrity promotion for vegan diets
B. The risks associated with animal foods
C. An increasing number of books on veganism
D. The scarcity of animal foods and food products

Here's How to Crack It

Choice B is correct because of the first sentence of paragraph 2, which lists the risks associated with animal foods as one of the reasons for the upsurge in vegetarian diets. The factors mentioned in other answer choices are not mentioned in the passage, so they must be incorrect.

THE TEST OF ESSENTIAL ACADEMIC SKILLS (TEAS)

About the Test

The TEAS is available as a paper-and-pencil exam or as a computer-based exam administered by the Assessment Technologies Institute (www.atitesting.com). The TEAS assesses basic knowledge of reading, math, science, and English/Language usage. Calculators are not allowed. The concepts tested on the TEAS are chosen because they test entry-level skills and knowledge of nursing program applicants.

The Breakdown

As just mentioned, the TEAS is divided into four sections: reading, math, science, and English/language usage. The entire test is made up of 170 multiple-choice questions that you must complete in 209 minutes. Here is the way these 170 questions are broken down:

- You must complete the 40 questions in the reading section in 50 minutes.
- You must complete the 45 questions in the math section in 56 minutes.
- You must complete the 30 questions in science in 38 minutes. This section covers high-school level biology, chemistry, human physiology, physics, and general science.
- You must complete the 55 questions in the English/language usage section in 65 minutes. This section covers grammar, spelling, punctuation, sentence structure, and vocabulary.

Here's all of the preceding information summarized in a chart:

Section of TEAS	Question Type	Number of Questions	Time	Content
Reading	Multiple-choice, with four choices per question	40	50 minutes	• Reading a passage or analyzing a graphic and then answering questions about the passage • Identifying the main idea • Drawing conclusions and inferences • Locating information • Applying conclusions to new information • Identifying the author's tone • Defining vocabulary in context • Following directions
Math	Multiple-choice, with four choices per question	45	56 minutes	• Numbers • Operations • Ratios and proportions • Fractions and percents • Basic algebra • Measurements • Graphs and diagrams.
Science	Multiple-choice, with four choices per question	30	38 minutes	High-school level sciences: • Biology • Chemistry • Human physiology • Physics • General science
English/ language usage	Multiple-choice, with four choices per question	55	65 minutes	• Grammar • Spelling • Punctuation • Sentence structure • Vocabulary in context

Scoring

If you take the TEAS, your results will be available 48 hours after completion of the test. You will receive a score for each of the four parts of the exam, as well as 16 subscores for specific content areas within those four sections. Like the NET, the TEAS doesn't have any official passing scores. Rather, nursing schools establish their own criteria for admission.

Take a Look

Here are a few questions that are similar to those you might see on the TEAS.

―――――――――○―――――――――

B cells form plasma cells. How does a plasma cell tag a virus for destruction?

A. By producing antibodies
B. By producing cytotoxic T-cells
C. By binding to the helper T-cells
D. By directly binding to the viral antigens

Here's How to Crack It

Choice A is the correct answer because plasma cells produce antibodies that bind to the antigens present over the virus. This tags the virus for destruction. Choice B is incorrect because plasma cells do not produce cytotoxic T-cells, nor do they bind to helper T-cells (choice C). Finally, choice D is wrong because plasma cells do not bind directly to the viral antigens. Plasma cells produce antibodies that bind to the antigens present over the virus.

―――――――――○―――――――――

Here's another one.

―――――――――○―――――――――

Biofuels are easily biodegradable and are safer to handle than traditional fuels, thus making spills less hazardous. Which one of the following words best describes *hazardous?*

A. Safe
B. Healthy
C. Manageable
D. Dangerous

Here's How to Crack It

You are probably already confident in your knowledge of the word *hazardous*, but let's assume you don't know what it means. Look carefully at the question where it says "safer to handle than traditional fuels." This phrase gives the clue to the meaning of *hazardous*. Choice D is the correct answer. Study that vocabulary!

―――――――――○―――――――――

THE NATIONAL LEAGUE FOR NURSING PRE-ADMISSIONS EXAM (NLN PAX-RN)

About the Test

The NLN PAX-RN is available only in paper-and-pencil format. It's administered by the National League for Nursing (www.nln.org). The NLN PAX-RN uses multiple-choice questions to assess verbal skills, mathematics ability, and science knowledge.

The Breakdown

The NLN PAX-RN is made up of 214 multiple-choice questions, and students have three hours to complete the exam. The verbal section includes 80 questions, which test both word knowledge and reading comprehension. You have 60 minutes to complete that section. The word knowledge questions are about vocabulary in context, and the reading comprehension passages are about 400–500 words, with associated questions. The math section is comprised of 54 questions which cover basic calculations, word problems, algebra, geometry, conversions, graphs, and applied math. You have 60 minutes to complete that section also and you may not take a calculator into the exam. The science section is comprised of 80 questions which cover general biology, chemistry, physics, and Earth science. You have 60 minutes to complete that section as well. So you have one hour per section, but not a consistent number of questions per section. Let's break it down in a chart.

Section of NLN PAX-RN	Question Type	Number of Questions	Time	Content
Verbal	Multiple-choice, with four choices per question	80	60 minutes	• Vocabulary (word knowledge) • Synonyms and antonyms • Reading comprehension
Math	Multiple-choice, with four choices per question	54	60 minutes	• Basic calculations • Word problems • Algebra • Geometry • Conversions • Graphs • Applied math
Science	Multiple-choice, with four choices per question	80	60 minutes	• General biology • Chemistry • Physics • Earth science

Scoring

Similar to the NET and the TEAS, the NLN PAX-RN doesn't have an official passing score. You will get a raw score for each section based on the number of questions you answer correctly. You will answer 214 questions, but your raw score is not based on 214 points. Only 160 of the questions you answer will actually be graded—the others are experimental questions. Since you don't know which questions are experimental and which are the real thing, work your hardest on all questions. The highest possible scores are

> Verbal: 60
> Math: 40
> Science: 60

You will receive a composite score that is a weighted combination of your three section scores. The composite score ranges from 0 to 200. You will also receive a percentile rank for each section and for the test as a whole, showing where you fall among other test takers. According to NLN data, percentiles ranging from about 40 to 60 are in the average for the exam.

Take a Look

Here are a few questions that are similar to those you might see on the NLN PAX-RN.

For clinical purposes, why are digital thermometers more commonly used than mercury thermometers?

A. Mercury thermometers are not accurate enough to be used for clinical purposes.
B. Digital thermometers are more environment-friendly and hazard-free.
C. Digital thermometers are more durable than mercury thermometers.
D. Mercury thermometers are more expensive than digital ones.

Here's How to Crack It

In your chemistry classes, you should have learned about the toxic nature of mercury (specifically its vapor). So choice B might look like a strong choice, but take a look at the other choices to be sure. Choice A must be incorrect because mercury thermometers are extremely accurate and are still used for careful measurement in the science world. Choice C is also incorrect because mercury thermometers are actually more durable, if used properly, than digital thermometers, but aren't very expensive (so choice D must also be wrong). Let's go back to choice B. Mercury vapor's toxicity means that it may pose environmental and health hazards. Go with choice B.

Here's another:

A man buys 12 two-ounce packs of soup for $14.40. If he now makes packs containing four cups of this soup, how much would each pack cost?

    A. $4.80
    B. $9.60
    C. $14.40
    D. $19.20

Here's How to Crack It

Unit conversion questions will definitely come up on your nursing school entrance exam, so be sure to brush up on your conversion. See our helpful conversion list on page 257 and the table on page 258. The first thing you should do to tackle this problem is convert ounces to cups. The man has 12 two-ounce packs of soup, so he has 24 ounces total, which converts to 3 cups (because 1 cup has 8 ounces). He bought this quantity for $14.40, so divide $14.40 by 3 to find out the cost per cup ($4.80). But you're not done yet, so don't fall for choice A. You need to calculate the cost of a pack that contains 4 cups of soup, so multiply $4.80 by 4 ($4.80 × 4 = $19.20). Choice D is correct.

MOVING ON

Now you have a clear idea of what you will see on the TEAS, NET, and NLN PAX-RN. Before we introduce test-taking strategies and jump into content review, let's explore nursing as a career.

> ### NSEE
> Throughout this book, you'll see the acronym NSEE (nursing school entrance exams). We use this term to refer to the TEAS, the NET, and the NLN PAX-RN as a group.

Chapter 2
Nursing as a Career

NURSING AS A CAREER

Perhaps you have always known that you would someday pursue the important career of nursing. Perhaps this is a second career and you have sought it later in life. Either way, you have made an exciting choice and are about to embark on a rewarding career path. With the current challenges and changes in health care, there is a demand for nurses and that demand isn't waning anytime soon. Schooling, training, and preparation will all be part of your journey to become a nurse. You want to help, and your patients need you! That's why you are here and that's why you are preparing for your nursing school entrance examination.

Congratulations on making it this far in your journey to become what many people consider an angel on Earth. You are on a path to become the voice for those who cannot speak for themselves, and an advocate for the lives, health, and well-being of others. Nurse, visionary, educator and mystic, Florence Nightingale put it beautifully: "Nursing is an art: and if it is to be made an art, it requires as exclusive a devotion, as hard a preparation, as any painter's or sculptor's work; for what is the having to do with dead canvas or dead marble, compared with having to do with the living body, the temple of God's spirit? It is one of the Fine Arts: I had almost said, the finest of Fine Arts."

Are you ready? Your shift is about to start.

A LOOK INTO YOUR FUTURE

You have prepared for your nursing school entrance exam with this Princeton Review book. You have applied for admission to one or more accredited schools, rearranged your life for the next four years, carefully created a disease-free environment (no time for sick visits), prepared roughly 4,383 meals (and frozen them), and purchased four years' worth of undergarments for the family (because there will be no spare time to cook or do laundry). You had a physical examination and rechecked your immunization status with titers. You filled up your Starbucks and Dunkin Donuts gallon coffee card and invested in Kleenex (with aloe). You were accepted into an accredited nursing program. You are 97 percent happy, and 3 percent scared (or maybe more like 60/40). Your family and friends are proud of you. You attend classes (day and night), you study (day and night), and you pass all your exams. You've written several term papers and care plans. You can now think like a nurse. Looking back, you see that some courses were more difficult than others. You learned that some things in life are very different than the way textbooks portray them, and life doesn't always follow the rules we were brought up to believe. People suffer unfairly and unjustly sometimes. And in between witnessing the happy moments of nursing, bad things happen and sometimes people die. But you learned, studied, absorbed, and applied. You made a difference and did your very best. You gave it your all. Wow. You graduated and are now a graduate nurse! (50 percent excited, 50 percent scared). You need a vacation, but you can't yet. Next stop: NCLEX review. You have to study for the NCLEX-RN in order to become an official registered nurse (RN). (Might we recommend a book? *Cracking the NCLEX-RN* from, who else, The Princeton Review.) You begin your exciting career as a nurse in a major teaching hospital setting, most often a medical-surgical unit, to gain the most experience. Some of you may go right into a specialty such as pediatrics, psychiatry, neonatology, or even critical care. You pass your RN exam and are now ready to undertake the greatest responsibility ever—caring for your patients: newborn to one hundred years old.

NURSES ARE IMPORTANT

Disease affects the mind, body, and spirit, and illness alters continuity of homeostasis. A change in one body system affects the rest of the body systems. When there is change or illness, there needs to be healing and regeneration, sometimes guidance, and oftentimes lifestyle modification. Change creates stress and disorder and affects the entire patient system (which includes everything that comes along with that patient system: the spouse, the ex, the new significant other, the ex-significant other, the parent, the child/children, the sibling, the neighbor, the neighbor's ride, and so on). It's a big feat to take on patient care and be mindful of the entire support system who will assist in patient care once the patient leaves the hospital. Factor in the addition of or change in medications or treatments and their related side-effects. Monitoring the patient and the associated treatment or medication can add stress and anxiety to both patient and family. Because of that, there is the need for patient education—hence, the nurse. Nurses will always be in demand.

BEING A NURSE

The Reality

Being a nurse is not at all taken from an episode of *Grey's Anatomy, Scrubs,* or even *St. Elsewhere.* There's no Luke and Laura happy ending in the world of nursing at a real General Hospital. There's just the reality of nursing and the daily responsibilities and tasks. Providing care as a nurse is not just carrying out doctors' orders, emptying out bedpans, and memorizing algorithms for cardiac arrests. It should be providing life-saving care and comfort, while working in collaboration with other health care professionals for the good of the patient. Providing top-notch nursing care means looking at the bigger picture, while using your foundation: the nursing fundamentals. Drawing from your experience, knowledge, skill, and theoretical framework while applying critical thinking to every decision made. It means checking medication dosages (twice), knowing the side effects and how to recognize them, understanding how to intervene when side effects happen, knowing what drugs interact with others, and being able to identify which drugs will cross the blood brain barrier. It means managing emergency situations and facilitating an urgent admission for a septic child, hanging chemotherapy, monitoring for extravasations, adjusting bicarbonate drips, dipping urines, taking vital signs (and interpreting them), assisting a spinal tap, feeding an infant, changing a pain patch, giving morphine to a terminally ill patient, timing a seizure, assisting a cardiac arrest situation, documenting your assessments, taking blood for analysis, hanging antibiotics in triple form, hanging blood for transfusions, intervening when there is a blood transfusion reaction, interpreting blood gases, paging residents to give them the blood gas results, managing a ventilator machine, changing central line dressings, preparing IV solution bags and rapidly infusing colloids, intervening when you believe your patient is having a stroke, obtaining an EKG, placing an IV line (sometimes twice), helping a new mother breast feed, consoling a grieving family, and even wheeling or carrying a deceased patient to the morgue—all in a day's work. There's no closet McDreamy smooching or cafeteria proposals—it's life and a remarkable career.

It takes a special person to be a nurse. Nurses don't leave their inner nurse behind at the hospital when the shift is over. Nurses assist at the scenes of motor vehicle crashes, tend to people collapsed in restaurants, respond to incidents on airplanes, and help little kids when they are injured in parks. Nurses are always on duty. That's why we often hear: "Ask Kristen, she's a nurse, she will tell you what to do," or "Call Jake, he's a nurse, he can explain it to you." Be careful to maintain boundaries and be mindful of burnout.

Patient Advocacy

Being a nurse means being an aggressive patient advocate, too. Your professional nursing role might be assisting in the miracle of birth, working in the delivery room as the newborn baby is passed into your arms. Nurses and proper nursing interventions can assist in birth and throughout life, to keep patients alive and healthy. Or sadly, when disease cannot be fought any longer or even after a horrible accident, your role will be to prepare and honor the dead by assisting with family grieving and preparation for burial. The nurse might be asked to bathe the patient one last time and remove breathing tubes, machines, wires, sutures, lines, IVs, catheters, dressings, and remnants of hospitalization. Your nursing interventions can save a life, just as a decrease in nursing acuity, skill, or care can contribute to the loss of a life. Nurses can help patients become healthier (keeping in mind different belief systems, social mores, disabilities, barriers in communication, and cultural differences). Nurses who are skilled at keeping patients free from pain, minimizing suffering, and ensuring safety will always be noticed. Patient care and patient prioritization is not a job for the faint of heart. The most effective nurses have an equal balance of brain and heart. They can stack 'em, pack 'em, and rack 'em in the emergency rooms, but once on the floors they want to get 'em healthy, happy, whole, and on a road to go home. That is just one of many mantras said by nurses. Nurses are trained to think strategically, beyond the care plan for the day, and to always expect the unexpected. On the day of admission, nurses are already planning for the anticipated discharge and everything between today and that day. The nursing process is quite a process!

Patient Privacy

Part of a nurse's job is to assist the patient through his or her time of need, then preserve the privacy of that patient. This is of utmost importance, as nurses are privy to extremely personal and private information about their patients. In 1996, the U.S. Congress enacted the **Health Insurance Portability and Accountability Act (HIPAA)**, which, among other things, outlines clear privacy and security rules for the health care industry. The Privacy Rule of HIPAA establishes regulations for the use and disclosure of protected health information (PHI). An individual's medical records and payment history are considered protected health information, and thus these items are to be protected by the Privacy Rule of HIPAA.

A nurse or caretaker who is in violation of a patient's right to privacy or who is disseminating a patient's protected health information is engaging in what is called an **invasion of privacy** and **intrusion of solitude**. Those are serious **criminal torts** in the legal system and allow the victim (person violated) to seek justice through the legal system on both the federal and civil levels. Known HIPAA violators will have charges brought against them as a person and as a professional with the **State Office of Professional Discipline**. The offending person may lose his or her license, be fined a large sum of money (depending on the maliciousness of her or his acts), and may even serve time in jail. Equally, the institution (hospital, nursing department, doctor's office, and so on) is liable as well. In addition to the HIPAA violator, another guilty party would be the person in a nursing leadership role who refuses to investigate a legitimate verbal and written complaint by a patient. She or he will face equally harsh HIPAA law violation charges, as the obligation to investigate was neglected.

As a nurse, you are responsible to report abuse, neglect, and harassment, not just with children and local protective services, but with adult patients, too. Abuse can occur in the nursing profession, just like anywhere else, unfortunately. If you have something happen to you, or if you hear something suspicious or witness something inappropriate, you are morally and professionally obligated to communicate your concern to the appropriate higher-ups. And if you get nowhere, communicate to the next appropriate higher level. Be an aggressive patient advocate and advocate for your rights as well.

CAREER PATHS IN NURSING

Let's explore what you can do as a nurse. There are many pathways that you can take and specialties that you can pursue.

Many Types of Positions

You might love the idea of working in a large teaching facility or medical center, or perhaps you would prefer work in a smaller town hospital. You may have interest in an inner city hospital, a school-based clinic, or a burn center. There are full-time, part-time, and locum tenens positions available. (A locum tenens employee fills in for a full-time employee who must be off work for a period of time.) Nursing shifts can be days, evenings, nights, and days with rotation to nights. Most hospitals offer 8-hour, 10-hour, and 12-hour shifts. As you can see, there are many options across an assortment of career specialties, schedules, and shifts.

Nursing Opportunities Within a Hospital and Outside a Hospital

Within a hospital, there are many in-patient units and departments. As a nurse, there are myriad departments where you can work: emergency room, radiology suite, nuclear medicine departments, MRI department, rehab units (pediatric or adult), pre-surgical testing suite, out-patient lab, blood donor room and/or blood bank, operating room, recovery room, critical care (pediatric or adult), step-down unit, telemetry, geriatrics/eldercare department, coronary care unit, stroke unit, short stay post-op unit, maternity ward, labor and delivery, post-partum, newborn nursery, special care nursery, neonatal intensive care unit (NICU), general pediatrics, pediatric intensive care unit (PICU), medicine units, psychiatry, general surgery, oncology, oncologic surgery, hematology-oncology, and transplant units. Phew! But wait—there's more.

Some hospitals also employ nurses as lactation consultants, child birth advocates, sign language interpreters, foreign language interpreters, infusion therapy specialists, and wound care specialists. There are ambulatory surgical suites with recovery rooms and out-patient offices and clinics, including primary care (pediatric and adult), pulmonary, ob-gyn, high-risk obstetrics, infertility, specialties such as neurology (pediatric and adult), ophthalmology (pediatric and adult), psychiatry (adolescent and adult), neuro-psychology (pediatric and adult), dermatology (pediatric and adult), and oncology (pediatric and adult). Each of these specialties might have subspecialties within that include dermatologic, urologic, breast, hematologic—all of whom need RNs (registered nurses).

Other out-patient clinic practices include radiology, plastics, reconstructive surgery, neurosurgery, spine and orthopedic, bariatric, gastroenterology (GI), genitourinary (GU), minimally invasive urologic units (MIUU), endocrine, renal, nephrology, and hematology. Nurses can assume transport roles, IV team roles, and phlebotomy roles both in the hospital as well as in out-patient lab settings. If you feel inspired to work with addiction, many drug and alcohol rehabilitation centers and clinics hire on-site nurses. There are specialists who work in private office settings, too. Surgical nurse coordinators are used in both in- and out-patient settings. Hospitals and clinics utilize infection control nurses due to the ongoing rising infection rates from poor provider hygiene and resistant bacteria strains. Out-patient cardiac rehab-exercise physiology suites need nurses on site, as well as vascular suites where minor sclerotherapy injections and microphlebectomies are performed. Believe it or not, a nurse who pursues medical aesthetics education and training can eventually administer Botox, perform dermal fillers, and do micro dermabrasion in medi-spas (and on cruise ships!). There are endless possibilities.

Nursing Opportunities in Education

If bedside or floor nursing isn't of interest to you, you can consider going into an educational role. There are positions as a nurse educator, diabetes educator, and heart health educator in hospitals, in out-patient facilities, or through community agencies. You can be an administrator, manager, or assistant nurse manager in a hospital, an ambulatory center, or private office. There are nursing opportunities in correctional facilities (juvenile or adult), hospice centers, palliative services, and visiting nurse services, as well as nurse-staff recruiter positions.

As far as employment opportunities completely outside of a hospital, you can teach in a nursing school or other academic setting. You can volunteer as a Red Cross nurse. You can work in a school-based clinic in an elementary school, a secondary school, a high school, or a college setting. You can become a traveling nurse and take 4–12 week assignments and travel the world. (Travel nurse positions are neat because your travel is reimbursed and housing is provided for you.) You can be a nurse overseas in a military or non-military setting. You can work for your local Department of Health or the Center for Disease Control. Pharmaceutical, nutritional, and medical device companies are enthusiastic about hiring RNs to represent their products and educate their clients.

Nursing Opportunities in Law and Compliance

Nurses can go on into the legal world, too! Perhaps you aren't familiar with such positions as a nurse paralegal, a nurse expert, or a medical legal nurse consultant. With a computer background, a nurse can easily assume the role of an IT specialist and educate staff on computer charting (as hospitals are increasingly moving away from paper charts and toward computerized charts). That job highlights yet another employment opportunity—a nurse compliance officer.

Earlier in this chapter, we discussed HIPAA laws in relation to patient privacy and the obligation of an assisting nurse to preserve that privacy. Let's briefly talk HIPAA in relation to nursing opportunities. Patients have a right to privacy. Violating a patient's privacy right is a federal crime punishable by law in both the civil and federal court systems. HIPAA laws and hospital codes of conduct are intended to protect patients and hospital employees from intrusive individuals who illegally obtain private health information. The role of the nurse compliance officer (and the nurse hospital administrator) is to be vigilant in attempting to prevent this type of atrocity from ever happening, and to formally investigate any complaints within a specific time frame. It's an extremely important job within the health care industry.

Other Nursing Opportunities

Risk mangers/quality assurance specialist positions (in hospitals or out-patient facilities) are often filled by registered nurses. The responsibilities in these positions include investigating complaints, concerns, risks, infection rates, morbidity and mortality rates, falls, fatalities, and planning performance improvement modules for staff. Managing this information helps facilities prepare for Joint Commission surveys and surprise visits from the Department of Health, so that they can remain operational and in good standing. Nurses can act as mock survey consultants and serve on Joint Commission Boards. Case mangers for hospitals, agencies, and insurance companies are oftentimes nurses, also. Insurance companies often hire nurses to administer physicals and blood and urine tests for potential new policyholders. Medical research foundations, foster care agencies, child protective services, paramedicine, homecare agencies, nursing homes, assisted living centers, sub-acute care centers, nonprofit organizations, and crisis centers—all need nurses. Some nurses enjoy policy and procedure issues and advocacy and fare well as organizational leaders and lobbyists, nurse association liaisons, or department chairs with the State Licensing Board and the Office of Professional Disciplines.

Nursing Opportunities with a Master's Degree

Once you become a registered nurse, whether you obtained your bachelor's (BSN) or associate (AAS) degree, you will have to get a master's degree if you want to become a nurse practitioner, a clinical nurse specialist, or a nurse administrator. Programs that lead to a master's degree are offered in a variety of settings and there are myriad health-related, specialty, and business tracks from which to choose.

First things first, though—nursing school. Let's dive into the content review for your nursing school entrance exam. We'll introduce some helpful test-taking strategies for you to utilize, whether you're tackling the NET, TEAS, or NLN PAX-RN. Then we'll jump into content review to brush up your knowledge of key science, math, and verbal concepts.

KEY TERMS

Health Insurance Portability and Accountability Act (HIPAA)
invasion of privacy
intrusion of solitude
criminal torts
State Office of Professional Discipline

Chapter 3
General Strategies

USING THE PRINCETON REVIEW APPROACH TO CRACK THE SYSTEM

At The Princeton Review, we teach effective test-taking strategies for you to crack the test, be it the TEAS, NET, NLN PAX-RN, or any other exam. The score that you achieve on a standardized test isn't a reflection of your intelligence—it's a reflection only of how well you take that test. So we're going to give you tons of strategies to help you tally up as many points as you possibly can. Many of our strategies are based on common sense—for example, using mnemonics such as "ROY G. BIV." (Remember that one? It's the mnemonic for red, orange, yellow, green, blue, indigo, violet—the colors of the visible spectrum.) Others are not so common-sensical. In fact, we're going to ask you to throw out much of what you've been taught when it comes to taking standardized tests.

There are seven strategies that we'll ask you to apply come test time:

- Strategy 1: Pacing Yourself
- Strategy 2: Applying the Three-Pass System
- Strategy 3: Using Process of Elimination (POE)
- Strategy 4: Aggressive Guessing
- Strategy 5: Word Associations
- Strategy 6: Mnemonics
- Strategy 7: Ballparking

Let's take a look at these strategies of The Princeton Review.

Strategy 1: Pacing Yourself

When you used to take tests in school, how many questions would you answer? Naturally, you would try to answer all of them. You would do this for two reasons: (1) Your teacher told you to, and (2) if you left a question blank, your teacher would mark it wrong. However, that's not necessarily the case for the exam that you are going to take for nursing school admission.

One of the reasons that taking tests is so stressful is the time constraint, which determines how much time you have for each question. For the NLN PAX-RN, you have 3 hours (180 minutes) to complete 214 questions, which breaks down to less than one minute per question. Yikes. For the NET, you have about one minute per question, and for the TEAS, you have just a bit more than a minute to complete each question. Gee, thanks. If you had all day to complete your exam, you would probably ace it. We can't give you all day, but we can do the next best thing: encourage you to slow down and scoop up points methodically.

Slowing down and selecting which questions you will answer is the best way to improve your score. Rushing through questions in order to finish will always hurt your score. When you rush, you're far more likely to make careless errors, misread, and fall into traps. Keep an eye on the clock (or an eye on your watch) to be sure that you are moving along and not getting stuck on particularly difficult problems. This strategy is a perfect lead-in for our next strategy.

Strategy 2: Applying the Three-Pass System

We're going to encourage you to do something that might seem counterproductive: Skip the most difficult questions.

The TEAS, NET, and NLN PAX-RN cover a wide range of topics. There's no way, even with our extensive review, that you will know everything about every topic presented on your exam. So what should you do?

Do the Easiest Questions First

If you can skip around on your exam, you will definitely want to do that. The best way to rack up points is to focus on the easiest questions first. Many of the questions on the test are straightforward and require little effort. If you know the answer, nail it and move on. Other questions, however, are not presented in such a clear, simple way. Therefore, as you read each question, decide if it's easy, medium, or hard. During a first pass, do all the easy questions. If you come across a problem that seems time-consuming or completely incomprehensible, skip it. *Remember:* Easier questions count just as much as harder ones, so your time is better spent on shorter, easier questions.

Save the medium questions for the second pass. These questions may be time-consuming, or they may require that you analyze all of the answer choices (that is, the correct answer doesn't pop off the page or screen).

If you come across a question that makes no sense from the outset, save it for the last pass. You're far less likely to fall into a trap or settle on a silly answer if you wait until the end to do these difficult questions.

Watch Out for Those Bubbles!

If your exam is a written exam (as opposed to a computer-based exam), you can easily skip around, but you must be careful not to make mistakes when bubbling in your answers. One way to accomplish this is by answering all of the questions on a page and then transferring your choices to the answer sheet. If you prefer to enter the answers one by one, make sure that you double-check the numbers beside the ovals before filling them in. We'd hate to see you lose points because you filled it in for the wrong question.

So then, what about the questions that you don't skip?

Strategy 3: Using Process of Elimination (POE)

On most tests, you need to know the material backward and forward to get the right answer. In other words, if you don't know the answers beforehand, you probably won't answer the questions correctly. This concept is particularly true for fill-in-the-blank and essay questions. You've probably been taught to think that the only way to get a question right is by knowing the answer. However, that's not the case on the NET, the TEAS, or the NLN PAX-RN because all questions on these exams are multiple-choice. You can get a perfect score on any one of these tests, even without knowing a single right answer...provided you know all the wrong answers!

What are we talking about? Since process of elimination is perhaps the most important technique in terms of multiple-choice questions, let's take a look at an example:

> The structure that acts at the sites of gas exchange in a woody stem are the
>
> **A.** lungs.
> **B.** gills.
> **C.** lenticels.
> **D.** lentil beans.

Now, if this were a fill-in-the-blank-style question, you might be in a heap of trouble. Lucky for you, the only questions on the NET, the TEAS, and the NLN PAX-RN are multiple-choice questions. Let's take a closer look at this question. You see "woody stem" in this question, which leads you to conclude that the question refers to plants. Right away, you know the answer is not choice A or B, because plants don't have lungs or gills. Now you've got it narrowed down to either choice C or choice D. Notice that these choices are very similar—lenticels and lentil beans. Obviously, one of them is a trap. At this point, if you don't know what "lentil beans" are, you have to guess. However, even if you don't know precisely what they are, it's safe to say that lentil beans have nothing to do with plant respiration. Therefore, the correct answer is choice C, lenticels.

Although our example is a little goofy, it illustrates an important point:

Process of Elimination is the best way to approach multiple-choice questions.

Even if you don't immediately know the right choice, you'll surely know that two or three of the answer choices are not correct. What then?

Strategy 4: Aggressive Guessing

All of your exam questions will be multiple-choice with four choices. The moment you have eliminated a couple of answer choices, your odds of getting the question right, even if you guess, increase greatly. If you can eliminate as many as two answer choices, your odds improve enough that it's in your best interest to guess.

Strategy 5: Word Associations

Another way to rack up points on the NET, the TEAS, or the NLN PAX-RN is by using word associations in tandem with your POE skills (from Strategy 3). Make sure that you memorize the words in the Key Words lists at the close of each chapter of this book. Know them backward and forward. As you learn them, make sure that you group them by association. Let's use the terms *mitosis* and *meiosis* to illustrate how word associations work.

There are a number of terms associated with mitosis and meiosis. For example, *synapsis, crossing-over,* and *tetrads* are words associated with meiosis but not mitosis. We'll explain more about what these words mean in Chapters 4 and 5. For now, just take a look at this question:

Which one of the following typifies cytokinesis during mitosis?

A. Crossing-over
B. Formation of the spindle
C. Formation of tetrads
D. Division of the cytoplasm

This might seem like a difficult problem. But let's think about the associations we just discussed. The question asks us about mitosis. However, choices A and C mention events that we've associated with meiosis. Therefore, they are out. Without even racking your brain, you've managed to get this down to two answer choices. Not bad! For the record, the correct answer is choice D, division of the cytoplasm.

Once again, don't worry about the science for now. We'll review it later in the book. What is important to note is that by combining the associations we'll offer throughout this book and your aggressive POE techniques, you'll be able to rack up points on problems that might have seemed difficult at first.

Strategy 6: Mnemonics—the Biology Name Game

Chapters 4 and 5, which cover, biology and human anatomy and physiology, are the most important chapters in this book (as you can tell by the size of those chapters versus other chapters). These subjects are all about names: the names of body organs and body parts, chemical structures, processes, theories, and so on. How are you going to keep all of these names straight? A great tool for memorizing them is mnemonics. A mnemonic, as you may already know, is a convenient device for remembering something.

For example, one important issue in biology is taxonomy—that is, the classification of life forms, or organisms. Organisms are classified in a descending system of similarity, leading from domain (the broadest level) to species (the most specific level). The complete order runs as follows: domain, kingdom, phylum, class, order, family, genus, species. Don't freak out yet. Look how easy it becomes with a mnemonic: **Dumb Kings Play Chess On FiberGlass Stools.**

Dumb	Domain
Kings	Kingdom
Play	Phylum
Chess	Class
On	Order
Fiber	Family
Glass	Genus
Stools	Species

Learn the mnemonic and you'll never forget the science! Mnemonics can be as goofy as you like, as long as they help you remember.

Strategy 7: Ballparking

We've covered a lot of strategies for verbal content on your exam, but what about helpful math strategies? Fear not—here is a math tip to help you ace your exam.

Ballparking is The Princeton Review's take on estimation. You won't have a calculator with you during your exam, so estimation will save you time and help you avoid frustration. For many questions, calculating the exact answer is a waste of time when you can quickly ballpark and eliminate answer choices immediately.

Ballparking is extremely useful on NLN PAX-RN, NET, and TEAS math questions, especially geometry problems. For example, on many geometry problems, you will be presented with a drawing in which some information is given and you'll be asked to find some of the information that is missing. In such problems, you are expected to apply a formula or perform a time-consuming calculation. But you'll almost always be better off if you look at the drawing and make a rough estimate of the answer (based on given information) before you dive in to work out the problem.

Some useful estimates to memorize are

π = about 3
$\sqrt{1}$ = 1
$\sqrt{2}$ = about 1.4
$\sqrt{3}$ = about 1.7+
$\sqrt{4}$ = 2

In Chapter 10: Algebra, we'll cover metric versus U.S. units of measure in depth. On a few math questions, you'll need to convert units of measure from one system to another. Estimation will come in handy on those questions, too. The following are a few conversion estimates to memorize:

1 yard = about 1 meter
1 inch = about 2 1/2 centimeters
2+ lbs = about 1 kilogram
15 lbs = about 1 stone
1+ quart = about 1 liter
1 ounce = about 30 grams

WHEN TO START YOUR REVIEW

"All things in moderation," as the saying goes. For your nursing school entrance exam, that means you should study a little bit each day, as opposed to cramming for the test the night before. So if you can, start preparing for your nursing school entrance exam the year before you plan to take the exam. Make an appointment with yourself and schedule it on your calendar for weekly (or daily) review. The sooner you begin your review, the less anxious you'll be on test day. When you spread your studying over a long period of time, you have time to cover a multitude of subjects and have plenty of time for taking practice tests. If daily or weekly test-prep time for about 12 months doesn't work in your busy schedule, try to begin studying three to four months in advance. Anything short of that may be considered unwise. Attempt practice tests about one month prior to the exam date.

LET'S GET CRACKING!

Along the way, we'll highlight what's important in each area, from human anatomy to the water cycle, and everything in between. By helping you at each step, we take all the guesswork out of preparing for your test. In addition, you'll soon see that you don't need to be dull and long-faced when it comes to test preparation. You can have some fun while you learn and review.

Before you get started, let's take a look at a quick summary of the strategies you need to remember for your test:

- **Pacing:** Be mindful of the time—you have around a minute per question. Use your time wisely.
- **The Three-Pass System:** If you are taking an exam in which you can bounce around, be sure to focus your energy on the easy questions first—save the rest for later.
- **Process of Elimination:** Use POE to answer questions. *Remember:* You don't need to know the right answers to get the questions right.
- **Aggressive Guessing:** Guess after you've eliminated two or more answer choices—it's in your best interest.
- **Word Associations:** Learn the lists at the end of each chapter in this text. Know which words should be grouped together.
- **Mnemonics:** Use the ones we suggest, or invent your own.
- **Ballparking:** Use estimation skills to save time and avoid making lengthy calculations in which errors could be introduced.

If you're comfortable with these strategies come test day, your score is bound to improve. First, however, you need to review all of the different topics that you'll see on your test. Without any further ado, let's get moving!

Chapter 4
Biology

INTRO TO BIOLOGY

Chapter 4 is an extremely important review because it covers the basic structure of living organisms, along with their organization and function on the cellular level. This review is in preparation for the bigger picture in Chapter 5: Human Anatomy and Physiology. In turn, Chapter 5 then leads to the topics of health, pathophysiology (study of disease processes), pharmacology (study of medications), intervention (critical and noncritical thinking), re-evaluation of your nursing process and the patient's progress, teaching (the family, the patient, other nurses, and collaborative teams), revising patient-centered goals, and being healers or advocates for healing—in short, the art and science behind being a student nurse. Does all of this sound like a huge undertaking? Fear not—we'll lead you through a thorough review of the most important content.

Some of the greatest and most influential nursing theorists are Florence Nightingale, Dorothea Orem, and Martha Rogers. You won't need to be familiar with their names or even their work for your NSEE, but you will study and admire their work, once you are enrolled in your Nursing Degree Program.

The very foundation of nursing relies not just on body pieces and the sum of parts. Nursing is concerned with these parts, but it's also concerned with the integrated functions as a whole and their effects on the entire organism, its theoretical framework, and a belief that a change in one system causes a change in another. Of course, where there is change, there is stress, damage, and the need for repair, healing, and the nursing process. Where there is change, there is the need for you, the nurse. If you understand how something did function at the beginning, and on the cellular level (basic biology), you will certainly be able to recognize either a change or a problem and then implement a strategy to fix the problem. An effective strategy will achieve balance, homeostasis (wellness), and optimal health for the entire organism (your patient), along with his or her family and loved ones. Whether providing direct patient care, promoting self-care, or running a department, your vocation as a nurse is to promote healing and wellness according to the teachings and theoretical framework of nursing role models and educators who are recognized in the history of the science and art of nursing.

You will most definitely need to be savvy in your biology review if you are planning to take the **NLN PAX-RN (National League for Nursing Pre-Admission Examination)**. That exam contains 80 science questions, which cover biology, chemistry, physics, and Earth science. If you're preparing for the **TEAS (Test of Essential Academic Skills)**, you'll face these same subjects, just in a smaller number (30 science questions total). If you're preparing for the **NET (Nursing Entrance Test)**, you don't need to worry about reviewing this content at all! (Although a lot of it is interesting, nonetheless—we swear.)

As far as the science questions in the NLN PAX-RN and the TEAS, no one knows the exact ratio of biology to chemistry to physics to Earth science, but you should mentally prepare yourself for about 18–25 questions (meaning correct test answer points) to be based on biology. In this chapter, you're going to complete a high-level review of a ton of biology concepts that you'll need to know for any nursing school entrance exam.

BIOLOGY: LET'S GET GENERAL

Biology is the study of life and **organisms** (living things). These organisms can be tiny (such as **bacteria**, which are single-celled organisms) or large (such as human beings, which are multicelled organisms).

Living Things

All living things—animals and plants—are composed of **cells** that originated from a pre-existing cell. We know that cells are the smallest unit of a living thing, and they carry out all of the activities necessary for survival. The theory that cells are life's most basic units of structure and function is known as the **cell theory** (creative name, huh?). Cells have been studied with different types of microscopes, which we will discuss briefly in a moment.

How Are Living Things Organized?

There are many, many, many different organisms, all of which are organized into groups of **species**. Species are a group of closely related organisms that share the ability to interbreed and produce fertile offspring. Those closely related organisms are then grouped into a broader **taxon tier** called the **genus**. For the test, you should be able to recall the basic ascending organizational order from the species all the way up through the domain. The following list is the organizational order of all things:

Species
Genus
Family
Order
Class
Phylum
Kingdom
Domain

Remember the mnemonic for the groupings of species, from most general to most specific: Dumb Kings Play Chess On FiberGlass Stools.

RESEARCH OVERVIEW

The Scientific Method

The **scientific method** is important to understand within the realm of biology, as a means to test an event or phenomenon. This method uses the following steps: observing, developing questions, researching what other scientists have already done, creating a **hypothesis** that will predict the outcome of the questions, designing an experiment to test the hypothesis, collecting information and data, and finally forming a conclusion based on scientific research. A test is considered a reliable one if other scientists are able to get the same results—every time—by repeating the experiment.

Compound Microscopes

Compound microscopes are important essential tools in the study of biology too. You've probably worked with a compound microscope in a lab setting—it is a high-powered microscope with more than one lens. Refamiliarize yourself with this instrument and its basic parts. It is unlikely that there will be a diagram of a microscope on the exam; however, you may be tested on the way to prepare a slide and on the magnification capabilities of a microscope. These questions count as valuable test points, so give a look to the figure below.

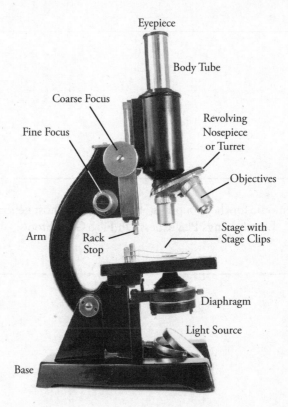

Microscope

MATTER AND ENERGY

The structure and organization of both living and nonliving things are derived from certain properties of matter and energy. **Matter** is anything that has mass (weighs something) and takes up space—it can be a solid, a liquid, or a gas. Matter is made up of many **elements**, which are the building blocks of matter. **Helium**, **oxygen**, **chlorine**, **nitrogen**, **potassium**, and **radium** are just a few examples of elements. The **periodic table** (see figure) is a chart of all known elements. Don't worry; you don't have to memorize these. Just be familiar with the ones we mention as we move along with the review. Most of this section will be discussed later in the chemistry section.

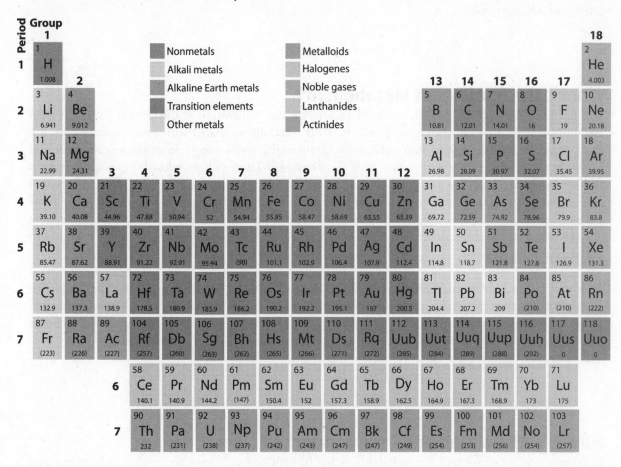

Periodic Table

Energy is the ability to do work, bring about change, or make things happen. Energy can change, shift, and be converted—but energy can't be created or destroyed. These principles are called the **law of conservation of energy**. Energy exists in many forms, such as light, heat, chemical energy, and electrical energy. Energy or conversion of energy is needed for cell life maintenance. We discuss laws of energy in Chapter 6: Physics.

HOMEOSTASIS

Homeostasis is the maintenance of equilibrium within an organism by a tendency to compensate for changes and disruptions. Organisms are living things that can sense and react to stimuli (change, stress, or disruption), reproduce (duplicate), grow and develop, essentially evolve, transform (utilize and convert) energy, and maintain internal balance (homeostasis). Organisms can be viruses, bacteria, parasites, fungi, plants, or animals. In order to live and survive, they need internal balance and cellular homeostasis.

Have you ever heard the saying "A happy wife is a happy life"? Well, in biology and nursing, "A balanced cell means a healthy being."

What's the Beef About Metabolism?

The survival of all organisms relies on metabolic activity and homeostasis at the cellular level. The term **metabolism** refers to all of the physical and chemical reactions associated with every aspect of cell life. These reactions include an organism's ability to obtain and convert energy from the environment and its ability to use that energy to maintain itself (homeostasis). These abilities allow for growth, evolution, and reproduction. Just as a plant cell converts the sun's light energy and uses it in the process of **photosynthesis**, other cells can convert energy via both **aerobic** and **anaerobic respiration**. Organisms can **synthesize** larger molecules from smaller molecules with a process called **anabolism**, and they can do the opposite—that is, they can break down products or digest them and transform them into energy with the process of **catabolism**.

With metabolism, **active** and **passive transports** occur within and in and out of the cells. Oxidative prosphorylation (or OXYPHOS, as the cool kids call it) also occurs to produce ATP, the molecule that supplies energy to metabolism. As a future student nurse, all of this review of metabolism builds to better prepare you for the bigger picture: looking at systemic maintenance, the effects of dilated coronary arteries, contractions of the major muscle groups, mineralization of bone, and so on.

How It's All Related and Interconnected

In homeostasis, a cell (or body) is in balance—that is, cells and cells of systems work in harmony and function in an ideal manner. It is the maintenance of a relatively stable or constant internal physiological environment. **Hormones** are chemicals in the blood that are responsible for homeostasis. **Negative** and **positive feedback** serve as adjuncts to maintaining homeostasis.

Later, you'll have a much greater review of anatomy and physiology, but for now, here's a sample of how we build upon cells, cell function, organism function, and homeostasis in life. Let's take a look at a few examples of negative and positive feedback in homeostasis within the human body.

Examples of Negative and Positive Feedback in Homeostasis

- When you eat a large meal, your blood sugar elevates, your **pancreas** produces a chemical hormone called **insulin**, which allows the liver to then remove the excess sugar from your bloodstream and store it as **glycogen**. Stored glycogen can make you fat, but those glycogen stores can be broken down later for use when your body needs it most.
- If you forget to eat lunch or intentionally skip a meal, your body begins to break down glycogen for energy. This process is called **glycogenolysis**. After this happens, your blood sugar comes down to normal balance, or homeostasis. Cells can't survive long term with a constant high sugar load, just as they can't survive long term if high levels of insulin are floating around in the absence of food (energy).
- Let's think about a woman in labor. The hormones secreted during labor tell the uterus to contract, causing increased pain. These contractions in turn cause dilation, thinning or effacement of the cervix, and increased force or contractions until the baby is birthed (the delivery). Once the baby is born, those hormones decrease and other hormones are secreted to prepare for the production of breast milk. Continued, less severe contractions help the body get back to the pre-pregnant state. If the mother chooses to nurse and the baby latches on well, milk will continue to be produced. If the mother is unable to nurse or chooses not to, the breast milk supply will diminish and dry up. All of this is thanks to positive and negative feedback, stimuli, and hormones.

DARWIN: WE ALL CAME FROM A PRE-EXISTING CELL

Who's Your Daddy, Now?

The characteristics found in all life begin at the cellular level (involving biology and chemistry) where there are very specific instructions contained in a cell's **DNA (deoxyribonucleic acid)**. DNA is a molecule that contains instructions, or blueprints, for the organism. DNA is essentially the molecule of inheritance. Its instructions for reproducing traits are passed on from the parent-ancestor cell to the offspring or daughter cells. There are two types of cell reproduction: mitosis (reproduction of all cells except sperm and egg) and meiosis (reproduction of sperm and egg cells). (You'll review reproduction later in this chapter.)

Examples of feedback control mechanisms include thermoregulation (body temperature stabilization), blood pressure control and heart rate regulation (vessel constriction and dilation), platelet aggregation (for clotting), and the primordial fight-or-flight survival mechanism.

Mutations: Problematic or Not?

Mutations in reproduction cause variations in the traits of an organism and allow new genes to enter a population and become part of the organism's gene pool. Mutations are heritable changes in the structure or number of DNA molecules in a cell. If a mutation is allowed to survive (through Charles Darwin's theory of survival of the fittest—**natural selection**), then it enables new characteristics to develop, which will contribute to diversity in any given population. Some mutations do not survive, however, if they are harmful or unable to withstand the stronger ancestor gene and/or the demands or functional responsibility of the organism. Therefore, mutations may die out if they are unable to reproduce—that is, if they are not "fit enough" to survive. (Genetics is discussed in later chapters that cover the reproductive system. For now, just remember that mutations enable new characteristics to develop in a population, and the environment can play a part in whether or not an organism is fit to survive.)

CELL BASICS

According to the cell theory, every living organism—plant, animal, or otherwise—is made up of cells that arose from pre-existing cells. Cells are the basic functional and structural units of all plant and animal life. The simplest organisms have one cell—they are **unicellular**. An example of a single-celled organism is bacteria. More complex, larger organisms (such as humans) are made up of countless trillions of cells—they are **multicellular**.

Within the cells are very talented, tiny, task-oriented **organelles**, **electric charges** (both positive and negative), DNA instructions (genes), **protein**, and fluid. Cells are arranged in **tissues**, which make up **organs**. Organs in turn make up **systems**, which make up **bodies**. Bodies make up **people**, people make up **populations**, and so on.

To understand biology, you must first understand the level of biologic organization, which begins with the sequence that traces organization in nature from the very simple to the very complex.

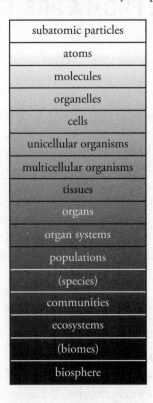

| subatomic particles |
| atoms |
| molecules |
| organelles |
| cells |
| unicellular organisms |
| multicellular organisms |
| tissues |
| organs |
| organ systems |
| populations |
| (species) |
| communities |
| ecosystems |
| (biomes) |
| biosphere |

Biologic Organization

REFRESHING THE BIO-BASICS

Let's continue to review the biology basics that you should be familiar with for your nursing school entrance examination. The information provided in these next several pages should help you to recall what you learned in biology courses—whether last year or even 20 years ago. This review will help you remember important information overall and feel comfortable and prepared on exam day. If you feel weak in certain review areas, it is normal. That's why you are reviewing.

As part of the biology basics, let's do a quick review of atoms, elements, molecules, and compounds.

That Sounds a Bit More like Chemistry

Don't worry; you'll study this content in more detail in the chemistry chapter later in this book. For now, let's review some introductory information.

Elements are substances made up of a certain number of **atoms** and within those atoms are subatomic particles called **protons**, **neutrons**, and **electrons**. Atoms are the fundamental units of the physical world. They have no **net charge**, but they can lose or gain electrons. Individual atoms combine in chemical reactions to form **molecules**.

Here's an example of a hydrogen molecule:

Hydrogen Atom + Hydrogen Atom = Hydrogen molecule

$$H + H \rightarrow H_2$$

As you can see from the diagram above, molecules are combinations of atoms. Molecules can react with other atoms or other molecules to form larger molecules.

Here's an example of hydrogen molecules and oxygen molecules coming together to make the compound water. The molecules of hydrogen and oxygen are held together by bonds denoted by the lines between H and O in the figure below:

Hydrogen + Oxygen (reactants) yields (gives) Water (compound)

$$2H_2 + O_2 \rightarrow 2H_2O$$

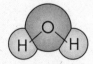

A molecule that contains different elements is called a **compound**. Because water contains two elements (hydrogen and oxygen), it's a compound. Another example of a compound is salt (NaCl). Salt is a compound because the molecule contains both **sodium** (Na) and **chlorine** (Cl).

Elements cannot be broken down into simpler substances by ordinary measures. Since salt is a compound, it can be broken down to sodium (Na) and chlorine (Cl), but sodium alone and chlorine alone cannot be broken down any further, since they are elements.

ELEMENTS ARE ELEMENTAL

There are 92 natural elements—check them our periodically on your periodic table (awful joke, we know). Just four of these elements (**carbon**, **hydrogen**, oxygen, and nitrogen) make up 96 percent of the mass of all organisms. Don't forget to look back at your periodic table of elements that you skipped over earlier in this chapter. Hold on to it, as it will be useful later on in the chapter on chemistry—and then when you're studying pharmacology in just a few more years (*yawn*).

C = carbon
H = hydrogen
O = oxygen
N = nitrogen

Carbon, hydrogen, oxygen, and nitrogen are the most abundant elements in an organism followed by **phosphorous** and **sulfur**.

P = phosphorous
S = sulfur

Calcium, **sodium**, **potassium**, **magnesium**, and **iron** are also among all organisms' chemical make-up, but in smaller or even trace amounts.

Ca = calcium
Na = sodium
K = potassium
Mg = magnesium
Fe = iron

Why Do Nurses Need to Know About Elements?

You will be responsible for reviewing and recognizing normal and abnormal lab values in your patients. You will be monitoring and replacing (or withholding) certain elements in the form of electrolytes through **intravenous (IV) access, enteric (oral) access,** or **parenterally** (which literally means "going around the gut" or "by way other than the gut") with replacement (nutritional) supplementation methods. TPN, **total parenteral nutrition**, is administered via **central venous access** (usually a central line not a peripheral line). Abnormal electrolyte levels cause stress in the cells → in the tissues → in the organs → in the body. For example, too high or too low a serum sodium level can cause seizures and dehydration. Too high or too low a potassium level can cause unstable and even fatal heart rhythms (**arrhythmias**).

Did you know that oxygen is considered a medication and needs a doctor's order so that it can be administered to a patient? Did you know that heliox is a combination of oxygen and helium that, when administered properly, reduces the work of breathing in certain types of respiratory situations in patients?

COMPOUNDS AND BONDS

The atoms of a compound are held together by **chemical bonds**. Chemical bonds are broken down into two types:

- Ionic bonds
- Covalent bonds

Much like a tug-of-war game, electrons can be pulled away from atoms or added to them.

Ionic bonds form between two atoms when one or more electron is transferred from one atom to the other. One atom loses electrons and becomes positively charged while the other atom gains electrons and becomes negatively charged. The charged forms of the atoms are called **ions**, and they are either positive or negative.

An example of an atom that lost an electron is Na^+ (it has the plus-positive charge sign added to it).

An atom that gained an electron is Cl^- (it has the minus-negative charge sign added to it).

$$Na \cdot \; + \; \overset{\displaystyle ..}{\underset{\displaystyle ..}{:Cl}} \cdot \; \longrightarrow \; Na^+ \; + \; \overset{\displaystyle ..}{\underset{\displaystyle ..}{:Cl:}}^-$$

Covalent bonds form when electrons are shared by atoms, not pulled away completely. If the electrons are shared equally between the atoms, the bond is **nonpolar covalent**. If the electrons are shared unequally, the bond is called **polar covalent**.

A third kind of bond, **hydrogen bond**, occurs when hydrogen bonds together to other hydrogen atoms of different molecules. Hydrogen bonds are weak chemical bonds that form when a hydrogen atom weakly interacts with a nearby hydrogen atom that is already part of a covalent bond. Water molecules are held together by hydrogen bonds. When water is in its liquid state, hydrogen bonds constantly break and reform.

Bonds are discussed in even greater detail later in the chemistry chapter.

WATER

Water plays an important role in life and nature. Life originates in water and the human body is made up of 70 percent water. Water is an inorganic molecule because it doesn't contain carbon. Human cells contain water, reactions happen in water, and water helps to sustain life and life functions. Keep in mind that water can have both positive and negative effects. Within your nursing career, you will learn how there can be too much of a (seemingly) good thing. Excess water can cause cell death—that is, excess amounts of fluid in cells can cause **edema**. Edema, if present in the lung tissues, can cause suffocation because gas exchange that is necessary in the work of breathing becomes stifled. Also, if there is too much fluid volume systemically, the heart muscle can become overtaxed and stretch out, a condition leading to heart failure. Conversely, absence of water can cause cell death. Too little water or volume loss due to disease or injury can cause dehydration. Dehydration can lead to cell membrane instability, electrolyte imbalance, shock, and subsequent organ failure. All things in moderation, as they say.

What Water Is and How It Functions

Water has two hydrogen atoms joined to an oxygen atom (H_2O). In water molecules, the hydrogen atoms exhibit a partial positive charge on one side, and the oxygen atom exhibits a partial negative charge on the other side, which makes water a **polar molecule**.

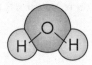

As you can see in the figure above, water molecules are held together by bonds. When two or more molecules of water in liquid phase bond, hydrogen bonds form between the hydrogen of separate molecules. The oxygen and hydrogen in H_2O are held together by covalent bonds. Different water molecules are held together by hydrogen bonds. Although hydrogen bonds are individually weak, they are collectively strong when present in large numbers. One function of water is that is can **dissolve** other polar substances—that is, water is a **solvent**. The things that dissolve in water are called **solutes**. A **solution** is a solute plus a solvent. For example, both salt and sugar are solutes because they dissolve in water. If you've ever had a sore throat, you're probably familiar with gargling salt water.

As previously mentioned, water molecules have a strong tendency to stick together. That is, water exhibits cohesive forces. These forces are extremely important to life. For instance, when water molecules evaporate from leaves, they "pull" neighboring water molecules. These, in turn, draw up the molecules immediately behind them, and so on, all the way down the plant vessels. The resulting chain of water molecules enables water to move up a stem.

Water molecules also like to stick to other substances—that is, they are adhesive. Have you ever tried to separate two glass slides stuck together by a film of water? They're difficult to separate because of the water sticking to the glass surfaces. These two forces taken together—**cohesion** and **adhesion**—account for the ability of water to rise up roots, trunks, and branches of trees. Water has a high **surface tension** because of the cohesiveness of its molecules. Surface tension results from the force of attraction among molecules in a liquid. It's an elastic-like force that tends to minimize the area of a surface.

Another remarkable property of water is its **heat capacity**—the ability of a substance to store heat. For example, when you heat an iron kettle, it becomes hot rather quickly. Why? Because it has a low specific heat. It doesn't take much heat to increase the temperature of the kettle. Water, on the other hand, has a very high heat capacity. You have to add a lot of heat to get an increase in the temperature of water. The amount of heat that it takes to increase the temperature of 1 gram of water by 1 Celsius degree is called a **calorie**. Water's ability to resist temperature change is one of the things that helps keep the temperature in the oceans fairly stable. It's also why organisms that are composed mainly of water (like you and me!) are able to keep a constant body temperature.

Finally, water assists in the breakdown of complex food molecules in the human body. The breakdown of a compound due to reaction with water is called **hydrolysis**.

Acids and Bases

Acids and **bases** are responsible for the management of **pH balance**, which affects homeostasis. pH is a value or measurement of the acidity or basicity of an **aqueous** (water-based) solution. Pure water has a pH of 7.0, which is neutral. Look at the pH scale below to see where different solutions stack up.

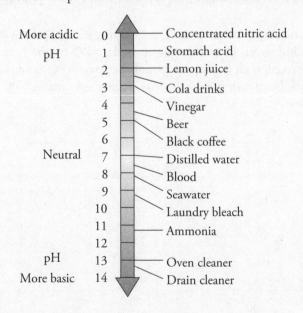

More acidic	0	Concentrated nitric acid
pH	1	Stomach acid
	2	Lemon juice
	3	Cola drinks
	4	Vinegar
	5	Beer
	6	Black coffee
Neutral	7	Distilled water
	8	Blood
	9	Seawater
	10	Laundry bleach
	11	Ammonia
	12	
pH	13	Oven cleaner
More basic	14	Drain cleaner

pH Scale

Acids release hydrogen ions in water (H^+). With a pH of 7, the solution's hydrogen ion concentration is equal to the hydroxide concentration and is considered to be equal (acid-base concentration is equal). Buffers help maintain the pH value. The normal pH value of human blood when in homeostasis is 7.35–7.45. The more acidic value is on the left of the hyphen, and the more basic value is on the right. As a nurse, you will find acid-base balance and imbalance while reading blood gases during respiratory emergencies and while managing a ventilated patient.

Let's look at a question about acidity and basicity:

A patient in the ER is complaining of stomach distress. After you obtain a thorough medical history including diet recall, you determine that her diet is far too acidic. Once the patient is medically cleared and medically able to eat, what would most likely be recommended that she drink with lunch that day?

A. Distilled water
B. Coffee
C. Beer
D. Lemonade

Here's How to Crack It
Choice D, lemonade, is a terrible idea if she needs to eliminate acid from her diet, so go ahead and cross out choice D. According to the pH scale you just saw, coffee has a pH of 5 and beer has a pH of about 4.5, while neutral is 7. So choice A is correct—distilled water with a pH of 7, neutral.

Note: This question is for test-taking purposes only. In real life, when a patient presents with any type of abdominal pain or stomach distress, he or she will be made **NPO** by the licensed health care provider until an evaluation is performed, with or without diagnostic tests. NPO is an acronym for the Latin *non per os,* which means nothing by mouth (food or drink). Patients are made NPO prior to any GI (gastrointestinal) procedure or surgery.

ORGANIC AND INORGANIC COMPOUNDS

Organic compounds contain carbon; **inorganic compounds** do not contain carbon, with the exception of carbon dioxide (CO_2). Carbon is important for life because it is a versatile atom. In other words, it has the ability to bind with other carbons as well as a number of other atoms. The resulting molecules are key in carrying out the activities necessary for life.

There are four classes of organic compounds that are central to life on Earth:

1. Proteins
2. Carbohydrates
3. Lipids
4. Nucleic acids

Let's review each one.

Proteins

Proteins are organic because they contain carbon. They are made up of several **amino acids**. There are 20 amino acids commonly found in proteins. (Don't worry. You do not need to memorize them for the test!) Amino acids are the building blocks of protein. A three-layer dimensional structure called a protein is formed when two amino acids form a bond between them (a **peptide bond**) and then form a string of bonded amino acids (**polypeptide chain**), which twists and folds on itself.

The image below illustrates the structural formula for a typical amino acid. The R in the molecule represents any saturated hydrocarbon. The shaded box on the left identifies an amine group—that's what puts the "amine" in "amino acid." The shaded box on the right identifies a carboxyl group, which makes the molecule an acid.

Proteins can be either **structural** or **globular**:

- Structural proteins are made of big, long filaments (such as **collagen**). Structural proteins make up hair, skin, and **connective tissues** such ligaments and tendons.
- Globular proteins are larger proteins or groups of proteins (such as **hemoglobin**, **antibodies**, and enzymes). Muscles in the human body are made of proteins.

When the shape of a protein is disrupted (weak bonds are broken), the protein is said to be **denatured** and it unwinds, untwists, and changes shape. The order of amino acids determines how a protein will fold up into its shape. The shape of a protein determines what it does.

Carbohydrates (AKA Carbs)

Carbohydrates are organic because—you got it—they contain carbon. Carbohydrates are made up of only carbon, oxygen, and hydrogen. The following is a list of some common carbohydrates:

- **Monosaccharides** (simple sugars), such as glucose and fructose
- **Disaccharides** (two sugars), such as sucrose, lactose (milk sugar), and maltose
- **Polysaccharides** (many sugars), such as glycogen (the form in which animals store glucose), **starch** (the form in which plants store glucose), and **cellulose** (a structural polysaccharide that forms the cell walls of plants)

Let's learn more about these sugars.

As you probably know, **saccharide** is a fancy word for sugar. The prefixes *mono-*, *di-*, and *poly-* refer to the number of sugars in the molecule. *Mono-* means "one," *di-* means "two," and *poly-* means "many." These saccharides serve as energy sources for cells. The two simplest of all sugars are glucose ($C_6H_{12}O_6$) and fructose (fruit sugar). When a person eats carbohydrates, they are broken down and then converted by the cells to give energy to that person's body. This energy can be used immediately or stored as glycogen for energy later.

Lipids

Lipids are organic, and like carbohydrates, they consist of carbon, hydrogen, and oxygen atoms but in a different ratio. Lipids are important because they function as structural components of cell membranes, sources of insulation, and a means of energy storage. Examples of lipids are fats, oils, waxes, phospholipids, and steroids. Fats contain three **fatty acids** and one **glycerol** molecule. **Triglyceride** is another word for "fat." The human body has both good lipids (**HDLs**, or **high-density lipids**) and bad lipids (**LDLs**, or **low-density lipids**). Too many bad lipids can lead to clogged arteries that can cause coronary diseases such as atherosclerosis and arteriosclerosis, which can cause heart attacks and cerebral vascular accidents, otherwise known as strokes.

Cholesterol

Cholesterol is a unique organic lipid composed of **hydrocarbon rings**. Cholesterol is necessary to build and maintain cell membranes, as it gives the cell membrane its plasticity so that it does not break. Cholesterol functions to produce steroid hormones (chemicals) and is found in animal bodies (vitamin D and sex hormones). See? Not all cholesterol is bad.

Nucleic Acids

Nucleic acids are biologically important organic macromolecules (large molecules) that are found in the **nucleus** of every cell. They too contain carbon, hydrogen, oxygen, and nitrogen but also contain phosphorous. Nucleic acid molecules are made up of simple units called **nucleotides**. Examples of nucleic acids are ATP (**adenosine triphosphate**) that provides energy, **coenzymes** necessary in transportation of protons and electrons from one reaction site to the next, and **deoxyribonucleic acid** (**DNA**) and **ribonucleic acid** (**RNA**), which store, transmit, and translate genetic information.

Two Kinds of Nucleotides

As previously mentioned, DNA contains genetic "blueprints" of all life—heredity. RNA is essential for protein synthesis (creation). DNA is a double-stranded molecule with a double helix that locks it into a specific shape. RNA is a single-stranded molecule, allowing it to assume various unique shapes.

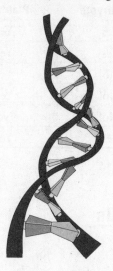

DNA Molecule

DNA and RNA are the nucleic acids that make life possible.

DNA and RNA decide what we will look like, how we will talk, if we limp or leap, the color of our hair, and much more.

CELLS AND STRUCTURE

There are two types of cells: **eukaryotic** and **prokaryotic**. A eukaryotic cell has a cell wall or a cell membrane (or both) forming its outer layer, cytoplasm within it where the organelles (tiny task-oriented organs) are located, and a nucleus where the DNA/RNA and **chromosomes** are located.

Plants, bacteria, and fungi have cell walls and cell membranes. Animal cells do not—they have only cell membranes. Know these differences in cells because you will probably be asked a question or two about them.

Prokaryotic cells are much smaller than eukaryotic cells and do not have a nucleus. Their genetic information (DNA/RNA) is found within a **nucleoid**. An example of a prokaryotic cell is bacteria.

We Are Eukaryotic

If you get stuck on a test question that asks you if humans are eukaryotic or prokaryotic, remember how it is pronounced: *Eukaryotic* is pronounced **you-karyotic**. This should help you remember the difference in the two cells. The "you" sound in eukaryotic stands for **you and me**.

Here's something for visual learners. To help you remember the differences among prokaryotic cells, plant cells, and animal cells, here is a nifty simple table:

STRUCTURAL CHARACTERISTICS OF DIFFERENT CELL TYPES			
Structure	Prokaryote	Plant Cell	Animal Cell
Cell Wall	Yes	Yes	No!
Plasma Membrane	Yes	Yes	Yes
Organelles	No!	Yes	Yes
Nucleus	No!	Yes	Yes
Centrioles	No!	No!	Yes
Ribosomes	Yes	Yes	Yes

Cell Membranes and Cell Walls

Animal Cells

Animal cells have outer envelopes known as **cell membranes**, or **plasma membranes**. These layers are made up of phospholipids and proteins. (They are organic molecules, because they contain carbon.) Cell membranes are so tiny that there would have to be stacks of thousands of them to be the thickness of a sheet of notebook paper.

The role of the cell membrane is to be the gatekeeper, or bouncer, by regulating movement (entry and exit) of substances into and out of the cell. The spot on the cell membrane where substances can move in and out is called the **pinocytotic vesicle**. This gatekeeper permits only certain substances, namely proteins, to pass through unaided. That is, it's **differentially permeable** (also referred to as **selectively permeable**). The lipid molecules in the cell membrane have their **hydrophilic** (water-liking) heads at the two most outer surfaces of the phospholipid bilayer. Their fatty acid tails that are **hydrophobic** (water-disliking) are in the middle (like a sandwich).

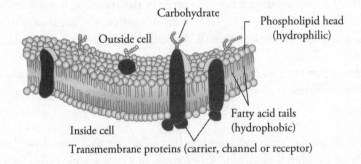

Cell Membrane

The watery substance within a cell is called **cytoplasm**. Cytoplasm helps maintain internal conditions like shape and concentration, which in turn helps maintain homeostasis.

Plant Cells

Plant cells differ from animal cells in that they are surrounded by **cell walls**, which are thick, rigid membranes made of cellulose fiber (a polysaccharide sugar). The cell walls give plant cells support and structure. Like animal cells, plant cells also have cell membranes, which are inside the cell walls. The cell walls of bacteria are made of peptidogylcan (protein and sugar), and the cell walls of fungi are made of chitin (a polysaccharide similar to cellulose).

Plant cells also have chlorophyll, which contain chloroplasts, the organelles required for photosynthesis. (Photosynthesis is discussed later.)

What's in a Cell?—Organelles

As you've already learned, organelles are the task-oriented parts of cells. A eukaryotic cell is like a microscopic factory. Let's take a tour of a eukaryotic cell and focus on the structure and function of each organelle. Here's a picture of a typical animal cell and its principal organelles:

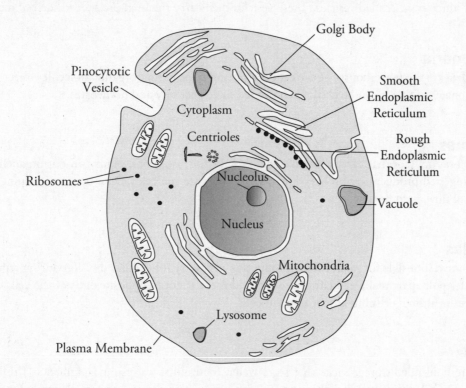

Animal Cell

Let's examine the organelles found in a typical eukaryotic cell.

Nucleus

The nucleus is the control center of the cell. It is the home of genetic information (DNA in the form of larger structures called chromosomes) and therefore responsible for the cell's ability to reproduce. Within the nucleus lies the **nucleolus**, which is where RNA is made and **ribosomes** are assembled. Ribosomes are the sites of protein synthesis (creation) and secretion.

Endoplasmic Reticulum (ER)

Endoplasmic reticulum (ER) is responsible for protein production and transportation. ER can be studded with ribosomes, which make it rough in texture. This rough texture inspires the name **rough ER**. Proteins made on the rough ER are the ones ear-marked to be exported out of the cell. ER without ribosomes attached is called **smooth ER**. The smooth ER breaks down toxic chemicals and makes lipids, hormones, and steroids.

Golgi Bodies

Golgi bodies also participate in protein synthesis by modifying, processing, sorting, and then packaging the final product in sacs called vesicles. These vesicles then carry the final product to the cell membrane.

Mitochondria

Mitochondria are the powerhouses of the cell, converting energy from organic molecules to ATP (adenosine triphosphate) so that it can be used when needed in cell activity and homeostasis.

Lysosomes

Lysosomes are tiny sacs that carry digestive enzymes. In the lysosomes, old, worn-out organelles, debris, and large ingested products are broken down. Lysosomes are the cell's clean-up crew, helping clear the cytoplasm of unwanted flotsam.

Centrioles

Centrioles are responsible for microtubule production necessary for cellular division during reproduction. Microtubules pull apart replicated chromosomes and move them to opposite ends of the cell. Centrioles are common in animal cells but absent in plant cells.

Vacuoles

Vacuoles are fluid-filled storage sacks that store water, food, salts, wastes, and pigments. Think of a vacuum cleaner to help you remember this one—a very strange and special vacuum cleaner where you store water, food, salts, wastes, and pigments. Or better yet, remember that in Latin, the term *vacuole* means "empty cavity," but these cavities are far from empty.

Peroxisomes

Peroxisomes, which are found in cytoplasm and responsible for detoxification, produce hydrogen peroxide (H_2O_2). They also contain enzymes responsible for the breakdown of hydrogen peroxide into oxygen and water. Peroxisomes are common in liver and kidney cells in animals.

Cytoskeleton

Cytoskeleton maintains the shape of the cell with a network of fibers called **microtubules** and **microfilaments**. Microtubules are made up of a globular protein called **tubulin**, which participates in cellular division and movement. Tubulin is an integral part of three structures: centrioles, **cilia**, and **flagella**. Cilia and flagella are thread-like structures located outside the cell. They're responsible for locomotion in single-celled organisms.

Did you know that tubulin is the target site for certain anti-cancer drug therapy, anti-gout medication, and anti-fungal treatment?

Cell Transport: Intracellular and Extracellular

Substances can cross a cell membrane in and out of the cell by methods of different transport phenomena. Some examples are diffusion, osmosis, facilitated diffusion, active and passive transport, and bulk transport. The ability to move across a concentration gradient or in and out of a membrane defines its permeability. The key is to know whether or not the method of transport needs energy to do so. Passive transport requires no energy; active transport requires an outside source of energy.

Diffusion

Diffusion is the passive movement of a substance from an area of higher concentration to an area of lower concentration—that is, the substance moves down what's called the concentration gradient. Diffusion describes a particle that randomly moves in an area of greater concentration to an area of lesser concentration. An example of diffusion is the scent of a perfume throughout a room. If you spray a bottle of perfume onto your neck, the scent is heavily concentrated as a mist that hits the nape of your neck. Once you walk away, the bit of perfume mist still in the room diffuses and moves to other parts of the room that do not have the perfume scent. Eventually, the room is filled with the scent.

Osmosis

Like diffusion, **osmosis** is a passive process and therefore does not require energy. One example of osmosis is water freely flowing in and out of a cell; another example is a plant's ability to draw water up from the soil. What's important to remember about osmosis is that a solvent (water) will travel from an area of higher concentration (called **hypertonic**) to an area of lesser concentration (called **hypotonic**) and that osmotic balance is an effort to achieve solute-solvent equilibrium.

Facilitated Diffusion

Facilitated diffusion is another type of passive transport in which the molecules require assistance from special membrane proteins to move substances across the cell membrane. Glucose and amino acids are examples of molecules requiring transport assistance. *Note:* Only small nonpolar molecules such as oxygen can diffuse easily across a cell membrane.

Active Transport

Active transport requires energy (good 'ole ATP—andenosine triphosphate) to move materials such as ions, salts, glucose, and amino acids from an area of lower concentration to an area of higher concentration.

An example of active transport is the sodium-potassium pump. Other forms of active transport include endocytosis, phagocytosis, pinocytosis, and exocytosis.

Bulk Transport

Bulk transport (also called **bulk flow**) involves the movement of larger molecules in one direction by pressure. It means that there is a one-way movement of fluids brought about by pressure until that which is transported fills a region to its bulk capacity. An example of bulk transport is the movement of blood through a blood vessel or movement of fluids in xylem and phloem of plants.

Enzymes

Enzymes are special proteins that act as **catalysts** to accelerate the reaction between specific substrates within a cell. **Substrates** are the substances acted upon by an enzyme. Examples of enzymes are vitamins, **cofactors** (non-protein chemical compounds that are bound to a protein to assist with the protein's biological activity), and coenzymes. You may be familiar with the coenzyme vitamin C. You'll read more about coenzyme A (CoA) in the material on cellular respiration.

Now, let's work on a problem:

The diagram below shows an experimental set-up of osmosis. A dialysis bag filled with glucose solution is placed in a beaker with distilled water. The experiment is performed for about an hour.

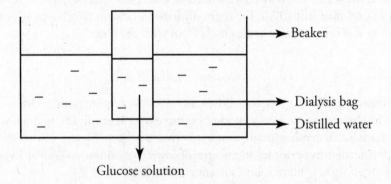

What will be the likely result after one hour?

A. Water from the beaker will move into the dialysis bag.
B. Glucose will move out of the glucose solution from the dialysis bag.
C. The glucose solution in the dialysis bag will become more concentrated.
D. No change will be observed in the set-up after one hour.

Here's How to Crack It

Choice A and choice D should jump out at you as "So right!" and "So wrong!" Choice D is wrong because osmosis is definitely going to happen in this experiment—things are not going to simply remain the same. Cross off choice D. Speaking of osmosis, choice A looks like a strong choice, since osmosis involves the transfer of solvent particles from a region of higher concentration to a region of lower concentration. Thus, water will move inside the dialysis bag. Keep choice A in mind, but let's check out choices B and C before we commit. Glucose molecules are large and cannot cross the semipermeable membrane of the dialysis bag, so choice B can't be the right answer. There is no way for the glucose solution in the bag to become more concentrated and, in fact, the opposite will happen. Water from the beaker will move into the dialysis bag because of osmosis. This reduces the concentration of the glucose solution in the dialysis bag. Eliminate choice C and confidently select choice A.

Cellular Energy

An important thing that you should understand is the law of conservation of energy: Energy in the universe remains constant. It cannot be created or destroyed, yet it can be converted from one form to another. Don't stress; we will review energy more in chemistry and physics in chapters to come.

Here's what you should know about **cellular energy**:

When a cell needs energy, it takes ATP (adenosine triphosphate), splits off (hydrolyzes with the presence of water) the third phosphate, and then forms **ADP** (**adenosine diphosphate**). A diphsophate has two phosphates instead of three. It loses one phosphate while releasing energy in the process.

$$ATP \rightarrow ADP + P + Energy$$

Photosynthesis

Photosynthesis will likely be mentioned in a few test questions. You should know that ATP comes from photosynthesis (plants use sunlight because sunlight = energy) and/or cellular respiration. Cellular respiration can either be aerobic (with the presence of oxygen) or anaerobic (without presence of oxygen).

Cellular Respiration

Cellular respiration is a series of chemical reactions that take place inside a cell to produce energy. It doesn't occur as single reaction, in a single step. Instead, cellular respiration occurs in a series of smaller steps designed to maximize the production of energy. The events that occur in cellular respiration are **glycolysis**, the **Krebs cycle**, **electron transport chain**, and **oxidative phosphorylation**.

- Glycolysis is the splitting of sugar, which results in ADP energy and **pyruvate** or **pyruvic acid**. It occurs in the cytoplasm of the cell without oxygen present.
- Pyruvate (the product of glycolysis) is transported to mitochondria where it enters into the Krebs cycle (also known as the citric acid cycle) once it is converted by an enzyme into a two-carbon molecule called acetyl coenzyme A.

- Coenzyme A enters the Krebs cycle where eight separate enzyme catalyst reactions occur and where energy and carbon dioxide are released.
- The final stage of cellular respiration, called the electron transport chain and oxidative phosphorylation, takes place in the inner membrane of the mitochondria. It is the final ATP conversion to ADP and then to oxygen. Oxygen is the final electron acceptor particle at the end of the electron transport chain.

What's Left?

When the energy-producing process of cellular respiration is completed, the cell is left with 30 molecules of ATP per glucose molecule.

Aerobic respiration is preferred over anaerobic respiration, as a substantially more useful amount of energy is released for the cell. With alcoholic fermentation (anaerobic), one of the major by-products is called ethyl alcohol. With lactic acid fermentation (anaerobic), lactic acid is one of its by-products.

Without oxygen present in anaerobic cellular respiration, **fermentation** occurs. Bacteria and yeasts are capable of fermentation. Bad yeast can manifest as a fungal infection in the diaper area of a baby or an older patient or even as a mycotic ball (also called a fungal ball) in the heart or brain. A yeast infection will often occur when a female patient is on a course of antibiotics, because antibiotic use can kill off both good bacteria (that keep yeast numbers in check) and bad bacteria (that cause the infection). Therefore, yeast can flourish, resulting in an uncomfortable yeast infection.

For your nursing school entrance exam, remember that photosynthesis involves the transformation of sun energy into chemical energy. Green plants take carbon dioxide, water, and energy in the form of sunlight and convert them to produce glucose for energy.

CELL REPRODUCTION

Cells need to reproduce in order to survive and maintain homeostasis. A cut in a person's skin will heal in time. Dead skin cells slough and flake off while new skin cells regenerate and grow. What cells do and how they do it is determined by the genetic information in the DNA in the cells. Every cell, except sex cells, has 46 chromosomes.

To understand how cells reproduce, you should first be familiar with the makeup of nucleotides.

Nucleotide Makeup

Nucleic acids (RNA and DNA) are made up of nucleotides, which are organic molecules. For the nursing exam, you should know the following information:

- DNA is a long polymer made up of repeating chemical units known as nucleotides.
- DNA is a double-stranded molecule, and RNA is single-stranded molecule.
- The three very important parts of nucleotides are (1) a five-carbon sugar (**deoxyribose** in DNA and **ribose** in RNA) made up of carbon, oxygen, and hydrogen; (2) a **phosphate group**, which is a chemical group made up of oxygen and phosphorous; and (3) a **nitrogenous base**, which is a chemical unit composed of carbon, oxygen, hydrogen and nitrogen, held together by a weak hydrogen bond. (*Note:* The specific arrangements of nitrogenous bases on the DNA chain make up the genetic code).

The nitrogen bases found in DNA are

- **adenine (A)**
- **cytosine (C)**
- **guanine (G)**
- **thymine (T)**

> In RNA, **uracil** replaces thymine.

In the double helix, thymine pairs with adenine (thymine-adenine, or T-A) and cytosine pairs with guanine (cytosine-guanine, or C-G).

RNA compliments DNA and is responsible for assisting protein synthesis (with three basic steps: transcription, RNA processing, and translation).

Genetic Mutations

Nursing school entrance exams often include a question or two about genetic mutations. Let's briefly review what can happen:

- **Deletion** is a type of chromosome mutation in which a section of a chromosome is deleted and missing.
- **Insertion** is a type of mutation in which one or more nucleotide base pairs are inserted.
- **Substitution** (or point mutation) occurs when a single-base nucleotide is replaced with another nucleotide of the genetic material.

Since cells come from pre-existing cells, mutations are passed on to every cell as well. If a mutation occurs in a **somatic cell** (a cell that makes up body tissues), then the mutation affects only that particular tissue. However, if the mutation occurs in a primary sex cell (that is, the egg or sperm cell), that mutation will be passed on to the offspring that results from fertilization or by the **gametes** produced from that primary sex cell division. In this instance, the mutation becomes **hereditary**. A gamete is a sex cell that has only 23 chromosomes. It unites with a gamete of the opposite sex to form a **zygote**.

MITOSIS AND MEIOSIS

Mitosis: How a Whole Cell Reproduces Itself

Mitosis is a type of cell division. Before we talk about mitosis itself, however, let's talk about what happens before mitosis occurs. To make things easy, we'll use a human cell as an example.

Most human cells (all, in fact, except for sperm and ova) have 46 chromosomes in their nuclei. The chromosomes are found in pairs, so we can say that the nuclei of the cells have 23 pairs of homologous chromosomes. Before a cell undergoes mitosis, every single chromosome in its nucleus replicates. In a human cell, all 46 chromosomes have to replicate.

The S Phase

The chromosome replicate during a portion of interphase called the S phase. "S" stands for "synthesis"—in this case synthesis (or replication) of DNA.

The purpose of mitosis is to produce daughter cells that are identical copies of the parent cell and to maintain the proper number of chromosomes from generation to generation.

Interphase

Interphase has three subphases, one of which is the synthesis phase (S phase) during which chromosomes replicate. There are also two growth phases (G phases) during which the cell carries out all of its normal activities. Interphase is sometimes called the resting stage of the cell—not because the cell is taking it easy, but because the cell is not actively dividing.

Once interphase is over, the cell has replicated every one of its 46 chromosomes. How many chromosomes does it have now? Well, the answer would seem to be $46 \times 2 = 92$. When a cell has finished interphase, you'd think it has 92 chromosomes, and more or less, you'd be right. But the terminology can get confusing.

> MiTosis—Remember the T for Two daughter cells with Two copies of each chromosome.

Watch Out for This Word: Chromatid

After interphase, each chromosome and the duplicate piece of DNA that was just made are held together at their center by a region called a **centromere**. The two chromosomes and the centromere make one united physical structure.

We look at the entire structure—the two chromosomes joined by a centromere—and call the whole thing a chromosome. The word **chromatid** is used to describe each of the individual chromosomes.

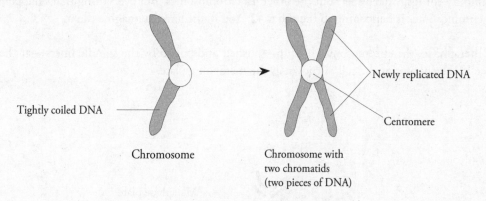

Tightly coiled DNA

Newly replicated DNA

Centromere

Chromosome

Chromosome with
two chromatids
(two pieces of DNA)

Chromosome vs Chromatid

When interphase is over, all of the cell's 46 chromosomes have doubled. We might *want* to say the cell has 92 chromosomes, but that's not the way it is described. Instead, we say the cell still has 46 chromosomes, each now consisting of two chromatids.

Let's examine each of the stages of mitosis.

After interphase, mitosis begins. Step 1 is called **prophase**. In prophase, the centrioles move away from each other to opposite sides of the cell. They form a bunch of fibers called the **mitotic spindle**. These fibers attach to the chromosomes at their centromeres and help to push and pull them around during mitosis. The chromosomes condense (coil up even tighter) and we can see them (under the microscope, of course). The nuclear membrane begins to break up, too.

Mitosis occurs in body cells to repair damaged tissue or to create new cells as an organism grows. One example of mitosis is skin re-growth after a sunburn or surgery. Another occurs as new red blood cells are made every 120 days or so—that's a lot of cell reproduction going on!

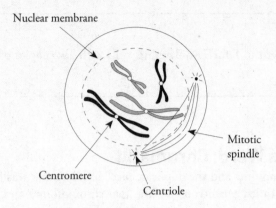

The Cell at Prophase of Mitosis

Note that in the drawing above, and in the ones that follow, the cell has only four chromosomes. That's okay. To simplify things, we have left out the other 42 chromosomes. But everything that's happening to these four chromosomes is happening to the other 42. You'll just have to imagine them.

In Step 2, **metaphase**, the chromosomes line up—pushed and pulled by the spindle fibers—at the equator of the cell. The equator of the cell is known as the metaphase plate.

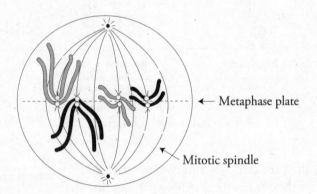

The Cell at Metaphase of Mitosis

In Step 3, **anaphase**, the centromere that joins each pair of chromatids splits in two so that each chromatid separates from its partner. And guess what? Now each chromatid is once again called a chromosome. So once the centromeres split, you have to admit that the cell briefly has 92 chromosomes. The newly separated chromosomes move toward opposite poles of the cell with the help of the spindle fibers.

Also during anaphase, the cell physically begins splitting in two. The area where it pinches inward is called the **cleavage furrow**.

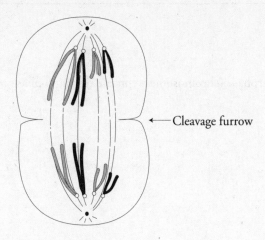

← Cleavage furrow

The Cell at Anaphase of Mitosis

During Step 4, **telophase**, a nuclear membrane forms in each new cell and two daughter cells result, each of which has 46 chromosomes. The cytoplasm then divides during a process called **cytokinesis**.

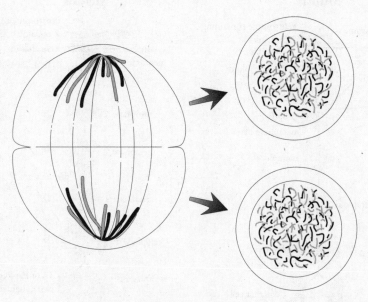

The Cell at Telephase of Mitosis

Then, of course, the two new daughter cells enter interphase.

The Order of Mitosis

So let's review the order:

- Before mitosis, interphase (chromosomes replicate during S phase of interphase)

- Mitosis:

    1. Prophase

    2. Metaphase

    3. Anaphase

    4. Telophase

Let's look at another diagram to review mitosis and introduce meiosis:

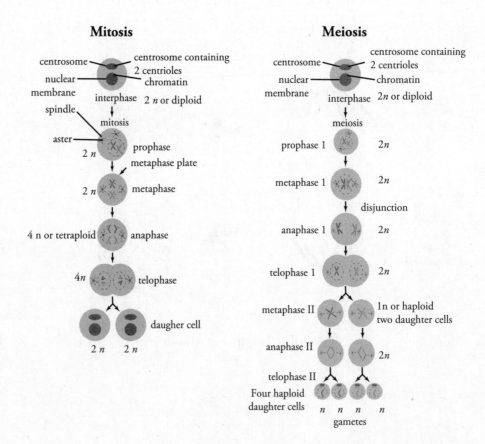

Mitosis vs. Meiosis

But How Will I Remember All That?

For mitosis, you may already have your own mnemonic. If not, here's a table with a mnemonic we created for you.

IPMAT	
Interphase	I is for **Interlude**
Prophase	P is for **Prepare**
Metaphase	M is for **Meet**
Anaphase	A is for **Apart**
Telophase	T is for **Tear**

Meiosis: The Formation of Gametes

Once again, you probably won't have to remember every stage of meiosis when you're working as a nurse, but you'll be expected to recall this information for any nursing school entrance exam.

> If you get stuck on a question and are confused about mitosis and meiosis,
> just remember the E in mEiosis. The E is used to make Egg and sperm.

The gametes—the sperm and ova—are the only human cells that are **haploid**. That is, each has 23 chromosomes. When a sperm and an ovum get together—when the sperm fertilizes the ovum—the chromosomes from the sperm join with the chromosomes in the ovum. The newly formed cell—the zygote—is diploid. The diploid zygote then undergoes mitosis to begin the new human's development. We'll look at the specifics of how a sperm is formed and how an ovum is formed in just a little while. But first let's go over the basics of meiosis.

During Meiosis

1. The cell undergoes DNA replication during interphase, just as it would if it were about to go through ordinary mitosis. All of the chromosomes replicate, and we're left with a cell that still has 46 chromosomes, each made up of two chromatids joined by a centromere.

2. The replicated chromosomes are split up in the course of two sets of divisions: prophase I, metaphase I, anaphase I, telophase I, and prophase II, metaphase II, anaphase II, and telophase II.

3. The differences between mitosis and meiosis are all found during the first set of divisions: prophase I, metaphase I, anaphase I, and telophase I.

Meiosis I

Meiosis I consists of four phases: prophase I, metaphase I, anaphase I, and telophase I. Remember that the chromosomes have already replicated and are found as two chromatids held together at the centromere. The biggest difference between these four phases and the four phases of mitosis is that at the very beginning, the homologous chromosomes pair up in a process called **synapsis**. This changes everything.

By the Numbers

Diploid number refers to the number of chromosomes a cell has when it's in a diploid state. For a human cell, the diploid number is 46. Haploid number means the number of chromosomes a cell has when it's in a haploid state. Naturally, the haploid number is always one-half the diploid number. For a human being, the haploid number is 23.

Prophase I

Synapsis occurs during **prophase I**. All the chromosomes have to find their homologous partner and pair up. Chromosome 1-A has to find chromosome 1-B, chromosome 2-A has to find chromosome 2-B, and so on. It takes a while, and prophase I is the longest phase of meiosis. When synapsis is complete, all the chromosomes are paired up with their partners. So instead of finding 46 replicated chromosomes floating around, we find *23 pairs* of replicated chromosomes. Because each pair consists of four chromatids (two chromatids per replicated chromosome, and two replicated chromosomes), this pair is also known as a **tetrad** (*tetra* = four). Notice that, in the drawings below, only four pairs of the 23 pairs are shown.

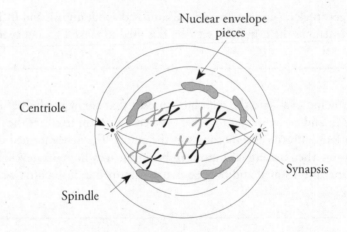

Prophase I of Meiosis

Crossing Over

Note that for simplicity in the drawings for meiosis, we are not showing crossing over. However, you can imagine that each one of the black chromosomes has a little bit of grey, and each of the grey chromosomes has a corresponding little bit of black. Also, the chromosomes do not necessarily line up with all the black on the left and all the grey on the right. It could be mixed up, with some of the black on the right and some of the grey on the left.

All of the other normal events that occur in prophase still happen. The spindle is formed, the chromosomes condense, and the nuclear membrane disintegrates. After synapsis occurs, an event called **crossing over** takes place. Basically, this means that like segments on homologous chromosomes are exchanged.

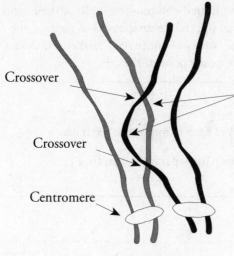

Crossover

Crossover

Centromere

These two segments would be
exchanged, so that the black
chromosome receives the gray
segment, and the gray chomosome
receives the black segment.

Crossing Over

Metaphase I

During metaphase of mitosis, the chromosomes line up on the equator of the cell. During **metaphase I** of
meiosis, the chromosomes also line up on the equator of the cells.

In meiosis, chromosomes *stay in their homologous pairs.* So instead of 46 individual
chromosomes lining up, there are 23 pairs of chromosomes.

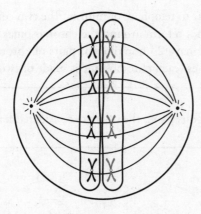

Metaphase I of Meiosis

Anaphase I

During anaphase of mitosis, the 46 replicated chromosomes split at their centromeres, and one chromatid goes to each of the opposite poles of the cell. In **anaphase I** of meiosis, the centromeres do *not* divide. Instead, the homologous pairs separate, with one entire replicated chromosome (a pair of chromatids and a centromere) moving to each of the opposite poles of the cell.

> ### During Anaphase
> - In mitosis, the chromatids of each chromosome separate.
>
> - In meiosis, the homologous pairs separate in anaphase I.

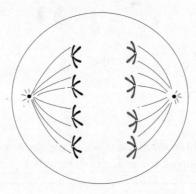

Anaphase I of Meiosis

Telophase I

Telophase I of meiosis is very similar to telophase of mitosis. The two cells finish dividing their cytoplasm (cytokinesis), and nuclear membranes reform around the chromosomes. But this leaves us with a strange situation. The two new cells do *not* have 23 homologous pairs of chromosomes (46 total chromosomes); they have 23 replicated chromosomes (each chromosome is made of two identical chromatids).

> Because there are no homologous pairs, the cells are considered haploid by Telophase I.

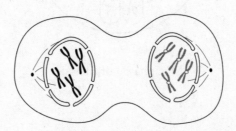

Telophase I of Meiosis

Meiosis II

Meiosis II is virtually identical to mitosis, in terms of how the chromosomes are moved and how they are split. However, because we're starting with the two cells formed in meiosis I, they have only half the number of chromosomes that a cell would have when undergoing mitosis. Remember that, in mitosis, the cell starts with 46 replicated chromosomes. The cells we're starting out with in meiosis II, because of meiosis I, have only 23 replicated chromosomes. But the phases and the chromosome movements are identical to those of mitosis. During prophase II the spindle forms, the nuclear membrane disintegrates, and the DNA condenses (of course, there is no pairing of chromosomes this time, because there is nothing to pair up with—the homologous partners were separated during anaphase I. During metaphase II, the chromosomes line up individually along the equator and, during anaphase II, *the centromere splits and the chromatids divide*. Then the chromatids are called chromosomes again. During telophase II, a nuclear membrane forms around the newly split chromosomes, and we are left with four haploid cells.

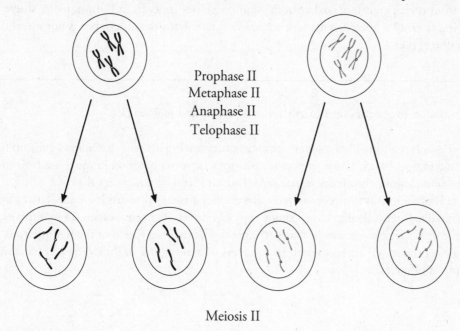

Prophase II
Metaphase II
Anaphase II
Telophase II

Meiosis II

The four haploid cells do not replicate any further unless fertilization triggers new cell cycles.

Differences Between Meiosis and Mitosis

A major difference between miTosis and mEiosis is that at the beginning of meiosis (in prophase), homologous chromosomes pair up to become tetrads (groupings of four chromatids) during a process called synapsis. This results in the change of linkage relationship (with formation of **alleles**) and therefore increases **variability**. The centromeres do not divide during anaphase of meiosis I, but rather the homologous pairs line up to separate into two cells.

In anaphase II of meiosis the centromeres divide (this is what attaches the chromatids), and this results in Telophase II, where four haploid cells with 23 chromosomes each form.

The cells that result from this process of meiosis will mature into specialized reproductive cells known as sex cells or gametes:

- **Spermatogenesis** is the gamete formation, through meiosis, of four haploid sperm cells from a single spermatogenium. (Remember that a spermato*goni*um is *gon*na become a sperm cell.)
- **Oogenesis** is the gamete formation, through meiosis, of a single haploid ovum from a single primary oocyte.

Recap

Meiosis is used for cell reproduction of eggs and sperm only. Each parent puts half of its genetic material into the offspring, giving the offspring two copies of each chromosome (one copy from each parent). Sexual reproduction combines traits from both parents, where the offspring resembles both parents (one sometimes more than the other), but is not identical to either one of them.

Before you move on to genetics, let's briefly recap meiosis I and meiosis II:

- In meiosis I, replicated homologous chromosomes (each with two chromatids) pair up to form a tetrad in prophase I. Crossing over leads to genetic recombination in prophase I. Recombined homologous chromosomes are separated into haploid daughter cells.
- Phase II of meiosis is similar to mitosis. Recombined sister chromatids are separated into haploid daughter cells that have a single copy of one set of chromosomes, 23 in humans.
- In humans, spermatogenesis in males (the process of making sperm in the seminiferous tubules of the testes) and oogenesis (the process of making ova in the ovaries) in females are examples of meiosis.

Genetics

It's unlikely you will be asked anything about DNA crossover or **segregation**. However, you should remember that a gene is a molecule of DNA (a segment of a chromosome) located on a chromosome; essentially it is a physical base for heredity.

An allele is one of the alternate gene forms—meaning more than one version of the same trait (such as eye color). There are two kinds of alleles: **dominant** and **recessive**.

When two alleles are in agreement (whether both dominant or both recessive), the organism is considered to be **homozygous** for that particular trait. An example is someone with sickle cell disease. He or she must have both abnormal alleles that cause the symptoms associated with the disease.

On the opposite end of the spectrum, when two alleles are not in agreement, the organism is considered to be **heterozygous** for that trait. An example is someone who has only one abnormal allele for the sickle cell disease. Because this person holds only one abnormal allele, he or she is considered a carrier.

If a baby is born with the sickle cell trait, he or she carries one abnormal allele and is considered a carrier, as just mentioned. If he or she marries a person also carrying the sickle cell trait, that couple has a 25 percent chance of having a child who will carry both abnormal alleles and actually have sickle cell disease.

Co-dominance means that a heterozygote expresses a mixture of the traits of both alleles (for example, with the blood type AB). Here's a **Punnett square** that shows a monohybrid cross—both parents have genotype Bb:

Female

	B	b
B	BB	Bb
b	bB	bb

Male

A Punnett square can be used to predict the genotype of the offspring of two particular genes. It could be used to predict eye color, hair color, blood type, and more. The genotype probabilities that are predicted by this Punnett square are that 75 percent of the offspring will have dominant traits (BB or Bb or bB) and 25 percent will have recessive traits (bb).

> You won't be predicting blood types on any nursing unit, trust me. A confirmed blood type will have already been processed (in some places twice) during a routine or emergency hospital admission.

Some alleles are passed from generation to generation only on the **sex chromosomes**. Sex chromosomes are one of the 23 pairs of chromosomes in humans that determine the gender of the offspring. A **sex-linked trait** is a trait whose allele is carried on one of the sex chromosomes. Color blindness, hemophilia, and baldness are sex-linked traits. All other chromosomes are called **autosomes**.

Here is some more useful test information (but not really for your nursing career):

- **Pedigrees** are diagrams that show the presence of phenotypes (the observable constitution of organisms) in several generations of a family.
- When discussing phenotype, you look at an organism's trait.
- When discussing genotype, you look at the genes responsible for those traits.
- **Hybrid** refers to the offspring produced when two different species breed.

A BRIEF TOUCH ON TAXONOMY

Jump in the Gene Pool

Taxonomy refers to the science that deals with the description, identification, naming, and classification of organisms. We briefly discussed the organization of species from genus to domain in the beginning of this chapter. Each individual in a population has his or her own set of genes. When these gene combinations are all added together, the result is called a population's **gene pool**. The gene pool is ever-changing, thanks to evolution. **Natural selection** (sometimes referred to as **Darwinism**) is a theory of evolution in which better competitors are more likely to survive and therefore continue to reproduce in future generations. **Fitness** is an organism's ability to contribute to the next generations' gene pool. If two individuals are members of two different species, they cannot produce viable offspring.

Organization

Species can be classified according to an organizational scheme. As mentioned at the beginning of this chapter, this organization scheme, from most specific to least specific, is domain, kingdom, phylum, class, order, family, genus, and species. Organisms have been classified into three different domains: Bacteria, Archaea, and Eukarya. (Humans fall into the domain Eukarya.) Further, the domain Eukarya has been divided into four kingdoms: Protista, Fungi, Plantae, and Animalia. (Humans fall into the kindom Animalia.)

Let's look at the full breakdown for humans:

Domain: Eukarya
Kingdom: Animalia
Phylum: Chordate
Class: Mammalia
Order: Primates
Family: Hominidae
Genus: Homo
Species: sapiens

> The four types or microorganisms that you need to remember are protists, fungi, bacteria, and viruses.

Protists are eukaryotes that contain organelles and a true nucleus. They can be unicellular or multicellular and they can form colonies. Examples of protists include the amoeba and algae. Most fungi are multicellular eukaryotes. Yeasts are unicellular fungi. Fungi can reproduce by asexual spores, by sexual spores, by vegetative growth, or by budding.

Bacteria are prokaryotes. Some bacteria are **autotrophs** (organisms that produce their own organic compounds from inorganic chemicals) and others are **heterotrophs** (organisms that obtain food energy by consuming other organisms or products created by other organisms). Some bacteria supply soil with nitrogen to help plants grow properly, which is good. There is good bacteria (such as the bacteria naturally found in our guts—when it stays in our guts) and bad bacteria (such as the ones that cause strep throat and methicillin-resistant staph aureus).

VIRUS

Viruses are not cells, and they are not alive. You should be familiar with them for all types of nursing school exam-taking purposes, and to understand the importance of viruses and how they affect people's lives with infection (both acutely and chronically).

Virus Defined

A virus is a nonliving, noncellular nasty infectious organism. Viruses are enclosed in a lipid layer (a **capsid**) and consist of a nucleic acid core and a protein coat. A virus cannot reproduce itself, but can replicate its genetic material once it enters a host cell (one of us or someone we love) and uses our (their) internal equipment to take over or kill the cell (make someone ill).

The Virus Life Cycle

The two methods in which viruses reproduce are the **lytic cycle** and the **lysogenic cycle** (*they both sound bad, huh?*). In the lytic cycle, the virus kills the host cell. Once the viral genes are inside a cell, they are transcribed to make proteins. Then, they replicate and are packaged into new viral envelopes, or capsids. Finally, the host cell is broken open (lysed) and the new virus escapes to infect new host cells (definitely a vicious cycle). Think of **influenza** (the flu) and **varicella** (chicken pox), both of which are viral illnesses. With these diseases, individuals become ill almost immediately. With flu exposure, they may become symptomatic 3–5 days after becoming infected with the virus. With the chicken pox virus, they may become symptomatic within 10–14 days of exposure.

In the lysogenic cycle, genetic information is not immediately transcribed, translated, and replicated. Instead, it's integrated into the host's genome, where it remains **dormant** (resting). The virus will then rear its ugly head during routine mitotic cell division. In this cycle, a virus enters a gene and remains quiet indefinitely, but does not kill its host. Much like an unwanted dinner guest, or that annoying someone who is intrusive or does not respect boundaries, this virus makes you sick or perturbed eventually over time, but doesn't kill you right then and there. That's the curse of the lysogenic cycle.

The lysogenic cycle is a bit different than the lytic cycle. During the lysogenic cycle, the virus becomes part of the host cell. Then when it attaches itself to a bacteriophage receptor, it becomes what's called a **provirus** and is copied by the host cell and replicated during normal mitotic cell division. That's right, during mitosis, the virus transmits to the daughter cells. The virus replicates with the cell. It remains dormant indefinitely, and then at any time thereafter, enters the lytic cycle where it proliferates, kills the host cell, and makes you become ill with symptoms.

Here's an example of a virus in the lysogenic cycle. Suppose an individual has the virus that causes **infectious mononucleosis,** or **mono.** It remains dormant in that person's body for several months to many years before it reactivates and makes him or her ill. Symptoms can include extreme fatigue, sometimes accompanied by a sore throat and even an enlarged spleen.

Another example of a virus in the lysogenic cycle is herpes simplex type I. This virus can enter your system and remain dormant for years, until it is activated. When activated, painful fever blisters appear on your skin. This formerly dormant virus activates when a person is run-down or overtired, often after too much sun exposure. It may also occur when an individual is stressed (perhaps while studying for a nursing exam?).

Finally, some viruses are **oncogenic.** These viruses often cause the formation of tumors and may lead to cancer.

Viruses are never good. Be sure you know how they work both for your nursing exam and for your future day-to-day tasks as a nurse. Remember that proper hand washing helps prevent the spread of disease, including those viral in nature.

RELATIONSHIPS

Here is some coverage of the many types of biological relationships that you may encounter in your nursing career and on your exam.

Parasitism is a type of symbiotic relationship between two organisms of different species in which one organism (the **parasite**) benefits at the expense of the other (the **host**). Examples of parasitic disease in health care include malaria, scabies, pinworms, amoebic dysentery, and cysticercosis.

Unlike parasitism, **mutualism** is a relationship in which two organisms biologically interact and both benefit. There is no harm, no fowl, no pathology, and no disease. An example of mutualism is the bacteria that we harbor in our guts (also called gut flora). These helpful little gut-bugs aid in digestion and in the production of vitamin K (as previously discussed), and they help maintain the integrity of the gut, preventing the overgrowth of harmful bacteria and yeast.

Symbiosis (often confused with mutualism) describes a close and often long-term interaction between different biological species. An example is lactobacilli in our guts and those found in yogurts that promote healthy digestion. Over-the-counter acidophilus is often recommended for persons undergoing antibiotic treatments. Acidophilus promotes normal intestinal activity and prevents the overgrowth of harmful bacteria and yeast.

Commensalism is a type of relationship between two organisms in which one organism benefits but the other is neutral (no harm or benefit). An example is ivy or moss that attaches to and grows up a tree, but does not harm or benefit the tree. Another example is a barnacle that attaches to a scallop shell and has a place to reside, without affecting the scallop or competing for food.

Neutralism is a concept difficult to prove, but it is used in tests. Neutralism describes an interaction or relationship between two species in which the interactions affect neither organism. Think about the roommate that you never see or hear but you know he or she is there.

Amensalism refers to the interaction between two species in which one species is unaffected while it impedes, stifles, or eliminates another. An example is the Juglans nigra (the black walnut tree), which secretes a chemical that is harmful to neighboring plants. Killing off neighboring plants allows the Juglans nigra plant to get all the sunlight and water it needs to survive, having eliminated competitive plants nearby.

ECOLOGY

If you are planning to take the NLN PAX-RN or the TEAS, you'll definitely want to familiarize yourself with cycles in nature: the water cycle, the carbon cycle, the nitrogen cycle, and the phosphorous cycle. You should also review the functions of sulfur, the greenhouse effect, ozone depletion, acid rain, environmental toxins, and pollution. These topics are often found in questions about Earth science. Let's briefly review these topics as a refresher.

FOOD CHAINS AND FOOD WEBS

All living things can be classified by how they obtain food. You might recall that plants are capable of making their own food through photosynthesis, and that some animals (for example, mice) eat plants. Some animals (for example, humans) eat both plants and animals, and some animals (for example, wolves) eat only other animals. A few pages back, you learned that there are two fancy terms that are normally used to describe these broad categories of organisms: Autotrophs are those organisms that can produce their own organic compounds from inorganic chemicals, while heterotrophs obtain food energy by consuming other organisms or products created by other organisms.

Finally, as unpleasant as it might be to think about, some animals feed only on the remains of other plants and animals! All of these different types of living things fall into specific categories—and you will definitely need to memorize all of these terms before the test, if you don't already know them!

Producers

Producers are organisms that are capable of converting radiant energy or chemical energy into carbohydrates. The group of producers includes plants and algae, both of which can carry out photosynthesis. The unbalanced overall reaction of photosynthesis is shown below.

$$H_2O + CO_2 + \text{solar energy} \rightarrow CH_2O + O_2$$

While most producers make food through photosynthesis, a few autotrophs make food from inorganic chemicals in anaerobic (without oxygen) environments, through the process of chemosynthesis. Chemosynthesis is carried out by only a few specialized bacteria, called **chemotrophs,** some of which are found in hydrothermal vents deep in the ocean. This unbalanced reaction is shown below.

$$O_2 + H_2S + O_2 + energy \rightarrow CH_2O + S + H_2O$$

Consumers

Consumers are organisms that must obtain food energy from secondary sources, for example, by eating plant or animal matter. There are a number of different types of consumers, and we've listed them below.

- **Primary consumers:** This category includes the herbivores, which consume only producers (plants and algae).
- **Secondary consumers:** Organisms that consume primary consumers are secondary consumers.
- **Tertiary consumers:** Organisms that consume secondary consumers are tertiary consumers.
- **Detritivores:** The organisms in this group derive energy from consuming nonliving organic matter such as dead animals or fallen leaves.
- **Decomposers:** These are bacteria or fungi that absorb nutrients from nonliving organic matter such as plant material, the wastes of living organisms, and corpses. They convert these materials into inorganic forms.

Note that one organism may occupy multiple levels of a food chain. By eating a hamburger with toppings, you are both a primary consumer, because you are eating tomatoes and lettuce, and a secondary consumer, because you are eating beef.

Let's move on and talk about how energy flows through all of these different types of organisms in ecosystems.

Food Chains

Energy flows in one direction through ecosystems: from the Sun to producers, to primary consumers, to secondary consumers, to tertiary consumers. In an ecosystem, each of these feeding levels is referred to as a **trophic level**. With each successive trophic level, the amount of energy that's available to the next level decreases. In fact, only about 10 percent of the energy from one trophic level is passed to the next; most is lost as heat, and some is used for metabolism and anabolism. Interestingly enough, this is why food chains rarely have more than four trophic levels.

Food chains are usually represented as a series of steps, in which the bottom step is the producer and the top step is a secondary or tertiary consumer. In food chains, the arrows depict the transfer of energy through the levels, and in fancier food chains, the relative **biomass** (the dry weight of the group of organisms) of each trophic level will often be represented. Here's a simple food chain.

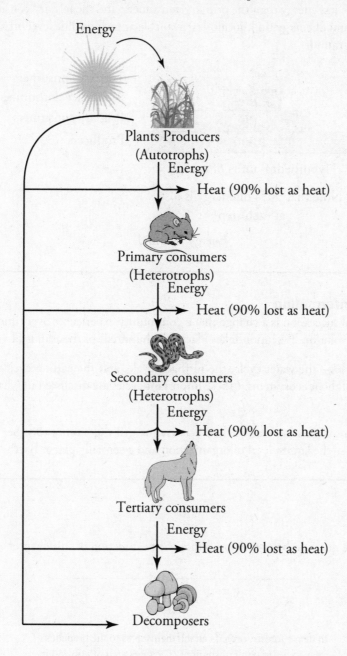

Energy

Plants Producers
(Autotrophs)

Energy

Heat (90% lost as heat)

Primary consumers
(Heterotrophs)

Energy

Heat (90% lost as heat)

Secondary consumers
(Heterotrophs)

Energy

Heat (90% lost as heat)

Tertiary consumers

Energy

Heat (90% lost as heat)

Decomposers

Food Chain

What we're showing here is a typical terrestrial food chain, but keep in mind that there are aquatic food chains as well, with algae and different types of fish.

One final note about food chains: In a food chain, only about 10 percent of the energy is transferred from one level to the next. The other 90 percent is used for things like respiration, digestion, running away from predators—that is, it's used to power the organism doing the eating! In other words, the producers have the most energy in an ecosystem; the primary consumers have less energy than producers; the secondary consumers have less energy than the primary consumers; and the tertiary consumers have the least energy of all. The amount of energy (in kilocalories) available at each trophic level organized from greatest to least is an **energy pyramid**.

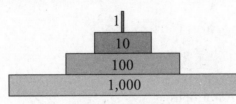

1	Tertiary consumers
10	Secondary consumers
100	Primary consumers
1,000	Producers

Hypothetical units of energy

Note that 90% of energy is lost
at each step

Energy Pyramid

Last-Minute Information

1. Ecological succession is a change that a community experiences over time. It is not the same as evolution. Evolution takes place over hundreds of thousands of years.

2. Three cycles—the water cycle, the nitrogen cycle, and the carbon cycle—move nutrients throughout ecosystems. (These important cycles are discussed in Chapter 8: Earth Science.)

3. Biomes are large areas classified by ecosystems. All the biomes together make up the biosphere—the largest level of organization and essentially planet Earth.

Let's take on a practice question before we jump into the next section of this chapter.

In dense forests, orchids attach themselves to the branches of trees to get maximum sunlight. The trees are not affected in any way by this. What relationship is displayed between the tree and the orchid?

A. Parasitism
B. Mutualism
C. Symbiosis
D. Commensalism

Here's How to Crack It

The most important part of the question stem is this: "The trees are not affected in any way by this." Therefore, you know that the relationship between the orchid and the trees is not toxic or parasitic, so you can eliminate choice A immediately. From your review of relationships, you know that mutualism is the way in which two organisms biologically interact and each individual derives a fitness benefit. From the question stem, we know that the trees are not getting any benefit from this relationship, so eliminate choice B also. Choice C is a tricky distractor—symbiosis is a broad term describing interactions between biological species. It's not specific enough to describe what is happening here, so eliminate choice C also. That leaves choice D, commensalism. Commensalism is a class of relationship in which one organism benefits and the other is neutral, which is just what we are looking for. Go with choice D.

PLANTS

Leaves

You won't need to be a florist to work as a nurse in a hospital, but on your nursing exam you will surely be asked a question or two relating to plants, leaves, or photosynthesis.

Let's begin by reviewing the parts of a plant leaf shown in the cross section below.

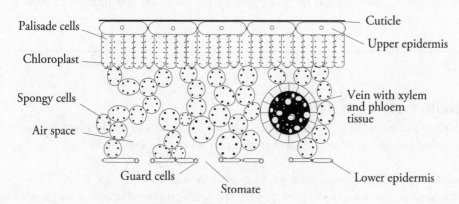

Cross Section of Plant Leaf

Cells of leaf plants stick together "wall to wall." Cell walls of plants are made up of cellulose. Cell walls give shape, structure, and protection to plant cells.

Leaves provide surface area that collects the energy from the Sun to make food—remember when we discussed photosynthesis? Tiny openings in the leaf structure allow for gas exchange—CO_2 and O_2—to move in and out of the plant while having control over the amount of water lost (remember cellular respiration?).

Did you ever wonder why people talk to plants? The carbon dioxide that people exhale nourishes the plant and in return, the happy plant converts that carbon dioxide into oxygen for people to breathe.

Most plants are made up of many cells. Plants make their own food through the process of photosynthesis. Plant cells contain a chemical called **chlorophyll**, which gives plants their green color. The growth process of plants depends on the seasons. Chlorophyll is depleted and relatively scarce during the fall and winter months. Leaves turn colors and fall from trees, which are leafless during the dreary and cold winter months. In the spring, vibrant green plants and flowering trees emerge once again, as chlorophyll stores are once again plentiful. Trunks protect trees because of their wood structure, allowing survival in the cold winter months.

Photosynthesis is the process in which green plants use energy from the Sun to produce food (sugar).

Photosynthesis occurs in the part of the plant that sunlight is most likely to hit—the leaves.

Photosynthetic reactions take place in the chloroplasts of a plant cell.

Plants take in carbon dioxide, water, and energy and use them to produce glucose and release oxygen.

The summary equation for photosynthesis is

$$6\,CO_2 + 6\,H_2O + energy \longrightarrow C_6H_{12}O_6 + 6\,O_2$$

Two types of reaction occur in the process of photosynthesis: light-dependent reactions and light-independent reactions.

Minerals, water, and nutrients are transported within a plant by vascular tissues xylem and phloem. Xylem takes nutrition from the ground up the plant and phloem transports back down.

Brief Review of Tropism

Tropism is a plant's response to an environmental stimulus. It results when the plant grows in a particular way. The list below is a review of each type of tropism found in the plant world:

- **Phototropism** occurs when a plant grows toward the light.
- **Geotropism** occurs when roots grow toward the earth and the shoots/flowers grow toward the sky.
- **Thigmotropism** occurs when plants curl around an object that touches them.
- **Hydrotropism** occurs when plant roots grow toward a water source.
- **Chemotropism** occurs when roots grow toward the presence of certain chemicals.

PLANT REPRODUCTION

Not for the Nurse, But for the Exam

For plant reproduction, you should recall that a flowering plant reproduces in the following manner:

- Grains of **pollen** fall on the stigma.
- During germination, the pollen tube grows down through the **style** to connect to the **ovary**.
- The two sperm (from the pollen) travel down the **pollen tube** to enter the ovary and the **ovule**, where they undergo a double fertilization: one sperm fertilizes one egg while the other sperm combines with the polar bodies.
- The fertilized egg becomes the plant embryo and the polar bodies become **endosperm**. Endosperm is a food-storing tissue that surrounds the plant embryo.
- The entire ovule (which contains the embryo and the endosperm) develops into a seed, and the ovary develops into a fruit. The fruit protects the seed and helps it disperse by wind or animals.
- The seed is released (the fruit drops, the plant is eaten, and so on), and when it finds a sustainable environment, that seed develops into a new plant.

Pretty cool, huh?

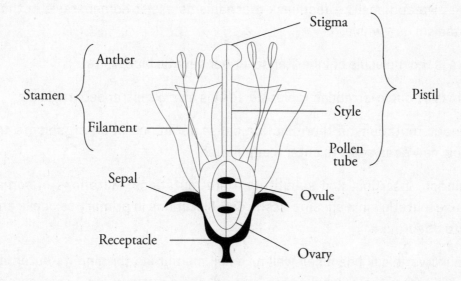

Parts of a Flowering Plant

A Breakdown of the Parts

The **stamen** is the plant's male component. It consists of the **anther** and the **filament**. The filament supports the anther, which produces the pollen. Pollen is made from little cells called **microspores**, and mature pollen grains contain a cell that can divide to form two sperm cells.

The **pistil** is the plant's female component. It consists of the **stigma**, style, ovule, and ovary. Inside the ovary is the ovule, which forms cells, called **megaspores**. Megaspores can divide to form eggs and polar bodies.

SUMMARY

- Biology is the study of life and living organisms.

- All living things are composed of cells that came from a pre-existing cell.

- The scientific method tests a hypothesis and forms a conclusion that other scientists will achieve every time.

- The structure and organization of both living and nonliving things are derived from certain properties of matter and energy.

- Homeostasis is the maintenance of equilibrium within an organism by a tendency to compensate for changes and disruptions.

- Metabolism refers to the basic processes of organic functioning and operating. These are all of the activities (physical and chemical) associated with life.

- Hormones are chemicals released into the bloodstream that are responsible for homeostasis.

- Negative and positive feedback mechanisms assist homeostasis in the cell and organism as a whole.

- DNA is the molecule of inheritance, or our genetic blueprints.

- DNA is a double-stranded molecule; RNA is a single-stranded molecule.

- Genetic mutations in reproduction cause variations in an organism's traits and allow new gene pools to enter a population.

- Deletion, insertion, and substitution are mutations. Mutations in somatic cells cause mutation in a specific tissue cell. Mutations in primary sex cells are passed onto offspring.

- A eukaryotic cell has a cell wall or a cell membrane forming its outer layer cytoplasm, where the organelles are located, and a nucleus, where the chromosomes are located.

- The organelles of a eukaryotic cell are found in the cytoplasm.

- Organelles are tiny task-oriented structures within a cell, responsible for a specific function or functions in cell life.

- Water is a polar molecule.

- Pure water has a pH of 7.0, which is considered neutral.

- Organic compounds have carbon while inorganic compounds do not.

- Plant cells have cell walls and cell membranes.

- Cellular transportation is both passive and active. Active forms of transport require energy.

- Cellular respiration is a series of chemical reactions that take place inside a cell to produce energy. It occurs in a series of smaller steps designed to maximize the production of energy. The events that occur in cellular respiration are glycolysis, the Krebs cycle, electron transport chain, and oxidative phosphorylation.

- All cells, except egg and sperm cells, undergo cell division through mitosis.

- In the final stage of mitotic cell division, there are two daughter cells with 46 chromosomes each.

- Gametes form during a process called meiosis.

- Spermatogensis is the formation (through meiosis) of four haploid sperm cells from a single spermatogonium.

- Oogenesis is the formation (through meiosis) of a single haploid ovum from a single primary oocyte.

- Ova and sperm have only 23 chromosomes each.

- An allele is an alternate form of a gene.

- Punnett squares can be used to predict the phenotype and genotype of the offspring.

- Pedigrees are diagrams that show the presence of phenotypes in several generations of a family.

- The two main methods of reproduction of a virus are the lytic cycle and lysogenic cycle.

- Food chains, food webs, and food pyramids show the movement of material and energy from one group of organisms to another.

- Photosynthesis is the process by which green plants use energy from the Sun to produce food. It occurs in the chloroplasts of plant cells.

KEY TERMS

NLN PAX-RN (National League for Nursing Pre-Admission Exam)

TEAS (Test of Essential Academic Skills)

NET (Nursing Entrance Test)

biology

organisms

bacteria

cells

cell theory

taxon tier

genus

domain

kingdom

phylum

class

order

family

species

scientific method

hypothesis

compound microscope

matter

elements

helium

oxygen

chlorine

nitrogen

potassium

radium

periodic table

energy

law of conservation of energy

homeostasis

metabolism

photosynthesis

aerobic respiration

anaerobic respiration

synthesize

anabolism

catabolism

active transport

passive transport

hormones

negative feedback

positive feedback

pancreas

insulin

glycogen

glycogenolysis

DNA (deoxyribonucleic acid)

mutations

natural selection

unicellular

multicellular

organelles

electric charges

protein

tissues

organs

systems

bodies

people

populations

atoms

protons

neutrons

electrons

net charge

molecules

compound

sodium

carbon

hydrogen

phosphorous

sulfur

calcium

sodium

potassium

magnesium

iron

intravenous (IV) access

enteric (oral) access

parenterally

TPN (total parenteral nutrition)

central venous access

arrhythmias

chemical bonds

ionic bonds

ions

covalent bonds

nonpolar covalent

polar covalent

hydrogen bonds

water

edema

polar molecule

dissolve

solvent

solutes

solution

cohesion

adhesion

surface tension

capillary action

heat capacity

calorie

hydrolysis

acids

bases

pH balance

aqueous

NPO (non per os) (nothing by mouth)

organic compounds

inorganic compounds

amino acids

peptide bond

polypeptide chain

structural protein

globular protein

collagen

connective tissues

hemoglobin

antibodies

denatured

carbohydrates

monosaccharides

disaccharides

polysaccharides

starch

cellulose

saccharide

lipids

fatty acids

glycerol

triglyceride

HDL (high-density lipid)
LDL (low-density lipid)
cholesterol
hydrocarbon rings
nucleic acids
nucleus
nucleotides
ATP (adenosine triphosphate)
coenzyme
DNA (deoxyribonucleic acid)
RNA (riboneucleic acid)
eukaryotic cell
prokaryotic cell
chromosomes
nucleoid
cell membrane (plasma
    membrane)
pinacytotic vesicle
differentially permeable
    (selectively permeable)
hydrophilic
hydrophobic
cytoplasm
cell walls
nucleolus
ribosomes
endoplasmic reticulum (ER)
rough ER
smooth ER
Golgi bodies
mitochondria
lysosomes
centrioles
vacuoles
peroxisomes
cytoskeleton
microtubules
microfilaments
tubulin
cilia
flagella
diffusion
osmosis
hypotonic
hypertonic
facilitated diffusion

bulk transport (bulk flow)
enzymes
catalysts
substrates
cofactors
cellular energy
ADP (adenosine diphosphate)
cellular respiration
glycolysis
Krebs cycle
electron transport chain
oxidative phosphorylation
pyruvate
pyruvic acid
fermentation
deoxyribose
ribose
phosphate group
nitrogenous base
adenine (A)
cytosine (C)
guanine (G)
thymine (T)
uracil
deletion
insertion
substitution
somatic cell
gametes
hereditary
zygote
mitosis
interphase
centromere
chromatid
prophase
mitotic spindle
metaphase
anaphase
cleavage furrow
telophase
cytokinesis
haploid
meiosis I
synapsis
prophase I

tetrad
crossing over
metaphase I
anaphase I
telophase I
meiosis II
alleles
variability
spermatogenesis
oogenesis
segregation
dominant allele
recessive allele
homozygous
heterozygous
co-dominance
Punnett square
sex chromosomes
sex-linked trait
autosomes
pedigrees
hybrid
taxonomy
gene pool
natural selection (Darwinism)
fitness
protists
autotrophs
heterotrophs
viruses
capsid
lytic cycle
lysogenic cycle
influenza
varicella
dormant
provirus
infectious mononucleosis (mono)
oncogenic
parasitism
parasite
host
mutualism
symbiosis
commensalism
neutralism

amensalism
producers
chemotrophs
primary consumers
secondary consumers
tertiary consumers
detritivores
decomposers
trophic level
food chain
biomass
energy pyramid
chlorophyll
tropism
phototropism
geotropism
thigmotropism
hydrotropism
chemotropism
pollen
style
ovary
pollen tube
ovule
endosperm
stamen
anther
filament
microspores
pistil
stigma
megaspores

Chapter 5
Human Anatomy and Physiology

QUICK REVIEW OF HUMAN ORGAN SYSTEMS

Tissues are composed of cells (that came from pre-existing cells) that have similar structure and function. Organs are composed of two or more tissues that are integrated to do a similar function. Organs make systems. Let's start with an overview of the major organ systems of the body and their functions.

- The **digestive system** is comprised of the mouth, the stomach, small and large intestines, and more. It uses enzymes to break down the food that we eat in order to release it into the bloodstream and have it absorbed into the cells. It rids the body of undigested food that did not enter the bloodstream (in the form of feces or stools).
- The **respiratory system** is made up of the nose, the mouth, the trachea, and the lungs. This system is responsible for gas exchange and pH regulation. It removes CO_2 from the blood and exchanges it for O_2.
- The **circulatory system** is made up of the heart, blood vessels, lymphatics, and blood cells. This system is responsible for internal transport, pH maintenance, and temperature stability (sounds like homeostasis all over again). The circulatory system also delivers nutrition and oxygen to cells and carries waste products and carbon dioxide away from the cells.
- The **immune system** is a defense system that provides protection from foreign substance or particles when exposed. It is made up of white blood cells (fighter cells, memory cells, killer cells) and lymph nodes. The immune system maintains or restores homeostasis in animals. (Guard cells help to maintain homeostasis in plants.)
- The **excretory system** enables the disposal of metabolic wastes and the regulation of salts, fluids, and electrolytes. It also allows waste removal from the bloodstream via the liver, kidneys, urinary bladder (in the form of urine), skin (in the form of sweat), and lungs (in the form of carbon dioxide).
- The **integumentary system** (layers of skin) protects the internal organs. As the first line of defense, skin doesn't allow foreign bodies in. Skin also produces vitamin D (after sunlight exposure) and assists in excretion (we sweat to let off heat).
- The **musculoskeletal system** includes such body parts as the hips, the spinal column, deltoids, and quadriceps. It serves as protection, movement, support, and shape. It also supports the production of blood and serves as storage sites for some minerals. Muscles enable movement, strength, posture, and heat production. Musculoskeletal systems work together to move the body.
- The **nervous system** consists of the brain, the spinal cord, and nerves. This system integrates body function through nerves, detects stressors/change/stimuli, secretes chemicals and electrical signals, and controls other organ systems.
- The **endocrine system** is made up of the hypothalamus, the pituitary gland, adrenal glands, the pancreas, and the gonads. It integrates the body through chemicals (hormones released into the bloodstream). Cells use hormones to communicate with each other. Hormones are necessary to maintain homeostasis and life.
- The **reproductive system** is made up of the scrotum, testes, prostate gland, vas deferens, and penis in males; ovaries, fallopian tubes, uterus, cervix and vagina in females. It provides mechanisms for internal fertilization and production of new offspring.

This material on anatomy and physiology is important for your foundation as a future nurse. Therefore, we wrote this section in a way that you can share an in-depth understanding of the what, why, and how systems function together within the whole person. You may hesitate and wonder why there is so much detail in this section, and perhaps you are right to question. Keep in mind that you will be asked a number of anatomy and physiology questions if you are taking the NLN PAX-RN or the TEAS. Both exams have science sections that include many science questions. The information presented to you in this chapter will hopefully entice and impassion you. Our hope is that this section will confirm your desire to become a future healer and that this chapter is something you would consider to hold onto in the future, as anatomy and physiology is a course you will revisit in all academic settings in preparation for becoming a nurse. Let's begin!

PHYLUM TALK

Remember dumb kings play chess on fiberglass stools from Chapter 4? Well let's talk about the phylum in that statement—specifically **phylum Chordata**. Phylum Chordata is divided into three subphyla:

1. **Urochordata**
2. **Cephalochordata**
3. **Vertebrata** (includes humans, fish, reptiles, amphibians, and mammals)

Why do you need to know this? Because it provides classification and differentiation from other organisms, and soon you will be moving forward with your exciting future nursing classes, clinical obstetric and pediatric rotations, and much more in due time.

Well, here's what you should know: Human beings (*us*) are called Vertebrata because, unlike the urochordates and cephalochordates, we have

- A column of bones (a back bone, a spinal column) and
- A tube-within-a-tube construction (Vertebrata have an outer tube formed by a body wall and an inner tube, the digestive tract.)

> Humans have bilateral symmetry—that is,
> the left side of body is a mirror image of the right side.

ANATOMICAL POSITION

We must first recognize the proper anatomical locators and descriptions as in body part location and proximity.

An example is "...to the left of the umbilicus."

Locations of tumors or body parts in question are described according to human anatomy and anatomical position, which means that which is near, around, above, below, or behind the backbone and inner tube parts. In this way, prepositions rule the day.

Anatomical position (also known as **supine position**) refers to the human body in a standing position with the palms facing forward. Conversely, when prone, the human body is positioned posteriorly so you have the back-side view. The following material defines terms used to describe positions within a body and presents an example for each one.

Want More?

For additional review, check out *The Anatomy Coloring Workbook* and *Essential Anatomy Flashcards* from The Princeton Review.

Superior and Inferior

Superior means toward the head end of the body. For example, the superior vena cava is above the inferior vena cava; the chin is superior to the shoulder.

Inferior means below or away from the head end of the body. The umbilicus (belly button) is inferior to the nose.

Anterior and Posterior

Anterior means nearer the front of the body. The nose is anterior to the buttocks.

Posterior means nearer the back of the body or behind. **Myocardial** tissue (the heart) is posterior to the **sternum**, or breast bone. Posterior wall myocardial infarction (heart attack) is the back wall of the heart, not the front wall.

Medial and Lateral

Medial means closest to the imaginary midline of the body. The great toe (big toe) is medial to the little toe.

Lateral means further away from the midline of the body. The appendix is lateral to the stomach.

Proximal and Distal

Proximal means toward or nearest the trunk or point of origin of a part. The proximal phalange (finger bone) is connected to the wrist bones.

Distal means away from or farthest from the trunk or the point of origin of a part. The finger nail is distal to the phalange. The distal portion of the femur bone is closest to the patella (knee) joint.

Superficial and Deep

Superficial means toward the surface of the body. A superficial laceration or cut on the skin is not very deep.

Deep means away from the surface of the body. A deep tissue massage focuses on deep layers of muscles, and a deep scalp laceration would require sutures (stitches).

Dorsal and Ventral

You may recall the terms *dorsal* and *ventral* to describe the anatomical position of the poor cat used for dissection in biology lab class, but occasionally these terms will still be referenced in nursing. Therefore, you should learn to recognize them in preparation for any NSEE.

Dorsal refers to the back, while **ventral** refers to the abdominal area. The body has two distinct cavities: dorsal and ventral.

The **dorsal cavity** contains the cranial and spinal parts.

The **ventral cavity** is the largest cavity in the body, filling the entire front section of the body. It contains the **thoracic cavity** (chest cavity) and the **abdominopelvic cavity**. Within the thoracic cavity are the left and right **pleural cavities**, which contain the lungs, and the **pericardial cavity** (which encases the heart). The abdominopelvic cavity contains the **abdominal cavity** and the **pelvic cavity**.

Remember that the dorsal section refers to the entire back section of the human body. For example, consider that mid-dorsal thoracic pain you are having from stooping over the table reading your NSEE prep book. It's the annoying upper back pain in between the shoulder blades.

Serous and Mucous Membranes

Serous membranes, such as the peritoneum, coat and form cavities within the body. **Mucous membranes** surround cavities that lead outside the body, such as the respiratory and digestive tracts.

Transverse and Longitudinal

Transverse represents horizontal (like the ground and horizon). **Longitudinal** represents vertical (up and down).

ANATOMY AND PHYSIOLOGY VOCABULARY: PREFIXES AND SUFFIXES

You're probably thinking, *Hey wait—sounds more like English class! <shudder, shudder>*. That's right! Prefixes and suffixes are utilized not just in the English language section but also in ALL aspects of nursing education, preparation, and careers (including advanced practice and medicine too). These word parts may be asked, referenced, or noted in the science section of your exam, and they will also help you with the English section on all nursing school entrance exams.

Prefixes Indicating Location or Direction

Prefix	Meaning	Examples
ab-	from, away	abnormal, hip abductors
ad-	to, near	hip adductors, adrenal gland
ante-	before	antenatal, antepartem
anti-	against	antiseptic, antibiotic
brady-	slow	bradycardia (slow heart rate), bradypnea (slow breath)
circum-	around	circumoral (around the lips), circumocular (around the eyes)
co-	with	coordination, comorbid, coenzyme
con-	with, together	congenital
contra-	against	contraindicated, contralateral, contradict
counter-	against	counterirritant, counter transferance
dis-	apart from	disarticulation, dismember, disarthria, disease, disadvantage
dys-	abnormal, impared	dysuria (painful urination)
ecto-	outside	ectonuclear, ectoderm, ectopic pregnancy
endo-	within	endocardium, endometrial
epi-	upon	epidermis, epigastric
ex-	out from	exhale, exogenous
extra-	outside, beyond	extradural (out from or above the dura)
hyper-	above	hypertension, hypervigilance, hyperglycemia
hypo-	under	hypodermic, hypoglycemia
im-	no	immature, impermeable (cell membrane), imperforate anus

in-	not	incurable, incorrect
infra-	under	infrapatellar (under the knee cap)
peri-	around	pericardium, periumbilical
post-	after	postmortem, postnatal, postictal (after a seizure)
pre-	before	prenatal
pro-	before	probiotics, prodrome (early symptom), prognosis
sub-	under	subgaleal (under the scalp)
super-	above	superior vena cava
supra-	above	supra-orbital rim (top of the brow bone), supratentorial (above the "tent" or tentorium of the brain), supraclavicular
sym-	with	symphysis pubis, sympathy
syn-	with	synarthrosis, synergy, synthetic
trans-	through	transesophogeal, transurethral, transvaginal, transdermal

Prefixes Denoting Organs and Structures

Prefix	Meaning	Examples
abdomin/o	abdominal	abdominal aortic aneurysm
acr/o	extremity	acrocyanosis
aden/o	gland	adenopathy
angi/o	vessel	angiogram
arthr/o	joint	arthroscopy
cardi/o	heart	cardiovascular
chol/e	gall bladder	cholesystitis
chondr/o	cartilage	costeral chondrditis
cyst/o	bladder	cystitis, cystoscopy
cyt/o	cell	cytoplasm
dent/o	teeth	dental, dentition
dermat/ or		
derm/o	skin	dermatitis
duodeno	duodenum	duodenal ulcer
enter/o	intestinal	enteric coated aspirin
gastr/o	stomach	gastritis, gastroenteritis
hepat/o	liver	hepatitis
laryng/o	larynx	laryngo spasm, laryngitis
my/o	muscle	myasthenia gravis
nephr/o	kidney	glomerular nephritis
neur/o	nerve	neurology, neurosurgery, neurogenic
ocul/o or		
opt/o	eye	oculist, ophthalmic drops
oste/o	bone	osteogenic sarcoma, osteotomy, osteoperosis
ot/o	ear	otorrhea
para	around, by one side	paraplegic, parasympathetic nervous system, paramedic
path/o	disease	pathology report, pathologic liar
pneumon/o	lung	pneumonia, tension pneumothorax, pneumonitis
pneumo	air	pneumocephaly (air in the brain)
rhin/o	nose	rinorrhea, rhinoplasty
stomat/o	mouth	stomatitis
thorac/o	thorax or chest	thorocotomy

More Examples

angio-	related to blood vessels	angioplasty (repair of blood vessels surgically)
auto-	self	autogulous, autonomy, autosomal recessive
colono-	related to large intestine (colon)	colonoscopy, colonic cleansing
colpo-	related to the vagina	colposcopy (procedure done after abnormal pap cells are obtained)
encephal-	related to the brain	cephalohematoma, encephalocele
hyster-	related to the uterus	hysterectomy
lamino-	related to vertebrae intervertebral disc	laminectomy, lamintomy
lapar-	related to the abdominal cavity	laparoscopic surgical procedure
mammo- and		
masto-	related to the breast	mammogram, mastoiditis
myo-	related to muscle tissue	myocardial infarction
onco-	relating to cancer	oncology, oncogenic
oophor-	related to the ovary	oophorectomy (removal of ovary)
orchio-	related to the testicle	orchioplasty (repair of undescended testical)
vas-	related to a duct, usually the vas deferns	vasectomy

Prefixes Denoting Number (Measurement)

uni-	one
mono-	one
bi- or bin-	two
di-	two
ter-	three
tri-	three
quad-	four
tetra-	four
poly-	many
macro-	large
mega-	great
micro-	small
oligo-	few (little)

Suffixes Denoting Relation to Something and Some Sample Conditions

-ac	related to	cardiac
-ious	related to	contagious
-ic	related to	pyloric
-ism	condition	mutism, alcoholism
-osis	condition	tuberculosis
-tion	condition	constipation, agglutination

-ist	agent	neurologist, opthalmologist
-or	agent	operator, dictator
-er	agent	primary examiner, ultrasonographer
-ician	agent	pediatrician
-centesis	to puncture	amniocentesis, paracentesis
-ectomy	to cut out excise	appendectomy, tonsilectomy
-desis	fusion of two parts into one, stabilization	arthrodesis
-oid	similar to	mucoid, schizoid
-opsy	looking at	biopsy
-oscopy	viewing of, normally with a scope	endoscopy
-ostomy	a surgical opening (stoma)	ileostomy, jejunosotmy feeding tube
-otomy	a surgical opening/incision into	tracheotomy, chrichothryoidotomy
-pexy	to fix, repair or secure	nephropexy
-plasty	to fix, repair, or reform	duraplasty
-graphy	to write or record	mammography
-rrhapy	to strengthen with a suture (a suffix not often used anymore-but why hold back?)	gastrorrhaphy

A Few More Suffixes

-algia	pain	arthralgia
-emia	of the blood	anemia
-gram	writing	encephalogram (EEG recording of electrical brain waves)
-itis	inflammation	otitis media (middle ear infection), proctitis (inflamed prostate gland), appendicitis
-ology	study of	cardiology, endocrinology
-orrhea	flow	rinorrhea (runny nose), otorrhea (purulent discharge from ears), diarrhea
-phobic or **phobia**	fear of	hydrophobic, astraphobia (fear of thunder and lightening storms)
-phylic	like to	hydrophilic

Phew! Believe it or not, you're now a master commanding the "body part and location lingo." Also, you've hit two birds with the same stone and advanced your English skills for the Verbal sections that we will cover later on. Bravo!

Now that you've reviewed the prefixes, suffixes, and vocabulary, let's get to the main event. The rest of the chapter will be an in-depth review of the organ systems. Here we go!

THE HUMAN DIGESTIVE SYSTEM

In the preceding chapter on biology, we reviewed the way in which cells obtain and convert energy for food. In this chapter, we cover the way we consume energy in the form of food, break it down to simpler compounds (simple sugars and amino acids) that can be absorbed to carry out cell function and maintain homeostasis, and then excrete the leftovers as waste.

The human digestive system consists of the **alimentary canal** and **accessory organs**. The alimentary canal is a long, muscular tube beginning in the **mouth** and ending at the **anus**. The digestive system consists of the mouth, **esophagus, stomach, small intestine, large intestine,** and accessory organs (**salivary glands, liver, pancreas,** and the **gall bladder**).

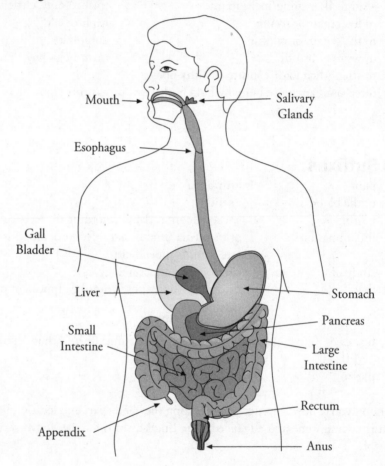

The Human Digestive System

The Digestive Process

The digestive process is comprised of five steps:

1. **Ingestion** is the process by which food enters the mouth or oral cavity, where it is met by **saliva** and a digestive enzyme called **amylase**. Amylase helps digest starch, which is a carbohydrate. Food is further chewed, broken down, and swallowed. **Peristalsis** is a series of rhythmic, wavelike contractions of the esophagus that pushes the food down to the stomach for further breakdown. (**Reverse peristalsis** occurs when someone **vomits** or **throws up**. The vomit, or what is thrown up, is called **emesis**.)

2. **Digestion** is the mechanical and chemical process that breaks down foods. The **pyloris** (stomach) is a thick muscular sac that temporarily stores ingested food, partially digests proteins, and kills bacteria because of its acidity (pH of 1–2). The hormone **gastrin** stimulates the stomach cells to produce gastric juice. The stomach secretes gastric juices, which contain enzymes and **HCl** (**hydrochloric acid**). When HCl is secreted, it lowers the pH of the stomach and converts **pepsinogen** into **pepsin**, which digests proteins. Once food is mechanically broken down with churning in the stomach, it is called **chyme**. The stomach lining is protected by its own mucous.

3. **Secretion** is the release of enzymes (hormones) and **bile** into the digestive tract. **Cholecystokinin** is a hormone that stimulates the secretion of pancreatic enzymes and the release of bile. The small intestine is the site of the most digestion of proteins and carbohydrates (*CARBS—yum!*) and absorption.
   When we discuss secretion, it's important to remember a few more things. Bile is stored and secreted by the liver and gall bladder. It functions to **emulsify** fat. When chyme enters the small intestine, it meets bile and mixes with the many enzymes that are secreted by the pancreas. The pancreas is special in that its enzymes are responsible for the further breakdown of proteins into **dipeptides**. It functions further to break down lipids into fatty acids and glycerol: carbohydrates into disaccharides and nucleic acids into nucleotides (*back to bio basics…?*).
   Note: **Secretin**, a hormone, stimulates the pancreas to secrete **bicarbonate** (a **base**) to help neutralize the acid from the stomach, so that the stomach doesn't digest itself (that is, the duodenum), as the food moves from the pylorus to the duodenum in route to the small intestine and beyond. The pH in the intestines is close to neutral.

4. **Absorption** is the movement of food (nutrient) molecules from the digestive tract into the blood. These nutrient molecules are absorbed into the blood by tiny fingerlike intestinal projections called **villi** and **microvilli**. Within each villi is a capillary that absorbs the digested food into the bloodstream and transports it directly to the liver for processing. If the digested food cannot be absorbed, a person develops **pernicious anemia**, which is fatal unless that person is receiving regular supplemental **vitamin B$_{12}$** injections. Also within the villi are **lymphatic vessels** called **lacteals**, which absorb fatty acids. The

The body cannot benefit from food ingested in its original form (that is, macaroni and cheese or avocado spread on multigrain bread), as its undigested form is not absorbable due to size and inability to dissolve in water.

Rennin, or *chymosin*, is produced by gastric chief cells in infants to curdle the milk they ingest, allowing a longer residence in the bowels and better absorption. It is produced in large amounts during infancy, but not as much during adulthood.

Did You Know?

The small intestine is longer than the large intestine, in that it measures about 19 feet.

Did You Know?

We absorb **vitamin B$_{12}$** in the small intestine. The role of vitamin B$_{12}$ is to help in the production of **red blood cells (RBCs)**.

capillaries from the intestines merge to form special veins called **portal veins**, which divide into **capillaries** again when they reach the liver. This system, called the **hepatic portal system**, is designed to deliver nutrients from the intestinal tract to the liver.

5. **Defecation** is the elimination of solid waste from the large intestines. The large intestine reabsorbs water and salts. It also harvests and houses harmless bacteria that are useful in breaking down undigested food and in that process, provides us with essential vitamins like vitamin K (responsible for clotting ability). The leftover undigested food (called **fecal matter, feces,** or **stool**) is then moved from the large intestine into the **rectum**, where it waits to be pushed out during defecation.

Let's review this content with a question that you might see on the NLN PAX-RN.

What is the function of the bicarbonate-rich fluid secreted by the cells in the pancreas?

A. It inactivates ingested microorganisms.
B. It controls acid secretion from parietal cells.
C. It activates pepsinogen to protease pepsin.
D. It prevents the stomach epithelium from auto digestion.

Here's How to Crack It

We know choice A is incorrect because bicarbonate ions are basic and act as buffers. The acid found in the gastric secretions inactivate microorganisms. You can rule out choice B because you remember that bicarb is produced by cells in the pancreas. It is not a hormone. It's an ionic base, so its function does not tell other cells what to do. Secretion of HCl is as a result of the hormone gastrin. Choice C is incorrect because in the presence of HCl, pepsinogen becomes pepsin which then aids in protein digestion. Choice D is the correct answer. The HCl produced in the lining of the stomach is a very powerful and caustic acid. Without a neutralizing agent (bicarb) secreted into the duodenum, the integrity of the entire stomach lining and intestinal track could be damaged. Bicarbonate serves as a buffer and neutralizes the acid so that the stomach does not auto digest.

Carbohydrate Digestion

Enzyme	Site of Production	Site of Function	Hydrolysis Reaction
Salivary amylase (ptyalin)	Salivary glands	Mouth	Starch → maltose
Pancreatic amylase	Pancrease	Small Intestine	Starch → maltose
Maltase	Intestinal glands	Small Intestine	Maltose → two glucoses
Sucrase	Intestinal glands	Small Intestine	Sucrose → glucose, fructose
Lactase	Intestinal glands	Small Intestine	Lactose → glucose, galactose

Protein Digestion

Enzyme	Production Site	Function Site	Function
Pepsin	Gastric glands (chief cells)	Stomach	Hydrolyzes specific peptide bonds
Trypsin	Pancreas	Small Intestine	Hydrolyzes specific peptide bonds, activates other zymogen proteases
Chymotrypsin	Pancreas	Small Intestine	Hydrolyzes specific peptide bonds
Carboxypeptidase	Pancreas	Small Intestine	Hydrolyzes terminal peptide bond at carboxyl
Aminopeptidase	Intestinal glands	Small Intestine	Hydrolyzes terminal end peptide bond at amino
Dipeptidases	Intestinal glands	Small Intestine	Hydrolyzes pairs end of amino acids
Enterokinase	Intestinal glands	Small Intestine	Converts trypsinogen to trypsin

THE HUMAN RESPIRATORY SYSTEM

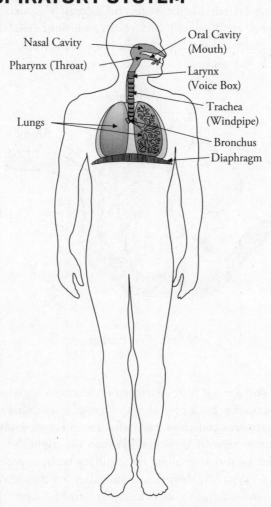

The Human Respiratory System

All cells need oxygen for **aerobic respiration**. Air enters our bodies through our **noses** (**external** and **internal nares**) and mouths. The nose cleans, warms, and moistens incoming air. The air then passes down through the **pharynx**, or throat, which is **stratified** (cells layered for protection) and **larynx** (voice box), where it enters the **trachea**, or windpipe. The trachea is made up of **cartilaginous rings** to help keep the air passage open as air rushes in. When food is swallowed, the **epiglottis** covers the trachea to prevent food from going down the respiratory tract instead of the digestive tract. Food may sneak by the epiglottis when a person is laughing or horsing around while eating. Food enters the **respiratory tree** and the individual chokes. Such a condition could end in a near-death experience, or the food could enter the lungs and cause **pneumonia** (**aspiration pneumonia**).

Did You Know?

The right bronchus is wider than the left bronchus.

The trachea branches into a **right bronchus** and **left bronchus**, which connect to the lungs where the passages become smaller tubes called **bronchioles**. Inflammation or infection of the bronchioles in children is often called **bronchiolitis**. Inflammation or infection in adults is often called **bronchitis**.

The little tiny air sacs where gas exchange occurs are the **alveoli**. These little sacs operate like balloons and increase the surface area of the lung to about the size of a tennis court. Alveoli are filled with **surfactant**, a substance that decreases surface tension and keeps the walls of the air sac from sticking together (like an uninflated balloon). This surfactant thus permits the sac to expand and fill with air.

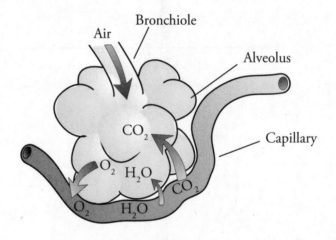

Alveolar Gas Exchange

In a premature infant, these sacs are not fully developed or functioning, which makes oxygenation often difficult for the first few weeks of life. Such newborns often need a **synthetic surfactant** administered into the lung to decrease the surface area and allow gas exchange. This procedure improves the symptoms of **respiratory distress**. Wow, there must be abnormal pH then too, right? Yes, exactly. Alongside the tiny grape-like sacs (called **alveolar sacs**) that sit along the **capillary beds**, oxygen and carbon dioxide diffuse across the membrane—how? Via passive diffusion. Remember bio basics? Another example of a surfactant is soap and water. Soap and water decreases the surface area between the fabric (that is, your dirty shirt) and the spillage (for example, ice cream dropping or oil from pizza). When you scrub with soap and water, the stain is removed.

By which process does the exchange of oxygen and carbon dioxide occur between the alveoli and blood?

A. Diffusion
B. Active transport
C. Passive transport
D. Osmosis

Here's How to Crack It

Choice A is correct because oxygen (a gas) and carbon dioxide (a gas) freely diffuse and cross the capillary beds sitting alongside the tiny alveolar sacs without the use of energy. But why are the others wrong? Choice B is incorrect because active transport requires energy in the form of ATP, to move molecules across the cell membrane. Passive transport is the movement of molecules across the cell membrane (with help of membrane proteins present in it) along their concentration gradient. Although diffusion is a form of passive transport, choice C is not the best choice and is therefore incorrect. Osmosis is the movement of molecules through a selectively permeable membrane, where the material goes from a region of higher concentration to a region of lower concentration. With regard to passive diffusion and gas exchange in respiration: O_2 and CO_2 gas exchange (diffuse) across the capillary beds regardless of the concentration gradient.

Let's discuss the physiology of breathing. The air we breathe contains oxygen and nitrogen. Nitrogen is harmless unless below sea level. **Room air** is considered to have 21% oxygen. When we breathe in, or **inhale**, (an **inhalation**), our bodies utilize only approximately 5% of the oxygen. Therefore, when we **exhale**, or breathe out (**exhalation**), we exhale carbon dioxide and the remaining unused portion of oxygen.

That is why **cardiopulmonary resuscitation (CPR)** or even **rescue breathing** is useful for providing rescue breaths for someone who is not breathing (they are said to be in **respiratory arrest**) or is breathing inadequately or insufficiently (**bradypnea**). When you give a breath to someone, that unused expelled oxygen from the upper portion of your lungs (be it only 16%) is better than none at all. **Apnea** is the absence of breathing—unfortunately, you will definitely see this situation as a nurse.

Many tools are involved in the work of breathing. When we breathe in, the **diaphragm** and **intercostals muscles** contract and our **rib cages** expand. This action increases the volume of the lungs, allowing air to rush in. The process of taking in oxygen is called inhalation or **inspiration**. When we breathe out and let carbon dioxide out of our lungs, that process is called exhalation or **expiration**. Our respiratory rate is controlled by **baroreceptors** (sensors located in our blood vessels) and **chemoreceptors**. When our blood pH decreases, chemoreceptors send nerve impulses to the diaphragm and intercostals to increase our respiratory rate. Oxygen is a base (basic)—too much oxygen, too much base, causes respiratory **alkalosis**. Carbon dioxide is an acid (acidic)—too much carbon dioxide causes respiratory **acidosis**.

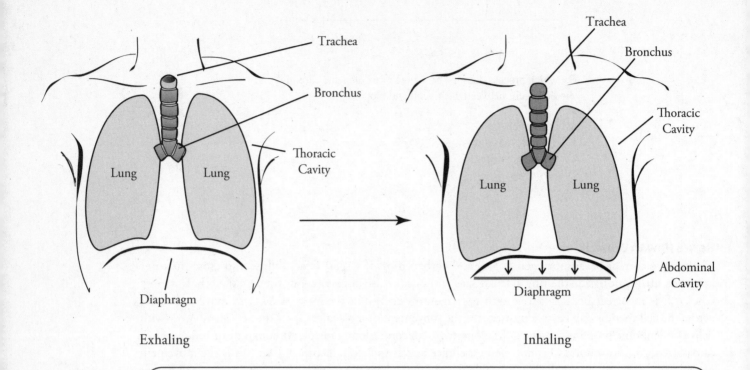

Exhaling

Inhaling

Oxygen and Carbon Dioxide Transport

Oxygen is transported through the body by the iron-containing protein **hemoglobin**, found in red blood cells (approximately 97%). A very small amount of oxygen (approximately 3%) is dissolved in the **plasma** (fluid portion of the blood). Carbon dioxide can travel out of the lungs through exhalation, or it may combine with blood cells and water to form **bicarbonate ions** (HCO_3), which is a **buffer** (utilized in the pH balance system to regulate acid-base balance of cells).

THE HUMAN CIRCULATORY SYSTEM

Meticulously designed to move blood and materials around the body, the circulatory system transports oxygen, carbon dioxide, glucose, hormones, waste products, lipids, and much more. At its most basic level, it is a **pump** (the **heart**), a network of tubing (the **blood vessels**), and fluid (the **blood**). It is divided into the pulmonary and systemic circulations. The **lymphatic system** filters out extra fluids from the cells, removes harmful products and disease, and prevents waste from returning to the blood for recirculation. **Lymph nodes** are concentrated areas of **white blood cells** (**WBCs**). When fluid passes through lymph nodes on the way back to the **veins**, the fluid is exposed to many white blood cells designed to help prevent infection and fight off harmful products by destroying them before they go back into circulation. **Lymphatic vessels** are similar to veins in that they have low pressure and do not have muscle, but contain valves. The fluid inside lymphatic vessels is called **lymph**.

The heart is a strong muscle that is divided into four **chambers**: the right **atrium**, **right ventricle**, **left atrium**, and **left ventricle**. The left and right sides of the heart are separated by the **septum**. Its atria and ventricles are separated by **valves**.

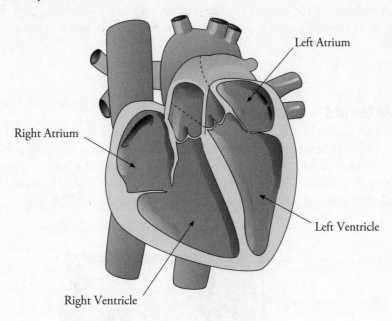

The Human Heart

The Broken Heart

You should know that the sac that goes around the heart is called the pericardial sac and it has TWO layers:

1. **Fibrous pericardium**
2. **Parietal serous pericardium**

The heart muscle itself has three layers:

1. **Epicardium**
2. **Myocardium**
3. **Endocardium**

Here's a Tip!

In the absence of illness or cardiac anomaly, the heart's apical pulse can be auscultated (heard) most clearly on the left side of the chest, 5th intercostals space, mid-clavicular line.

There's much more to the heart than just four chambers. Many heart problems don't affect the four chambers at all (excluding anatomical or congenital anomalies). For example, pericardial effusion affects the pericardial sac *around* the heart. **Endocarditis** is an infection/inflammation in the endocardial layer of the heart. The myocardium is the layer of the heart in which a heart attack happens. Perhaps it's depressing, but there are lots of potential problems outside of the heart's atria and ventricles.

Coronary Arteries

Coronary arteries are vessels that feed and nourish the heart muscle with oxygen-rich blood. Decreased oxygen supply is called **ischemia**. Ischemia causes **angina** (chest pain) and ultimately myocardial cell death (infarction or heart attack). You likely won't be asked to recall the coronary vessels on your exam, but they are important to know as a student, a nurse, a lay person, or a good Samaritan who takes a CPR class. Please familiarize yourself with these vessels and consider taking a CPR class.

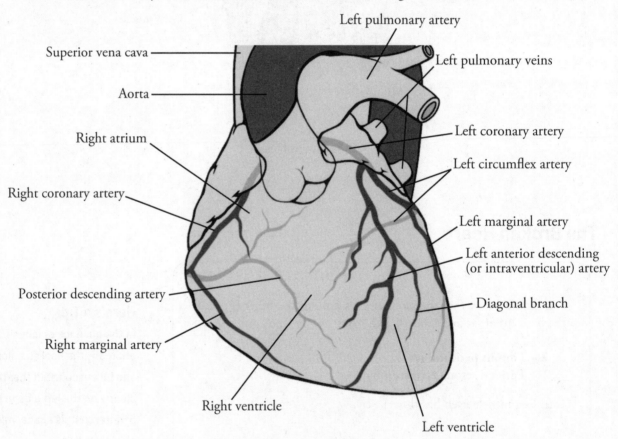

The Heart and Its Vessels

Left-Sided Coronary Vessels

- Left coronary artery
- Left circumflex artery
- Left marginal artery
- Left anterior descending (or intraventricular) artery
- Diagonal branch

Right-Sided Coronary Vessels

- Right coronary artery
- Posterior descending artery
- Right marginal artery

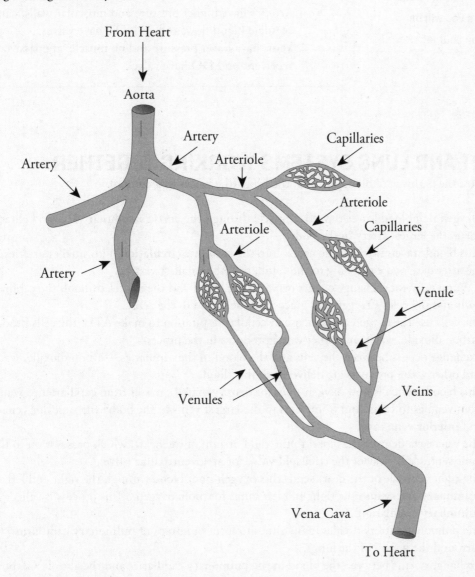

Blood Vessels

Varicose veins, **not** *varicose arteries*, happen to nurses. We know this, because arteries are muscular and thick-walled, but veins are not. Veins are thin-walled with no muscle, which means they get tired and sag. Gravity doesn't help, so invest in the suit of armor of support hose—you will need it with all the long hours you will be standing and running on your legs.

The Blood Vessels: A Quick Review

- Any vessel that carries blood away from the heart is an artery.
- Any vessel that returns blood to the heart is a vein.
- Arteries branch into smaller and smaller vessels, ultimately becoming capillaries.
- Capillaries are the sites of exchange between blood and tissues.
- Capillaries merge into larger and larger vessels, called veins.
- Arteries have higher pressure and muscular walls, can regulate blood flow, and do NOT have valves.
- Veins have lower pressure and no muscle, are passive receivers, and DO have valves.

HEART AND LUNG SYSTEMS WORKING TOGETHER

Let's retrace the pathway of blood through the body (the heart-lung combo).

1. Oxygen rich blood leaves the left ventricle through the **aortic semilunar valve** and enters the **aorta**, the largest artery in the body.
2. This blood travels through the aorta, into the **systemic circulation**, into smaller arteries, to the arterioles, and eventually to the capillaries (the smallest vessels).
3. Gas and nutrient exchange occurs between the blood and the tissues through the capillary walls and the cells. Oxygen and glucose are delivered to the cells.
4. The cells use the oxygen and glucose in cellular respiration to make ATP. The cells produce carbon dioxide, water, and other waste products in the process.
5. Exchange occurs between the cells and the blood in the capillaries. Carbon dioxide, water, and other waste products are delivered to the blood.
6. This blood, which is now oxygen-poor (or **deoxygenated**), passes from capillaries to venules, from venules to veins, and from veins to the largest veins in the body: the **superior vena cava** and **inferior vena cava**.
7. The vena cava delivers the blood to the right atrium of the heart, which passes it on to the right ventricle by way of the **tricuspid valve** (or **atrioventricular valve**).
8. The right ventricle of the heart sends this oxygen-poor blood through the right and left **pulmonary artery** into the right and left lungs for more oxygen. (This process is called **pulmonary circulation**).
9. The pulmonary artery divides many times to form hundreds of **pulmonary capillaries**, which surround the alveoli of the lungs.
10. Exchange occurs between the blood in the pulmonary capillaries and the alveoli. Carbon dioxide and water are delivered to the alveoli. (The other waste products are filtered out by the **kidneys**, which also play an important role in blood pressure. Blood pressure is covered later in this book.) Oxygen is delivered to the blood. Blood is now happily **oxygenated**.

11. The pulmonary capillaries merge to form pulmonary venules, which merge to form **pulmonary veins**, which merge to form the large left and right pulmonary veins.

12. The pulmonary veins carry this oxygenated blood to the left atrium of the heart, which passes it on to the left ventricle through the **bicuspid valve**, also known as the **mitral** (so called because it looks like a bishop's mitre.)

13. The left ventricle pumps the blood back out to the body's cells through the aorta and the whole cycle starts over again. (It doesn't miss a beat, now does it?)

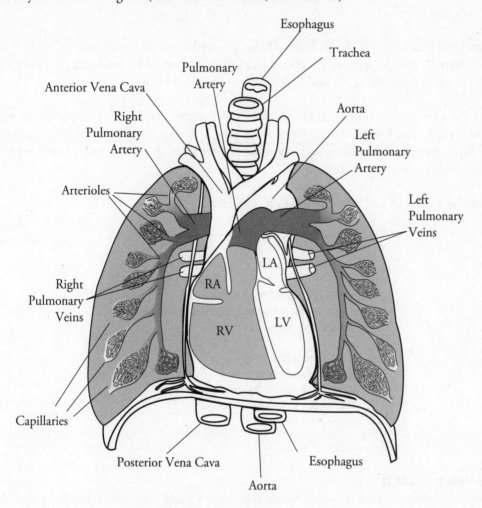

The Heart and Lungs Work Together

We Got the Beat: Conduction System of the Heart

A cardiac cycle is approximately 0.8 seconds long, allowing the heart to beat approximately 72–75 times per minute. (Young people and healthy athletes typically have a lower resting heart rate.) A special conduction system makes sure that the heart beats rhythmically. In the myocardium, specialized cardiac cells act like nerve tissue because they are able to transmit electrical impulses quickly.

The four components to the conduction system of the heart are as follows:

1. **Sinoatrial node (SA node)**, or the pacemaker of the heart
2. **Atrioventricular node (AV node)**
3. **Atrioventricular bundle (bundle of His)**
4. **Perkinje fibers**

The atria contract first.

The impulse to beat begins at the SA node, where the impulse travels down to the AV node. It is a delayed electrical impulse because it is not connected physically. It's more of an intangible, free-floating electrical impulse, unlike the bundle of His and Perkinje fibers discussed below.

Leaving the AV node, the impulse enters the ventricular system and follows its path, all the way down to the bundle of His and Perkinje fibers, which are located in both ventricular walls. The ventricles then contract. During ventricular contraction, blood is forced out through the systemic circulation and perfuses the entire body with oxygenated blood.

Let's take on a question that you might see on your exam.

While pumping blood, the heart makes a "dub" sound, which is the result of the simultaneous closing of some valves. Which valves are responsible for this sound?

A. Aortic and mitral valves
B. Tricuspid and mitral valves
C. Aortic and pulmonary valves
D. Pulmonary and tricuspid valves

Here's How to Crack It

You know that aortic and mitral valves do not close together and therefore do not make the "dub" sound, so choice A is wrong. Closure of the tricuspid and mitral valves (choice B) make the "lub" sound, which is the first sound you would auscultate. The "dub" sound comes from the closing of the aortic and pulmonary valves (so choice C is correct). And choice D is obviously wrong because the pulmonary and tricuspid valves do not close together.

Systole is the phase of a heartbeat when the heart muscle contracts, and **diastole** is the phase when the heart relaxes or rests. When you become a nurse and take a patient's blood pressure (BP), you will measure both the **systolic** and **diastolic pressures**. Systolic is the amount of pressure on a vessel with the added pressure when you squeeze the **sphygmomanometer**, or BP cuff. Diastolic pressure signifies the pressure of the vessel at rest once you release the added pressure from the tight squeeze.

For example, in your nursing career, you will often hear things like BP 120/80, BP 165/92, BP 90/60, and BP 110/70. The first number refers to the systolic pressure; the second refers to the diastolic pressure.

Another Thing

BP also indicates how well the kidneys are being perfused by the circulatory system.

Blood

Blood is made in the marrow of the bone. It begins as pluripotent **stem cells**, which mature to become a specific blood component:

- Erythrocyte (**red blood cell**)
- Leukocyte (**white blood cell**)
- Platelet

RBCs are made about every 120 days. You should remember that a red blood cell is anucleated—that is, it does not have a nucleus. RBCs also lack mitochondria and an endoplasmic reticulum. You may be asking yourself, "Then how do red blood cells survive for 120 days if they don't replicate and they don't have energy?" And that's a very good question.

Here's the answer and it's pretty neat:

RBCs do have cytoplasmic enzymes capable of metabolizing glucose and forming small amounts of ATP, which then is utilized to maintain the pliability of the cell membrane and the transport of ions. Metabolic activity of RBCs keeps iron in the preferred ferrous form, as opposed to the ferric form (which is useless because it cannot carry oxygen in this form) and also prevents oxidation of the protein in the RBC. This unique metabolic ability decreases over time, which causes the RBCs to become less active and more fragile until they are literally worn out. RBCs meet their demise when they rupture open while passing through tight circulatory spaces and then fragment in the spleen. Available iron from the hemoglobin is then transported back to the bone marrow, liver, and other areas to be stored in the form of ferritin.

One of the by-products of RBC destruction is *bilirubin*, which gives that orange-yellow bile color to many newborns' skin. If the bilirubin level is too high, many of those newborns are readmitted to the hospital for *phototherapy*, a light treatment that transforms the bilirubin in the skin into a product that can be excreted in urine and stool. Home methods include regular sunlight for twenty minutes t.i.d. (three times a day).

Plasma, the fluid component in the blood, is like lymph fluid, but it has more proteins. Red blood cells contain an iron-rich protein called hemoglobin, which binds to oxygen and carries it throughout the body. When you eat iron-rich foods or take an iron supplement (in the case of iron deficiency anemia), you increase your iron stores and increase your hemoglobin. With proper hemoglobin and iron stores, you will feel energetic and able to function without much fatigue. With depleted iron stores or abnormal hemoglobin, you may feel sluggish and may fatigue easily. You may even be pale or feel faint. When hemoglobin values are within normal range, all the cells in your body will meet homeostatic needs. The oxygen you breathe in will bind to adequate hemoglobin, and that iron-rich oxygen-rich blood will circulate and nourish your body. However, if those values are low, your entire body will react to the deficiency.

White blood cells fight infection in the body. WBCs consist of **phagocytes**, which "eat" bad material, and **lymphocytes**, which participate in defense cell immunity. **B-cells** are a type of WBC that produce antibodies against very specific foreign bodies or antigens. **Helper T-cells** help the B-cells and other T-cells reproduce. **Killer T-cells** kill cells that have been infected by a virus.

Note: The thymus, which is located in the chest wall near the heart, is included in the circulatory-blood-immune system. When **thymocytes** (**hematopoietic precursors** from the bone marrow) mature, they become the T-cells that are responsible for directing many facets of the adaptive immune system.

AIDS (acquired immune deficiency syndrome) is caused by **HIV** (human immunodeficiency virus), which infects and kills helper T-cells. Certain congenital genetic mutations result in immunodeficiency and the body's inability to fight infection. Without helper T-cells, the body cannot fight any infection.

Platelets are small cell fragments necessary for blood clotting. These platelets release a **clotting factor** substance that activates a chain of events that convert a soluble blood protein (**fibrinogen**) into insoluble **fibrin threads** (long protein molecules used to temporarily clot). Platelets must rupture in order to release the clotting factors. Remember that capillary walls are slippery and smooth until they are injured or poked, or if they are crusty with sharp plaque. Platelets float by and bump into the sharp capillary walls and then release clotting factors. Clot formation causes the lumen of the walls to become even smaller. A **thrombus** is a clot inside an artery. If the clot breaks off and floats around the body, it is then called an **embolus**. **Embolisms** are fatal when not found, treated, or blocked from travel. That thrombus will eventually settle in an area and block the circulation in the heart, lung, or brain, causing death. You may have heard of someone dying from a **pulmonary embolism**.

A thrombus could be a blood clot, an air bubble, a piece of fatty tissue, a mycotic ball, a foreign body, or tumor debris. When it breaks off and floats freely around in the bloodstream, it is called an embolism.

How Do We Clot?
Two chemical reactions must occur to make fibrin:

First, **prothrombin** (produced in the liver) activator converts prothrombin to **thrombin** (in the presence of calcium and intrinsic clotting factors found in blood). Second, thrombin converts fibrinogen (also produced in the liver) into fibrin threads, which strengthen and seal off a clot. This process requires calcium, vitamin K, and many other chemicals. Remember that vitamin K is a fat-soluble vitamin. If fat cannot be emulsified in the gut as part of digestion after meals, that phenomena will cause poor clotting. If someone is **hemorrhaging**, they are said to be **exsanguinating**. This can happen as a result of trauma, losing too much blood, being **coagulopathic** (a clotting abnormality from an infection), or having an underlying disease such as hemophilia.

Plasma is mostly water, protein (**albumin**, fibrinogen, and lipoproteins—all important proteins made by the liver used in clotting), glucose, hormones, ions, and gases. See the importance of bio-basics in NSEE preparation?

Which characteristic of a red blood cell prevents it from repairing itself?

- **A.** Biconcave shape
- **B.** Absence of nucleus
- **C.** Iron-containing protein
- **D.** Oxygen-binding capacity of hemoglobin

Here's How to Crack It

You can immediately cross off choice A, because cell shape isn't an indicator of the ability to repair itself. Choice C is equally wrong, as hemoglobin binds and carries oxygen through the circulatory system, but has no function in cell repair. Not does choice D have anything to do with cell repair—the oxygen-binding capacity of hemoglobin is the ability of blood to bind with oxygen and transferrin. That leaves choice B, which is the correct answer. RBCs lack a nucleus, mitochondria, and endoplasmic reticulum, which is responsible for protein synthesis. Without protein synthesis and DNA instruction, there is no replication or repair. The energy metabolized from glucose allows RBCs to function until they become worn out and die.

Brief Review of Blood Types

You may be asked a question about blood type and typing. There are four blood groups (A, B, AB, and O) based on the type of **antigen** (or antigens) found on the red blood cells.

Blood Type	RBC Antigen	Antibodies	Donates to	Receives from
A	A	Anti-B	A, AB	A, O
B	B	Anti-A	B, AB	B, O
AB	A, B	None	AB only	All
O	None	Anti-A, B	All	O

We talked a bit about foreign body recognition earlier. Your body contains antibodies that recognize, find, bind to, and destroy a foreign body. So if your body does not recognize the protein on the newly received RBCs (for instance, during a **transfusion**), the newly received RBCs will clump and be destroyed. The clumping of RBCs is called **agglutination** and causes fatality (shock, renal shutdown, and death). Know that Type O blood is considered the universal donor and AB is considered the universal recipient.

Rh factors are also antigens found on red blood cells. A person who does not have an Rh factor is said to be Rh– (Rh negative), and one who does have an Rh factor is said to be Rh+ (Rh positive). Rh factors are important for nurses to know, since they affect the blood that a patient can receive. If an Rh negative mother is pregnant with an Rh positive baby, the mother's blood can actually attack and kill the baby, unless she receives an immune globulin called **RhoGAM**.

> Blood type is determined by the membrane proteins that sit on the surface of RBCs.

THE HUMAN LYMPHATIC AND IMMUNE SYSTEMS

The lymphatic system is made up of a network of vessels that conduct lymph, a clear watery fluid formed from interstitial fluid (fluid that bathes and surrounds tissue cells). Plasma and interstitial fluid are very similar. Plasma, the major component in blood, communicates freely with interstitial fluid through pores and **intercellular clefts** in **capillary endothelium** (structural lining).

Lymph Vessels

Lymph vessels are found throughout the body along the routes of blood vessels. They play an important role in fluid balance, or homeostasis.

The lymph system has four functions:

1. Collecting, filtering, and returning fluid to the blood by the contraction of adjacent muscles (get lost plasma back)
2. Fighting infection using lymphocytes, which are cells found in lymph nodes (The lymph system produces lymphocytes, too.)
3. Removing excess fluid from body tissue through lymphatic ducts, which prevents **edema** (fluid overload)
4. Helping absorb fat from meals ingested so that fats won't clog the liver

Our tonsils belong to the lymphatic system. Sometimes a lymph vessel will form a node of tissue found along the course of a lymph vessel. A lymph node contains a large number of lymphocytes, which are important in fighting infection. Lymph nodes are found in the arm pits, the neck, under the chin, in the groin, and in the intestines. (When they are found behind the elbow, they can signify cancer.) They multiply rapidly when they come in contact with an antigen or foreign body recognized by the immune system. Lymph nodes swell or enlarge when they are fighting an infection. This swelling is called **adenopathy** (use those suffix and prefix skills on that one!).

Responsibility of Our Immune System

Our immune system is responsible for keeping us healthy and disease-free. If we are exposed or re-exposed to a disease, our immune system helps prevent spread of that disease with a series of events. Many different cells do this work:

- Phagocyte cells (**neutrophils, monocytes,** and **macrophages**) are activated and float around. They seek to engulf or "eat" the antigen, but more ATP is needed and produced, and there is an increase in lysosomal (digestive) enzymes. Gravitation toward the antigen for binding or engulfment is called **chemotaxis.**
- **Basophils** and **eosinophils** are cells that release inflammatory mediators. **Mast cells degranulate** (burst open and release chemicals), **histamine** is released, and clotting factors increase in number.
- Natural killer cells (NKCs) and tumor cells are released to go after the antigen.
- Molecules such as **complement proteins** (lyse the cell wall of the antigen), acute phase proteins, and **cytokines** and **interferons** (chemicals that inhibit viral replication and activate surrounding cells that have antiviral actions) are released.

Phagocytosis is an example of **innate immunity.** Others include anatomical barriers, mechanical removal, bacterial antagonism, pattern-recognition receptors, antigen-nonspecific defense chemicals, the complement protein pathways, inflammation, and fever (when our bodies mount a **febrile** response).

I Guess This Is Growing Up.

T-cells are made in the bone marrow but mature in the thymus.

Types of Immune Cells: T-Cells and B-Cells

T-cells fight infection and help B-cells proliferate.

B-cells (also known as B-lymphocytes) produce antibodies.

Your plasma membrane has complex markers that distinguish "self" and "non self." When T-lymphocyte cells encounter infected cells, they are activated and multiply. Some become memory T-cells; others become helper T-cells. Helper T-cells activate B-lymphocytes and other T-cells. Memory T-cells recognize bacteria and viruses that have been in your body before. Other T-cells (**cytotoxic T-cells**) recognize and kill infected cells. Activation of T-cells is referred to as a **cell-mediated response.**

With antibody-mediated immunity (**humoral immunity**), B-lymphocytes encounter antigens. They are activated and produce their own clones. Some B-cells become memory cells that can divide rapidly and produce plasma cells after an infection has been overcome. These plasma cells produce antibodies that bind to the antigens that originally activated them. Helper T-cells are also involved and produce interleukins. Both memory and memory B-cells are responsible for **long-term immunity.**

Types of Immunity

Active immunization is the induction of immunity after natural exposure to an antigen. It is a slow process. When antibodies are created by the recipient's immune systems and stored permanently, it is active immunization.

Conversely, **artificial active immunization** occurs when the microbe or antigen is injected into a person (not natural exposure). The antigen used has been treated or weakened and then parts of the antigen or dead antigen are used in this type of immunization. This weakened antigen is a treated toxin from the antigen, or it is synthetic (such as the **hepatitis B vaccine**), so that it won't harm the person receiving the vaccine. Some vaccines are live but attenuated (weakened), such as the **MMR** (**measles**, **mumps**, and **rubella**) as well as **varicella** (chicken pox) vaccine. Vaccines for measles, mumps, and rubella are no longer manufactured or available as separate immunizations. It's all in one—measles, mumps, and rubella—or none at all. Despite the current and ongoing discussions about early childhood vaccinations, most nurses, primary care providers, and parents opt to vaccinate. (Considering the number of highly communicable preventable diseases such as measles that have been reported this year alone, a pinch of pain may very well be worth a pound of performance).

In **passive immunization**, a body is provided with antibodies that protect against infection, and these antibodies give immediate, but short-lived, protection. For example, a pregnant woman passes along a tetanus antibody to her unborn child, which provides natural immunity to the newborn for several months until the antibody is degraded or lost.

Shots

A vaccine is composed of material from an antigen that is injected into or ingested by the patient or host to stimulate adaptive immunity to a disease. Vaccines can prevent or ameliorate the effects of specific infections caused by many harmful **pathogens**. Hence, a mandatory vaccine schedule has been developed, along with recommendations for schools, daycare settings, and most places of employment.

> Unless you are claiming religious exemption, nursing degree programs and almost all places of health care–related employment require serologic-laboratory titer proof of immunity against communicable diseases for the following: varicella, measles, mumps, and rubella.
>
> You should also have a current tetanus booster, which is now being offered as a vaccine called Tdap. This vaccine offers protection against pertussis (whooping cough).
>
> Hepatitis B vaccine is highly recommended but not mandatory. However, if you decline the vaccine, you must sign a waiver confirming your refusal to be protected against the preventable blood-borne pathogen disease. If you become infected through a work-related incident (a needle stick, blood splash, or bite), there is no foul on the part of the health care facility in which you work, and therefore no liability other than on yourself. Be educated in vaccination recommendations and be smart with your choices.

When our bodies need help fighting infection, an antimicrobial agent, or **antibiotic**, may be prescribed. **Antiviral drugs** may be administered within the first day or so of a viral infection or even during the **prodrome phase** when you think you are becoming ill but before the symptoms manifest. These drugs can shorten the longevity of the illness and help decrease the severity of the symptoms of the disease.

THE HUMAN EXCETORY SYSTEM

The organs of the excretory system include the kidneys (responsible for waste, urine production, and blood pressure control) and the skin (responsible for sweat and ridding of excess water and salt).

Waste products are filtered from the blood by the kidneys and eliminated as **urine**. Urine consists of urea (from amino acid destruction), **uric acid** (from breakdown of nucleic acids) and **creatinine** (waste product from muscle metabolism). Urine is made by three processes: **filtration, reabsorption,** and **secretion**.

Nephrons

Nephrons filter blood and remove nitrogenous-compound waste, excess water, and salts.

Urine produced in the **renal cortex** of the kidneys drains through **collecting ducts** and **pyramids** (**renal papillae**) in the area called **nephrons**—the functional units of the kidney. The human body has millions of nephrons.

Here's an illustration of a nephron:

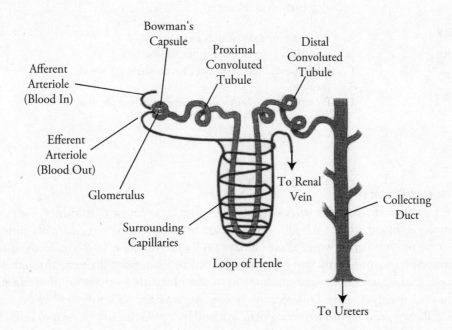

Nephron

The blood enters a nephron at the **Bowman's capsule** and is later filtered when it passes through the **glomerulus**. Small substances, such as ions, water, glucose, and amino acids, easily pass through the capillary walls; however, larger molecules, such as blood and proteins, cannot.

As the filtrate (plasma) moves through the tubule, some materials are reabsorbed. Tubular reabsorption occurs in the **proximal convoluted tubules, distal convoluted tubules,** and **loop of Henle.**

Tubular secretion occurs in the distal convoluted tubules, allowing some substances (such as drug byproducts, hydrogen, potassium and ammonium ions) to be secreted from the surrounding capillaries into the tubule, then into the **final collecting duct** where the substance is modified to become urine. The concentrated urine then moves from the collecting ducts into the **ureters**, down into the **bladder.**

Did you know that the bladder filling with urine and stretching stimulates neurons in the wall to send a message to the brain, which then sends a message to the internal and external sphincters making us feel the urge to void (urinate)? That urine is excreted through the **urethra** by way of a small opening called, the **urinary meatus.** The term **micturation** refers to the process of urination—that is, the voluntary opening of the external sphincter.

Here's a practice question.

More Practice!

For more questions like this one, check out your online companion tools at PrincetonReview.com/cracking.

How does the process of kidney dialysis help patients suffering from renal disorders?

A. By removing toxic wastes from the blood
B. By infusing oxygen and water into the blood
C. By reducing blood volume, thereby reducing blood pressure
D. By replenishing hormones produced by the adrenal glands

Here's How to Crack It

If you've ever seen the unintentional comedy *Rock Star,* you know that kidney dialysis removes toxic wastes from the blood (choice A). Dialysis is an artificial replacement for patients suffering from renal failure (acute or chronic) in which their kidneys no longer function properly. Dialysis is a complicated and time-consuming procedure that relies on diffusion of solutes and dialysate through a semipermeable membrane. Dialysis removes waste products from the blood that otherwise (if accumulated) could be toxic and even deadly. Choice D is patently wrong, as there are no hormones involved in renal dialysis. For choice B, oxygen is bound to hemoglobin in the RBCs, which carry oxygen to cells. Water is not isotonic and is never infused into a patient. Dialysis does not increase or decrease blood volume, so choice C is wrong. In theory, reducing blood volume (hypovolemia) will reduce blood pressure if not addressed or fixed, but the patient could go into shock from too much blood loss. Choice A is the right answer.

The Role of Chemicals in the Excretory System

Juxta glomerulosa is a gland in the kidney responsible for the production of two important hormones:

1. **Erythropoietin** is produced when the oxygen level in blood is low. This hormone goes into the blood and reaches the bone marrow and stimulates production of more red blood cells.
2. **Renin** is produced when blood pressure (BP) is too low. (*Note:* DO NOT confuse *renin* with *rennin* from the digestive system.) When renin enters the bloodstream, it combines with **angiotensinogen** (already sitting in the blood) and causes **angiotensin I** to convert to **angiotensin II,** which is a potent **vasoconstrictor** that can cause blood vessels to constrict and ultimately raise blood pressure. Angiotensin II also goes to the adrenal gland in the **zona glomerulosa** where it stimulates production of **aldosterone**, which causes the body to reabsorb sodium and water and also raises blood pressure.

During glomerular filtration in the Bowman's capsule, a decrease in pH of the blood constituents decreases the filterability of blood plasma and other organic constituents. This happens because a decrease in pH of the blood constituents

A. reduces the size of the blood constituents.
B. affects the charge of the blood constituents.
C. helps the blood constituents to diffuse easily through the lipid bilayer.
D. prevents the blood constituents from moving through the membrane proteins.

Here's How to Crack It

A decrease in pH of the blood affects the acidity of the blood, but it does not affect the size of the blood components, so choice A can be eliminated. The charge of the constituents of the blood is affected by the change in pH, so choice B is correct. As the pH of the blood decreases, cations release H^+ ions. Ionized particles require the presence of membrane proteins in order to pass through the cell membrane, since they cannot directly pass through the lipid bilayer. Choices C and D are incorrect because ionized particles cannot pass through the lipid bilayer directly. The ionized particles require membrane protein to pass through the cell membrane and they pass through the membrane with great difficulty.

The skin is an excretory organ that rids excess water and salt from the body. With over 25 million sweat glands and the ability to secrete water and ions through pores, the skin can regulate body temperature.

THE HUMAN INTEGUMENTARY SYSTEM

The integumentary system is composed of skin, hair, nails, and sebaceous and sweat glands. It has the following functions:

- Protecting the body from dehydration and mechanical injury
- Maintaining temperature control (for example, goose bumps and sweating)
- Producing vitamin D; excreting waste materials and toxins
- Reacting immunologically to microorganisms and chemicals

All cells in the body belong to four categories of tissues:

1. **Epithelial tissue:** classified by the different types of cells—**squamous** (flat, thin appearance), **cuboidal** (shape like a cube), and **columnar** (elongated like columns); each can be **simple epithelium, stratified** (multilayered) **epithelium,** or even **pseudostratisfied epithelium.**
2. **Connective tissue: dense connective** (bones, cartilage, blood) and **elastic connective** (ligaments)
3. **Muscle tissue:** skeletal, smooth, cardiac
4. **Nervous tissue:** main component of nervous system (brain, spinal cord, nerves)

The skin and all of its associated structures (including hair, nails, sweat glands, oil glands, and sensory receptors) are collectively considered an organ. The skin is the largest body organ and is the first line of the body's defense. Its function is to protect the body from abrasion (breakdown or damage), heat loss, water loss, infection, harmful sun, and UV radiation and to assist with vitamin D production, sensation, and thermoregulation.

Skin Makeup

The skin is made up of three layers of tissue:

1. The **epidermis** is a thin layer of cells at the surface of the body. Most of the cells in the epidermis are dead.
2. The **dermis** is a thick layer of dense connective tissue (bundles of collagenous fibers) underneath the epidermis. The dermis is vascular and innervated (meaning it's where nerve endings are located, so in this layer we have our sense of touch, heat, perception of pain). This layer contains hair follicles, sweat glands, and blood vessels. The upper layer of the dermis is called the **papillary layer,** which gives us fingerprints. Fibers from the dermis extend into the subcutaneous layer and anchor the skin.
3. The **hypodermis** is a deep layer of fat that helps protect and insulate the body.

Skin Deep

Now let's go even deeper. The first layer of skin, the epidermis, contains five layers within it. The diagram below illustrates the five layers of the epidermis:

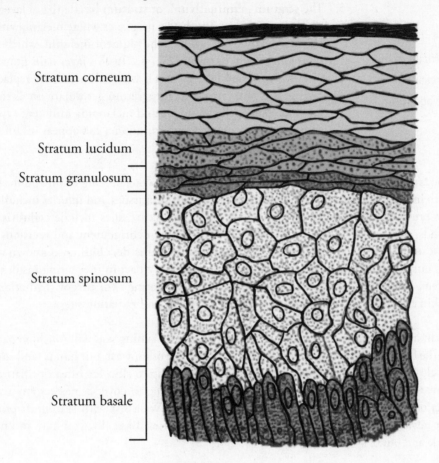

Stratum corneum

Stratum lucidum

Stratum granulosum

Stratum spinosum

Stratum basale

Layers of the Epidermis

1. The **stratum corneum** is the thickest, outermost layer of the epidermis. It is 25–30 rows deep. This layer contains **keratin**, a fibrous structural protein that keeps water from going in and coming out of our skin.
2. The **stratum lucidum** is a thin, clear layer of dead skin cells found only in areas of thick skin, such as the palms of hands and the soles of feet. This layer gets its lucid appearance because the **keratohyalin** found in the granulosum layer is transformed into another protein called **eleidin**, which gives a transparent appearance.
3. The **stratum granulosum**, the granular layer, is made up of 3–5 rows of cells found between the stratum lucidum and stratum spinosum. This layer is called granulosum because under the microscope you can see that the cells are filled with granules in cytoplasm. These granules are called keratohyalin. As a nurse, you will hear and see "granulating tissue," which is the tissue that replaces clots (scabs) when wounds are healing. A surgical incision will granulate to form a healing ridge. Over time it will become flatter and flush to the skin. In this layer, some cells are alive and some cells are dead.

4. The **stratum spinosum** is a thicker layer made up of 8–10 rows of cells that are alive. Its function is mostly protection. Some mitosis takes place in this layer. It is the layer in which keratinization begins. Also, some melanin is found in this layer.

5. The **stratum germinativum**, or **stratum basale** (basal layer), is a single layer of skin. It's the deepest layer where **melanocytes** are found. Melanocytes produce the pigment **melanin**, which shields individuals from harmful UV rays. In this layer nails grow. A lot of mitosis goes on here, so this is where skin cells are replaced. The cells in this layer are alive. The stratum germinativum is the layer in which basal cell carcinoma and melanoma (different types of skin cancer) occur, although melanoma can appear in different locations other than skin.

Melanin

Albinos have no melanin. African Americans have melanin present in all layers and can therefore adapt to UV rays.

You should be familiar with information about the skin both for your nursing exam and for your nursing career. In both instances, you will undoubtedly be faced with skin issues and injuries including sunburns, cuts, scrapes, bruises, acne, and minor trauma. More serious skin issues include **cellulitis, lacerations,** surgical wounds, **dehiscence,** and wound infections that require **debridement** and **revisions.** In geriatric or long-term care patients, you may see **decubidus ulcers** (plural is **decubidi,** also known as **bed sores**). Your role as a nurse will include making skin assessments as a key part in preventing insult to the integumentary system. Part of that skin assessment will include evaluating skin **turgor** (hydration status) and monitoring skin changes with chemotherapy, central catheters, and radiation sites.

Why is the skin important? Think about this. As a nurse, the first thing you will touch on patients is their skin. Skin is the body's first line of defense and protection. We often wash our hands (and some not often enough) to help prevent the spread of disease. We apply makeup to skin for fun in pediatric teen wards, and learn how to apply reconstructive makeup for those wishing to cover a mastectomy scar or a burn. We give injections **subcutaneously** and deep within a muscle. We assist with **skin graft** procedures and marvel at the advancements of necessary reconstructive surgeries. Basically, you have to know this skin material inside and out.

Let's try a practice question.

Which skin layer consists mainly of macrophages, fibroblasts, and adipocytes and attaches skin to the bones and the muscles?

A. Dermis
B. Hypodermis
C. Stratum corneum
D. Stratum germinativum

Here's How to Crack It

Choice A might stick out as obviously wrong, because the dermis is a thick layer of dense connective tissue (bundles of collagenous fibers) that is vascular, innervated, and has hair follicles and glands. It does not attach skin to bone. Choice C is also wrong, as stratum corneum is the outermost layer of the epidermis that contains keratin, the fibrous structural protein. That leaves choices B and D. Stratum germinativum is the innermost (deepest) layer of the epidermis (also know as the basale layer). It does not consist of macropahges, fibroblasts, and adipocytes; rather it is where melanocytes are found and where nails grow. Hypodermis is correct (choice B) because it's the deep layer of fat that protects and insulates the body, contains macrophages, fibroblasts, and adipocytes. It attaches skin to the bones and the muscles.

Scar tissue forms after normal skin has been insulted or damaged. Scar tissue initially appears to be reddened or more pinkish than normal skin, but after a year it becomes paler in color. It is very important to apply sunblock within the first year of a scar, as healing incision lines or scars tend to burn easily and become an unsightly darker pigment years later.

Fingernails grow about one millimeter a week, but toenails grow more slowly.

That's a Big Organ!

Our largest body organ, the skin, is waterproof and airtight. Sensors in the skin detect pressure, pain, and the temperature outside the body.

Which layer of the epidermis modifies to form nails?

A. Stratum corneum
B. Stratum lucidum
C. Stratum spinosum
D. Stratum germinativum

Here's How to Crack It

Here's another question for which there is no substitute for simply memorizing these key terms. Stratum corneum is the outermost layer of the epidermis that contains keratin, the fibrous structural protein. Nails do not form from this layer, so choice A can be crossed off. Choice B is another incorrect answer because stratum lucidum is the thin, clear layer of dead skin cells in the epidermis and is found only in areas of thick skin and it is not responsible for formation of nails. Choice C is also incorrect, as stratum spinosum is the prickly layer of epidermis where keratinization begins. There is no nail formation in this layer either. That leaves choice D. Stratum germinativum is the deepest layer of the epidermis and is also called the basale layer. In this layer, melanocytes are found and nail formation takes place, so choice D is correct.

Did You Know?

Sebaceous (oil) glands are located everywhere on the body except for the palms and soles. Sudoriferous (sweat) glands are found over the entire skin system but are most numerous in the palms, soles, forehead, and armpits.

We Cool?

The evaporation of perspiration cools the body. As water turns into vapor, the vapor draws off excess heat. "Dry fit" clothes are important for athletes so they don't overheat during a workout. A lot of heat is lost during the process of sweating, particularly from the hands and the tops of our heads. That's why winter athletes often run in shorts while wearing hats and gloves.

Here's a diagram of all those parts of skin:

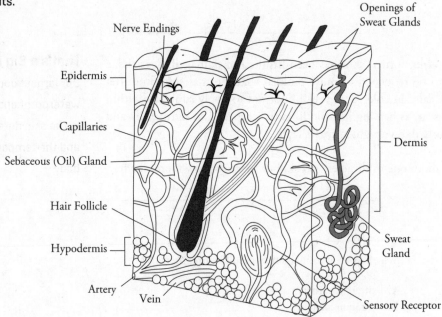

The Human Integumentary System

THE HUMAN MUSCULOSKELETAL SYSTEM

The skeletal system gives shape and support to the body and also protects internal organs. When muscles contract, the bones act as levers. Bones also store minerals (calcium and phosphorous) and have **hemopoietic** potential (the ability to produce red blood cells).

BONES (Not Starring David Boreanaz)

Bone ossification is the process in which new bone is made by specialized cells called osteoblasts. It's a continuing process that begins when an infant's skull is maturing, from baby skull bones that are no thicker than a potato chip to become thicker, firmer, and harder. There is a huge difference between the skull of a newborn and that of an infant three months old.

As a future nurse, you can expect to find bone ossification in an infant who is status post a craniectomy or osteotomy (that is, after a procedure to remove bone) to be anywhere from 4–12 months following surgery. You will see and feel nearly 95 percent bone re-ossificication as new bone is being formed, during the early part of the recovery period. For older or adult patients, sometimes bone has to be replaced by obtaining shaved bone from adjacent bone areas or even bone grafts to replace the area of lost bone due to trauma, surgery, or erosion from chronic disease.

Bone age X rays are often indicated when a baby or young child presents with secondary sex characteristics or who is short of stature. Bone age shows the clinician the stage of bone maturation.

Bone mineral density scans measure the amount of bone matter per cubic centimeter of bone. These scans may indicate osteopenia, osteoperosis, or future bone fracture risk.

The skeleton is made up of **bones** and **cartilage**. Bone is a rigid substance. It is connective tissue made up of **collagen** and calcium salts. Bones are short, irregular, flat, or long. They contain nerves and blood vessels. Cartilage is found in the early stages of embryonic development in all vertebrates. Cartilage doesn't contain nerves or blood vessels and it is later replaced by bone (except in the bridges of our noses, in external ear lobes, and on the ends of all bones and joints where cartilage acts as a shock absorber). Bone is continually being deposited by **osteoblasts** and continually being absorbed by **osteoclasts** (where they are active). The parathyroid hormone (discussed later in this chapter) controls the bone absorption activity of the osteoclasts with calcium and phosphorous absorption. Haversion canals contain capillaries and nerve fibers that supply nutrients for deposition or formation. Bone is deposited in proportion to the compressional load that the bone must carry (sort of like supply and demand). An example and application in nursing would be the observation of a patient who has an arm cast removed—the affected arm appears thinner than the unaffected arm due to bone decalcification.

Here's a diagram of a typical long bone showing both compact (cortical) and spongy (cancellous) bone:

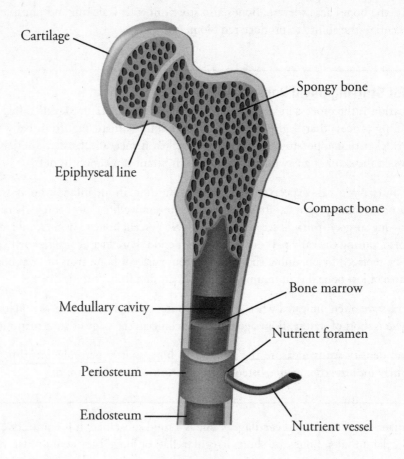

Cartilage

Spongy bone

Epiphyseal line

Compact bone

Bone marrow

Medullary cavity

Nutrient foramen

Periosteum

Endosteum

Nutrient vessel

Long Bone

Ligaments hold joints together, and **tendons** attach muscle to bone.

Let's try a few bone questions:

Which bone structure is made up of osteocytes?

A. Periosteum
B. Bone marrow
C. Spongy bone
D. Compact bone

Here's How to Crack It

This is another question that can be answered only by straight memorization. Osteocytes are cells found in compact bone, so choice D is correct. Let's review why the other choices are incorrect, though. Periosteum (choice A) is the tough outer membrane present over the bone. It's the first portion of bone you would see if you peeled back the skin. Bone marrow (choice B) is the tissue found in the inner part of the bone and it is the site of blood cell production. Choice C is incorrect—spongy bone is not made up of osteocytes.

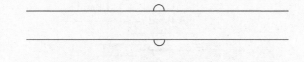

Which part of a bone provides the pathway for nerves and blood vessels to supply nutrients to the bone?

A.   Cartilage
B.   Periosteum
C.   Bone marrow
D.   Haversian canal

Here's How To Crack It

Let's simply go down the list of choices. Cartilage is flexible connective tissue and it doesn't contain nerves or blood vessels, so you can easily eliminate choice A. Periosteum is the tough outer membrane present over the bone mentioned in the previous test question. It is not innervated or vascular, so choice B is wrong. Choice C is also incorrect, because bone marrow produces blood cells—it is not a pathway for nerves or blood vessels. The Haversian canal contains capillaries and provides a pathway for nerves and blood vessels that supply nutrients to the bone. Choice D is the correct answer.

Muscle Types

There are three types of muscle tissue in the body:

1.   **Skeletal muscle** is attached to bones. It is a **voluntary muscle**—that is, the body has conscious control over its contraction and movement. Skeletal muscle is striated. The complex skeletal muscles of the head and neck are capable of rotation and powerful movements as well as the tiny coordinated actions that enable the expression of the slightest emotional changes in the face.

2.   **Cardiac muscle** is a striated muscle found only in the heart. Cardiac muscle tissue movement is **involuntary** and self-excitatory—that is it can initiate its own contraction.

3.   **Smooth muscle** is not striated. It is found in walls of organs, such as the stomach, walls of blood vessels, intestines, and bladder. Smooth muscle tissue movement is involuntary—that is, the body does not have the ability to control its contractions. The stomach churns and contracts without our control or command.

Did You Know?

There are nearly 700 muscles in the human body that contract.

> Muscles are made up of proteins, and proteins are made up of amino acids and nucleotides. The functional unit of the muscle cell is the **sarcomere** where there are two protein filaments: **actin** (thin filaments) and **myosin** (thick filaments).

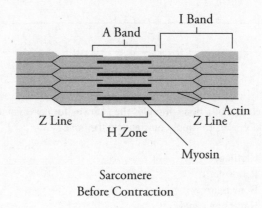

Sarcomere
Before Contraction

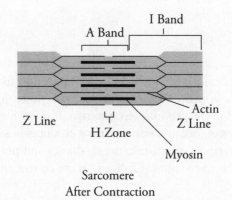

Sarcomere
After Contraction

How Do Muscles Contract?

You may be wondering why you need to know this. You won't need it for your career, unless you work in neurology (the study of nerve conduction and nerve damage), rehabilitative medicine, or a stroke unit. But you will need to be familiar with this content for your NSEE, which will most likely have a few questions about muscle contraction.

The following are the steps in the muscle contraction process:

1. Muscles can contract when a nerve impulse is sent to a skeletal muscle.
2. The neuron sending the impulse releases a neurotransmitter onto the cell muscle.
3. The muscle depolarizes.

4. Depolarization causes the **sarcoplasmic reticulum** to release calcium ions.
5. These calcium ions cause the actin and myosin filaments to slide past each other (**sliding filament theory**).
6. This sliding causes muscle contraction. (Don't forget that energy is required for muscle contractions—it's called ATP).

THE HUMAN NERVOUS SYSTEM

The smallest functional unit of the nervous system is the **neuron**. Neurons are excitable cells that conduct and transmit electrical impulses and convey information. They receive and send neural impulses that trigger an organism's response to the environment. A neuron consists of a **cell body (soma)**, **dendrites**, and an **axon**. A nerve impulse begins at the top of the dendrites, passes through the dendrites to the cell body, and then moves down the axon.

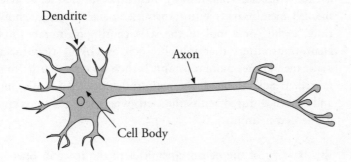

Neuron

Neurons are classified into the following three groups:

1. **Sensory (afferent) neurons** receive impulses from the environment and bring them to the body. For example, sensory neurons in your hand react to the stimulation of someone attempting to hold your hand.
2. **Motor (efferent) neurons** transmit impulses to muscles or glands to produce a response that causes either the contraction of a muscle or the secretion of a hormone.
3. **Interneurons (association)** are the links between sensory and motor neurons. They are found in the brain or spinal cord.

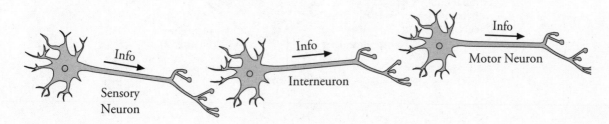

Three Types of Neurons

Polarized-Energized

Resting neurons are considered to be **polarized**—that is, they are more negative on the inside than on the outside. When an **action potential** comes along, the neuron transmits an impulse down its axon. First, **voltage gated sodium channels** open, allowing sodium ions to rush in (a process known as **depolarization**). The neuron becomes more positive on the inside and more negative on the outside. Sodium channels close and **potassium channels** open, thereby restoring the neuron's negative charge (a process known as **repolarization**). Then the neuron enters a **refractory period** (leave me alone, I am resting). The neuron re-establishes the ion distribution and returns to its resting polarized state in a process carried out by the **sodium-potassium pump**.

Did You Know?

Infants more than 12 months old require good sources of fat in their diets (for example, whole cow's milk instead of skim milk) because their brains grow a lot during the first three years of life—especially the first 12 months. Important brain development occurs during this time. Incorporating good sources of fat encourages brain growth and what's called **myelination** of the spinal cord. Myelination enables an infant to roll over and a toddler to talk, walk, jump, and even toilet train.

Myelin is a fatty insulator that increases the speed at which an impulse can travel down the axon. In some neurons, the axon is wrapped with special cells call **Schwann cells**. This wrapping of Schwann cells is called a **myelin sheath**. The spaces between the Schwann cells, the **nodes of Ranvier**, have no myelin.

When the action potential reaches the **terminal end** of the axon (at the bulb), it causes vesicles containing a **neurotransmitter** to be released and fuse with the cell membrane. Neurotransmitters, such as **acetylcholine** and **norepinephrine**, "excite," or stimulate, the cells, causing membranes to become depolarized. Neurotransmitters that inhibit, such as **GABA (gamma-amino-buteric acid)**, make membranes more resistant. It then becomes harder to get an impulse transmitted. If not inhibited, the neurotransmitter is released into the **synaptic cleft** and is then diffused across the cleft, where it binds to receptors on the dendrites of the *next* neuron.

This binding of the neurotransmitter to the receptor opens ion channels in the next neuron. If the ion channels allow sodium to enter the neuron, the neuron will depolarize. If the neuron depolarizes to threshold, voltage-gated channels open, causing an action potential to fire in that neuron, and the process can begin once again.

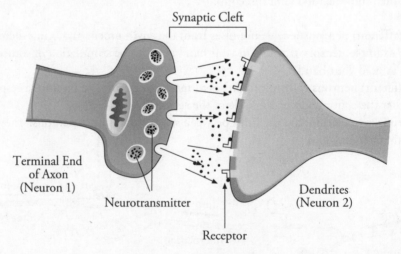

Passing of Impulse from Axon to Dendrite

The Nervous System Divided

The nervous system is divided in to two parts: the **central nervous system (CNS)** and the **peripheral nervous system (PNS)**.

Central Nervous System

- The central nervous system (CNS) consists of the brain and **spinal cord**, along with the **cranial nerves**. The CNS is known as the control center of the entire system. The brain is made up of the **cerebrum, cerebellum, midbrain, hypothalamus, medulla**, and **pons**.
- The cerebrum is divided into the right and left hemisphere by the **corpus collosum** and consists of outer **grey matter** and **white matter.** Grey matter makes up the outer cortex, and white matter makes up the inner cortex of the brain.
- The cerebrum is the area of conscious mind where we think, talk, remember, sense, move, and act. It is also referred to as the seat of emotions, revealing how we react. The cerebrum is even the area responsible for personality traits.
- The cerebellum is responsible for coordination and balance. In normal development, the cerebellum in infants under the age of 12 months enables them to pick up a Cheerio with the pointer finger and thumb (the **pincer grasp**) as opposed to the entire fisted swoop-scoop action that you generally see in infants 4–9 months old.
- The midbrain is the center for visual and auditory reflexes and many visceral or involuntary muscle activities.
- The hypothalamus monitors hormone levels and secretes hormones. It's responsible for electrolyte balance and temperature, and it also controls the pituitary gland, which regulates homeostasis. Of note, the hypothalamus is very close in proximity to visual pathways; therefore, a patient with a tumor in the area of the hypothalamus can present with visual abnormality.
- The medulla, which is an elongation of the base of the brain, joins with the spinal cord to control breathing, swallowing, heart rate, and the regulation of blood pressure.
- The pons connects parts of the brain with one another and contains the respiratory center or pneumotaxic center. Both the pons and the medulla comprise the **hindbrain**.
- The brain is the most complex and specialized organ of the body. It's covered and protected by three protective membranes (**pia mater, dura mater**, and **dura**) and **meninges** that extend downward to encase the spinal cord.
- The spinal cord is a long narrow bundle of nervous tissue that descends from the medulla at the base of the skull and enters into the protective canal formed by the vertebrae. The spinal cord has two important functions: to serve as the sensory motor mechanism for reflexes and to act as a two-way transmitter of electrical impulses, reactions and stimuli triggered by a variety of internal external conditions.

Did You Know?

The frontal lobe of the human brain is not fully developed until a human is approximately 18 years old.

More Review!

Check out more detailed diagrams of body parts in *The Anatomy Coloring Workbook* by The Princeton Review.

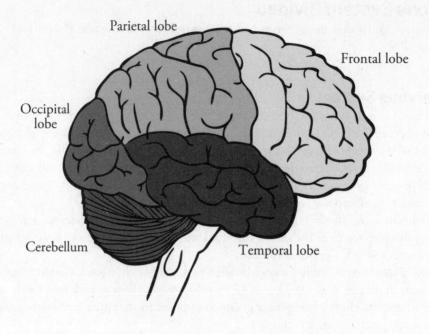

The Lobes of the Human Brain

The human brain has four lobes:

1. The **frontal lobe** is the site for motor function and speech.
2. The **parietal lobe** is the site for integration of sensory information from different body parts.
3. The **temporal lobe** is the site for memory and language.
4. The **occipital lobe** is the site where vision is processed.

The Spinal Cord

It's unlikely you will be asked anything about the anatomy and function of the spinal cord, including what areas innervate which part of the body; however, it would be good to be aware of the number of vertebrae and nerves present.

Here are the various parts of the spinal column:

Memorization Trick

One of the more fun but crass ways to remember this in school is C 3, 4, 5 keeps the diaphragm alive; S 2, 3, 4 keeps the wee wee off the floor.

• 7 cervical vertebrae and 8 cervical nerves: C1–C8
• 12 thoracic vertebrae and 12 thoracic nerves: T1–T12
• 5 lumbar vertebrae and 5 lumbar nerves: L1–L5
• 5 sacral vertebrae which is usually fused by maturity: S1–S5
• Sacral nerves testable on physical exam are S1, S2, S3, S4.
• A **coccyx bone**, also known as a **tailbone**

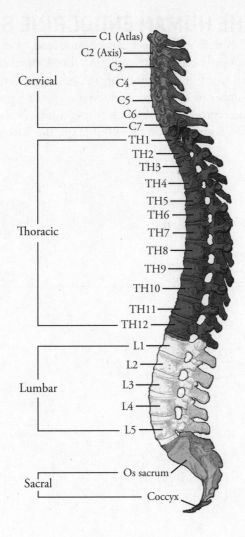

C1 (Atlas)
C2 (Axis)
C3
C4
Cervical
C5
C6
C7
TH1
TH2
TH3
TH4
TH5
TH6
Thoracic
TH7
TH8
TH9
TH10
TH11
TH12
L1
L2
L3
Lumbar
L4
L5
Os sacrum
Sacral
Coccyx

The Spinal Column

Peripheral Nervous System

The peripheral nervous system (PNS) consists of nerves that connect the CNS to all parts of the body. It is further broken down into two other systems:

1. The **somatic nervous system** controls voluntary activities such as waving.
2. The **autonomic nervous system** controls involuntary activities such as the heart beat and digestive system. The autonomic nervous system is further broken down into these two systems:
   a. The **sympathetic nervous system** controls individuals' "fight or flight" when they are confronted with a threat. A hormone called **epinephrine** is released into the bloodstream, causing a surge in heart rate, blood pressure, and blood glucose. In turn, the individual sometimes runs away, charges forward, hits back, freezes, or withdraws.
   b. The **parasympathetic nervous system** works opposite the sympathetic nervous system to restore homeostasis once a threat is passed and the body can go back to normal functioning.

THE HUMAN ENDOCRINE SYSTEM

Chemical messengers can be produced in one region of the body to act on target cells in another part. These chemicals, known as hormones, are produced in specialized organs called endocrine glands. Hormones have a number of functions, including regulating growth, behavior, development, and reproduction. First, let's take a look at the endocrine glands in the human body. Then, we'll examine specific hormones.

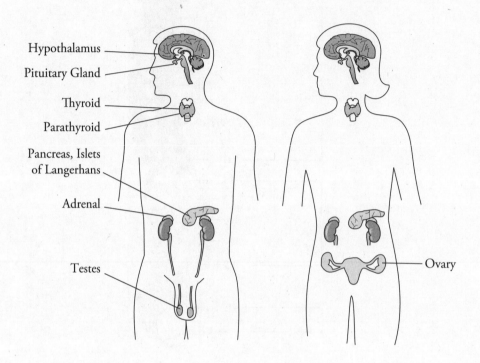

Hypothalamus
Pituitary Gland
Thyroid
Parathyroid
Pancreas, Islets of Langerhans
Adrenal
Testes
Ovary

The Human Endocrine System

Pituitary Gland

The **pituitary gland** is called the "master gland" because it releases many hormones that stimulate other glands to secrete their own hormones. The pituitary gland has two parts: the **anterior pituitary** and the **posterior pituitary**. Each part secretes its own set of hormones. The **hypothalamus** regulates the anterior pituitary by secreting neurohormones that can stimulate or inhibit the actions of the anterior pituitary.

The anterior pituitary gland makes and secretes the following hormones:

- **Growth hormone** (**GH**) targets all tissues and organs in the body and stimulates growth of organs throughout the body.
- **Thyroid stimulating hormone** (**TSH**) stimulates the thyroid gland to secrete thyroxine (thyroid hormone).

- **Adrenocorticotropic hormone (ACTH)** stimulates the **adrenal cortex** (its outer layer) to secrete hormones (**glucocorticoids** and **mineralocorticoids**).
- **Follicle stimulating hormone (FSH)** targets the **gonads** (male and female reproductive organs). In females, it stimulates the **ovaries**, prompting **mature eggs** and release of **estrogen**. In males, it stimulates the testes to make **sperm**.
- **Luteinizing hormone (LH)** targets the gonads. In females it stimulates the ovaries to release the **ovum** during **menstrual cycles**; in males it stimulates the production of **testosterone**.
- **Prolactin** is released only after a woman gives birth. The hormone stimulates **mammary glands** to produce breast milk.

The posterior pituitary gland stores and secretes the following hormones:

- **Oxytocin** causes the uterus to contract and prompts the release of breast milk.
- **Antidiuretic hormone (ADH)**, also known as **vasopressin**, is a powerful blood vessel constrictor. It causes nephrons in the kidney to retain water. It may also raise blood pressure.

Thyroid Gland

Located in the anterior portion of the neck, the **thyroid gland** secretes two hormones: **thyroxine** and **calcitonin**. Thyroxine contains iodine and is responsible for regulating the metabolic rate in your body tissues; calcitonin decreases blood calcium levels by removing calcium from the bloodstream and depositing it back into bone.

Parathyroid Gland

Located behind the thyroid gland, the **parathyroid gland** secretes parathyroid hormone, which increases blood calcium. Together with calcitonin, it regulates blood calcium level.

Adrenal Glands

The human body has two **adrenal glands** that sit on top of the kidneys. Each of these glands has two distinct parts: the **adrenal cortex** and the **adrenal medulla**.

- The adrenal cortex secretes glucocorticoids, which target the liver and promote the release of glucose. The adrenal cortex also secretes mineralocorticoids, which target the kidney and promote the retention of water. It also produces cortisol, which has widespread effects on metabolism.
- The adrenal medulla secretes epinephrine and norepinephrine, which increase and prolong the effects of the sympathetic nervous system. Epinephrine is needed for the fight-or-flight mechanism.

What is the function of noradrenaline produced by the adrenal medulla?

A. It dilates blood vessels.
B. It decreases blood pressure.
C. It decreases diastolic pressure.
D. It decreases insulin secretion.

Here's How to Crack It

Noradrenaline and epinephrine are vasoconstrictors, not vasodilators. They do not dilate blood vessels (choice A) or decrease blood pressure (choice B). When the sympathetic nervous system releases noradrenaline, the "fight or flight" mode kicks in. Choice C is also incorrect because noradrenaline acts on alpha receptors to increase (not decrease) the systolic and diastolic blood pressure. Noradrenaline is a hormone and neurotransmitter. It acts on α-receptors and increases blood pressure by increasing vascular tone. It triggers the release of glucose from energy stores so you have energy to fight or run fast and far. It also inhibits the secretion of insulin by the pancreas. (*Note:* If it acts on the β-receptors, noradrenaline can increase insulin availability.)

Pancreas

The **pancreas** secretes the digestive enzymes **insulin**, which lowers blood sugar, and **glucagon**, which raises blood sugar. Both insulin and glucagon are produced in the region of the pancreas known as the **islets of Langerhans**.

Gonads

The **gonads** are primary sex organs that are responsible for the production of estrogen, **progesterone**, and testosterone. They are responsible for the development of **secondary sex characteristics** that occur in puberty (the awkward change from childhood to teenager—we all remember those tough times). Estrogen and progesterone are released by the ovaries and regulate the menstrual cycle. Testosterone is the male hormone responsible for promoting **spermatogenesis** (the production of sperm).

Hormones

How Hormones Work

The way that hormones work depends on whether the hormone is a steroid, a protein, a peptide, or an amine. If the hormone is a steroid, then the hormone can diffuse across the membrane of the target cell. It then binds to a receptor protein in the nucleus and activates specific genes contained in the DNA, which, in turn, make a protein.

If the hormone is a protein, a peptide, or an amine, it cannot get into the target cell by simple diffusion. The hormone must bind to a receptor protein on the cell membrane of the target cell. This protein in turn stimulates the production of a second messenger called **cyclic AMP (cAMP)**. The cAMP molecule then triggers various enzymes that initiate specific cellular changes.

Here's a summary of the hormones and their effects on the body.

ORGAN	HORMONES	EFFECT
Anterior Pituitary	FSH	Stimulates activity in ovaries and testes
	LH	Stimulates activity in ovary (release of ovum) and production of testosterone
	ACTH	Stimulates the adrenal cortex
	Growth Hormone	Stimulates bone and muscle growth
	TSH	Stimulates the thyroid to secrete thyroxine
	Prolactin	Causes milk secretion
Posterior Pituitary	Oxytocin	Causes uterus to contract
	Vasopressin	Causes kidneys to reabsorb water
Thyroid	Thyroid Hormone	Regulates metabolic rate
	Calcitonin	Lowers blood calcium levels
Parathyroid	Parathyroid Hormone	Increases blood calcium concentration
Adrenal Cortex	Aldosterone	Increases Na^+ and H_2O reabsorption in kidneys
Adrenal Medulla	Epinephrine Norepinephrine	Increase blood glucose level and heart rate
Pancreas	Insulin	Decreases blood sugar concentration
	Glucagon	Increases blood sugar concentration
Ovaries	Estrogen	Promotes female secondary sex characteristics and thickens endometrial lining, oogenesis
	Progesterone	Maintains endometrial lining
Testes	Testosterone	Promotes male secondary sex characteristic and spermatogenesis

While the nervous system and the endocrine system work in close coordination, there are significant differences between the two:

- The nervous system sends nerve impulses using neurons, whereas the endocrine system secretes hormones.
- Nerve impulses control rapidly changing activities, such as muscle contractions, whereas hormones deal with long-term adjustments.

THE HUMAN REPRODUCTIVE SYSTEM AND EMBRYONIC DEVELOPMENT

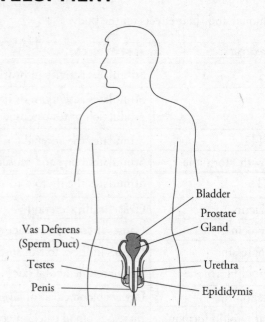

The Male Reproductive System

What to Know about HIS: The All-Boys Club

Sperm and male hormones are produced in the **testes**. The testes are located outside the body cavity in a **scrotum**, or **scrotal sac**. The function of the scrotum is to keep the testes slightly cooler than body temperature. The main tissues of the testes are the **seminiferous tubules**, where **spermatogonia** undergo meiosis, under the influence of FSH. The **spermatids** then mature in the **epididymis**, where they are stored.

The **interstitial cells** (also known as Leydig cells), which are supportive tissue, produce testosterone and other **androgens**. Sperm then travel through the **vas deferens** and pick up fluids from the **seminal vesicles** and the **prostate gland**. The seminal vesicles provide the sperm with fructose and nutrients for energy; the prostate gland provides a watery and alkaline fluid (**semen**) to neutralize acidotic vaginal fluids. Semen is transported to the **vagina** by the **penis**.

Unlike the female reproductive system, the male reproductive system continues to secrete hormones throughout the life of the male, thanks to hormones secreted by the anterior pituitary gland. FSH and LH are produced by the anterior pituitary gland in males and females. In males, FSH targets the seminiferous tubules of the testes, where it stimulates sperm production. LH stimulates interstitial cells (Leydig cells) to produce testosterone. In females, FSH stimulates follicles in the ovaries to grow.

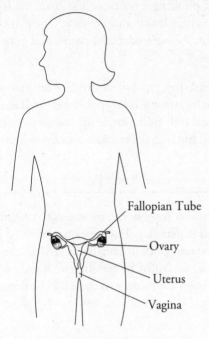

Fallopian Tube

Ovary

Uterus

Vagina

The Female Reproductive System

What to Know about HERS: Complex Lady Parts
- **Follicles** (and the **ova**) are contained in the ovaries.
- Hormones are released from the ovaries and pituitary gland.
- Ovaries produce gametes.
- **Fertilization** occurs in the upper third of the **fallopian tube**.
- The fertilized ovum implants itself in the **uterus** where it is fed, nurtured, and protected while it grows to term.

Reproduction in animals involves the production of egg and sperm. The testes manufacture sperm cells (spermatogenesis) in the seminiferous tubules by causing cells in the testes to start undergoing meiosis. The hormone secreted by the testes is testosterone, which is responsible for the development of secondary sex characteristics in males as well as for spermatogenesis.

> ### The Second(ary) Sex (Characteristics)
>
> In boys, secondary sex characteristics include a surge of hormones, broader shoulders, deepening of voice, facial hair (peach fuzz), axillary (armpit) hair, further growth and development of their below-the-belt parts, pubic hair, courser chest, arm and leg (and sometimes back) hair. During this stage, boys are often lanky and ape-like. Their arms may be longer than their torsos until growth evens out. Arm pit odor and sweat, plus acne and emotions, make for an awkward time for these fellows!
>
> In girls, secondary sex characteristics include a surge of hormones, the development of breast buds (**thelarche**), axillary hair, arm pit odor, pubic hair (**adrenarche**), changes in girl parts including transition of cervical cells from simple squamous to columnar, discharge, the period, acne, mood swings, increased hip size, fewer meals and more heels. Ahh—to be THAT young again.

In the ovaries, ova are manufactured (**oogenesis**) by meiosis. Ovaries secrete estrogen and progesterone (sex hormones) that are found in females. The hormones secreted by the ovaries are involved in the development of secondary sex characteristics in females as well as the initiation of the **menstrual cycle**. To better understand reproduction, you must be familiar with the menstrual cycle. **Menarche** refers to the age at which a female goes through the menstrual cycle for the first time (the first of many throughout her child-bearing years).

Menses: The Period

The following paragraphs describe the time frame for a typical menstrual cycle:

- On day 1, bleeding begins and lasts 5–8 days. Estrogen and progesterone levels are low at this point. FSH (remember follicle-stimulating hormone?) from the anterior pituitary stimulates the growth of a follicle in the ovary (so this phase is named the **follicular phase**), which secretes estrogen as it grows.
- After day 5, the rising estrogen levels stimulate the uterus to grow a new inner lining (the **proliferative phase**) and the egg matures. As the egg matures, the uterine lining thickens. During this phase, many women experience a bloating sensation, their clothes may be tighter, and they may experience mood swings and headaches.
- By day 14, the uterine lining is thick. A surge in LH (remember luteinizing hormone?) from the anterior pituitary gland causes the release of the egg and some of the follicular cells from the ovary. This process is called **ovulation**. This egg moves into the fallopian tube or oviduct and begins its journey toward the uterus. During ovulation, women often experience **middleschmertz**, abdominal pain that results from irritation of the peritoneum by bleeding from the ovulation site. It's also known as **intermenstrual pain**.
- LH causes the remaining follicular cells to form a yellow blob called the **corpus luteum**, which is made of cell and debris. During what is called the **luteal phase**, the corpus luteum secretes progesterone and estrogen. These hormones further enhance the lining of the uterus (the **secretory phase**).

- By days 14–28, estrogen and progesterone are secreted and the uterine blood supply increases and is almost engorged. An increase in progesterone helps the body prepare for **implantation** of the fertilized ovum. Progesterone is responsible for readying the body for pregnancy by promoting blood vessels to develop in the **endometrium**. Progesterone is necessary in maintaining a pregnancy and preventing the menstrual cycle from happening again, beginning with the "day 1."

If fertilization and implantation do not occur, the corpus luteum degenerates after 14 days and the drop in progesterone and estrogen causes the lining to degrade and slough off (shed), and bleeding occurs, with muscle cramping and pain which then starts the next cycle all over again.

When fertilization and **pregnancy** do occur, the tissue of the **fetus** releases **human chorionic gonadotropin** (**HCG**), which helps maintain the uterine lining (hence the "pregnancy test" or beta HCG test). HCG can be detected in blood and urine after implantation, which means about 6–12 days after fertilization. **Early pregnancy factor** or **early conception factor tests** can detect a pregnancy with the plasma portion of the blood fewer than 48 hours after fertilization. This test is time-consuming and costly, so it won't be readily available at your local drugstore and won't be mentioned on your nursing exam.

Embryonic Development

You may have no interest in becoming a parent or going into nursing related to obstetrics, labor and delivery, or pediatrics, but for any nursing exam, you should understand how everything happens, where it happens, why it happens, and when it happens.

Embryogenesis is the process by which an embryo forms and develops, until it becomes a fetus. Traditionally, parents get together, sperm reaches the egg, and fertilization occurs in the upper third of the fallopian tube. The fertilized egg plus sperm form a diploid cell called a **zygote**. (*Note:* In this NSEE preparation text, we do not discuss alternate assisted methods of conception such as in vitro fertilization (IVF) and surrogacy.)

The **zona pellucida** (the strong membrane around the ova) is dissolved by an enzyme called **hyaluronidase**, and the tail of the sperm is shed. The nucleus in the sperm head then becomes a **pronucleus**, a cell nucleus with a haploid set of chromosomes (23 chromosomes in humans) resulting from meiosis (**germ-cell division**). The male pronucleus is the sperm nucleus after it has entered the ovum at fertilization, but before fusion with the female pronucleus. The female pronucleus is the nucleus of the ovum before fusion with the male pronucleus.

So the female pronucleus + male pronucleus → segmentation nucleus → zygote.

This one cell now has 23 chromosomes from each parent: 46 total.
It contains the genetic blueprint for every detail of human development.

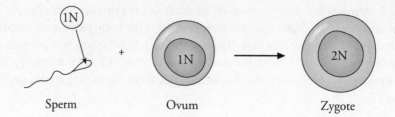

Formation of a Zygote

Fertilization triggers the zygote to go through a series of rapid mitotic cell divisions called **cleavage** (by day 3 it is already sixteen cells). The zygote keeps dividing until it forms a solid ball called a **morula** (by day 5).

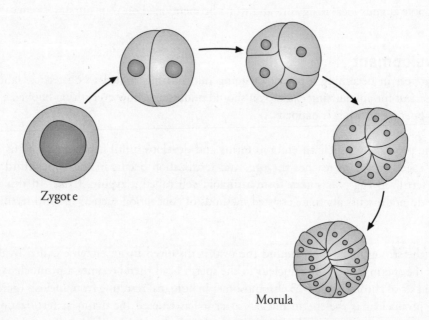

Formation of a Morula

Six days after fertilization, the zygote becomes a hollow ball called a **blastocyst** and the **blastula phase** begins. During the blastula phase, cells continue to divide and press against each other and produce a fluid-filled cavity called a **blastocoel**. The blastocyst attaches to the endometrium on day 7. **Ectoderm** secretes an enzyme that enables the blastocyst (**trophoblast** and inner cell mass) to penetrate the endometrium and implant in the **fundus** (body or lumen) of the uterus where it is protected, fed, and allowed to grow to term (the full pregnancy).

During a period called the **gastrulation phase**, the zygote begins to change shape and cells migrate to the blastocoels where they **differentiate** (**differentiation**—which parts of the human body are derived from each other is important information to know) to form three germ layers:

1. The **ectoderm** produces the skin (epidermis), eyes, and nervous system.
2. The **endoderm** produces the inner linings of the respiratory tract, digestive tract, and accessory organs (pancreas, gall bladder, and liver).
3. The **mesoderm** gives rise to everything else, including the peritoneum, muscles, bones, and other connective tissues, along with the excretory, circulatory, and reproductive systems.

That's cell differentiation in a nutshell. Or a nut cell.

In addition to these three primary germ layers, some animals have extraembryonic membranes. There are four extraembryonic membranes: the yolk sac, amnion, chorion, and allantois. The **yolk sac** provides food for the embryo while **amnion** forms a fluid-filled sac that protects the embryo and secretes **amniotic fluid**. **Allantois** is the membrane involved in gas exchange. Secretion of ectoderm becomes **chorion** (the outermost fetal membrane).

During pregnancy, hormonal and placental chemicals (progesterone and HCG) prevent the mother's body from having another menstrual cycle. The LH level stays high throughout the pregnancy because the human chorionic gonadotrophin hormone is produced by the placenta (feedback) and sends a message to the pituitary gland to keep the LH level high. So basically, throughout the duration of her pregnancy, the mother remains in day 15, or the post ovulatory phase of the menstrual cycle.

Organogenesis is the stage during which the development of the nervous system is well underway. The **neurula stage** (also known as **neuralation**) begins with the formation of two structures: the **notochord** and the **neural tube**, which develop into the nervous system. Fascinating, huh?

See how it all ties together now from the beginning? Remember the reason why humans are organized in the phylum chordate and subphylum vertebrata?

Since state preparation and nursing school entrance exams may have some questions on pregnancy gestation, cell differentiation in early development, and birth weight, we've included a bit of information in this section for you to review. The following chart describes the developmental milestones of a fetus. The entire pregnancy gestation period is 280 days (9 months).

Pregnancy Gestation	
Time	**Stage of Development**
By day 20	Foundations of the brain spinal cord and nervous system are already established.
By day 21	The heart is beating.
By day 28	The backbone and muscles are forming; arms, legs, eyes, and ears begin to show.
By 4 weeks	A transvaginal ultrasound may be able to pick up the heartbeat.
By day 30	The zygote is 10,000 times larger than the first fertilized single cell, blood is pumping and circulating, and the placenta forms a barrier to separate mother and baby blood, allowing food and oxygen to pass through.
By day 35	There are five fingers on each hand and five toes on each foot.
By day 40	Brain waves can be detected and recorded.
By week 6	The liver takes over production of blood cells, and the brain controls movements of muscles and organs.
By week 7	The embryo can move, the jaw and teeth form, and the eyelids seal closed.

By week 8	The fetus is almost 8 inches long and his or her pieces and parts all present now. The stomach produces digestive enzymes, the kidneys function, 40 muscle systems operate in conjunction with the nervous system, and the fetus responds to touch.
By week 9	Fingerprints are evident in the skin.
By week 10	The uterus has doubled in size.
By week 11	The fetus is 2 inches long. Urine is produced, and the face assumes a "baby's pro-file." Coordinated muscle movement occurs.
By week 12	Fetal sleep-wake cycles occur. Hand gripping, head turning, and mouth movement are apparent.
By week 13	Hair growth occurs, and sexual differentiation is apparent. (A sonogram can help the mother decide to buy pink or blue.)
By month 4	The baby is 8–10 inches long and weighs one-half pound or more. The baby has the ability to hear.
By month 5	The fetus is about 12 inches long, and fetal movement can be detected by the mother.
By month 6	Oil and sweat glands function, a "cheesy" protective skin coat (called **vernix**) is present, and the baby makes breathing movements.
By month 7	The senses of vision, hearing, taste, and touch are all working. Eyes open and close at about week 27 or 28, and the suck-swallow coordination develops.
By month 8	The skin thickens with "brown fat," which provides insulation and nutrition. Maternal antibodies build up and are transferred to the baby; amniotic fluid is absorbed and replaced.
By 9 months	*Almost ready?* He or she now weighs about 5.5 to 9 pounds, and the heart pumps 300 gallons of blood per day.

Did You Know?

During the first 2 months of gestation, the baby is called an embryo. During the third to ninth month, the baby is called a fetus (from the Latin route word meaning "young one" or "offspring").

Premature and Preterm Delivery

Sometimes babies come early, whether due to infection, trauma, distress, or just for unknown reasons. Their care is unique, special, and delicate, as they are below birth weight, fragile, and still developing. They require time to grow and develop in an incubator in place of their mother's womb. If they were full-term babies, they would be of normal birth weight, be fully developed, and have the maternal antibodies and iron that transfer from the mother to the baby during the third trimester of the pregnancy.

Preterm and premature deliveries of infants will be discussed in great detail once you begin your studies as a nurse. Find solace in knowing that neonatal medicine has advanced with practice and technology over the years. Thirty plus years ago, premature babies did not often survive, and if they did, their longevity and prognosis was often said to be grim. Today, these little early bundles of joy thrive and do well throughout life thanks to the dedicated nurses and neonatologists who truly care. So, if you are considering a career in a neonatal intensive care unit (NICU), you will soon share in the marvel of many little and big success stories and be a specialty in nursing where there is great demand.

Stages of Labor and Delivery

Here are the stages that occur during labor and delivery of an infant:

1. During the first stage of labor, the cervix becomes completely dilated and effaced. These cervical changes differentiate true labor from **Braxton hicks**, a false "practice" labor.
    a. Rupture of amniotic sac or **rupture of membranes**
    b. Dilation of cervix to 10cm (centimeters)
    c. 100 percent **effacement** (thinned)
2. During stage 2, the cervical dilation is complete and the baby is expulsed, or delivered.
3. During stage 3, powerful uterine contractions expel the **placental afterbirth** a few minutes after delivery.

SUMMARY

- The digestive system manages the process of eating, digesting, and absorbing foods.

- The circulatory system transports oxygen, carbon dioxide, glucose, hormones, waste products, and other materials around the body. It consists of the heart, a series of blood vessels, and blood.

- The lymphatic system recaptures and filters fluids from the tissues and returns it to the bloodstream.

- The respiratory system works to exchange oxygen and carbon dioxide with the blood. It also helps regulate body pH.

- The urinary system eliminates nitrogenous waste products from food digestion. It also helps in water and electrolyte balance and blood pressure regulation.

- The integumentary system supports and protects the organs in the body and helps in thermoregulation.

- The skeletal system, which is a mineral storage site, holds a body together in some regular shape, protects various organs, and produces blood cells.

- The musculoskeletal system supports, protects, and moves the body.

- The nervous system carries impulses between body parts.

- The endocrine system controls the body through the use of hormones.

- The reproductive system is responsible for the passing of genetic information to future generations.

- A single-celled egg develops into a complex multicellular organism by dividing and going through many stages in a process called embryogenesis.

KEY TERMS

digestive system
respiratory system
circulatory system
immune system
excretory system
integumentary system
musculoskeletal system
nervous system
endocrine system
reproductive system
phylum Chordata
Urochordata
Cephalochordata
Vertebrata
anatomical position
    (supine position)
superior and inferior
anterior and posterior
myocardial
sternum
medial and lateral
proximal and distal
superficial and deep
dorsal and ventral
dorsal cavity
ventral cavity
thoracic cavity
abdominopelvic cavity
pleural cavities
pericardial cavity
abdominal cavity
pelvic cavity
serous membranes
mucous membranes
transverse and longitudinal
alimentary canal
accessory organs
mouth
anus
esophagus
stomach
small intestine
large intestine
salivary glands
liver
pancreas

gall bladder
ingestion
saliva
amylase
peristalsis
reverse peristalsis
vomit (throw up)
emesis
digestion
pyloris
gastrin
HCl (hydrochloric acid)
pepsinogen
pepsin
chyme
rennin (chymosin)
secretion
bile
cholecystokinin
emulsify
dipeptides
secretin
bicarbonate
base
absorption
villi
microvilli
pernicious anemia
vitamin B_{12}
lymphatic vessels
lacteals
portal veins
capillaries
hepatic portal system
red blood cells (RBCs)
defecation
fecal matter (feces) (stool)
rectum
aerobic respiration
noses
nares
pharynx
stratified
larynx
trachea
cartilaginous rings

epiglottis
respiratory tree
pneumonia
aspiration pneumonia
bronchus
bronchioles
bronchiolitis
bronchitis
alveoli
surfactant
synthetic surfactant
respiratory distress
alveolar sacs
capillary beds
room air
inhale (inhalation)
exhale (exhalation)
cardiopulmonary resuscitation
    (CPR)
rescue breathing
respiratory arrest
bradypnea
apnea
diaphragm
intercostals muscles
rib cages
inspiration
expiration
baroreceptors
chemoreceptors
alkalosis
acidosis
hemoglobin
plasma
bicarbonate ions
buffer
pump
heart
blood vessels
blood
lymphatic system
lymph nodes
white blood cells (WBCs)
veins
lymphatic vessels
lymph

chambers
atrium
ventricle
septum
valves
fibrous pericardium
parietal serous pericardium
epicardium
myocardium
endocardium
endocarditis
coronary arteries
ischemia
angina
varicose veins
aortic semilunar valve
aorta
systemic circulation
deoxygenated
superior vena cava
inferior vena cava
tricuspid valve (atrioventricular
    valve)
pulmonary artery
pulmonary circulation
pulmonary capillaries
kidney
oxygenated
pulmonary veins
bicuspid valve (mitral)
sinoatrial node (SA node)
atrioventricular node (AV node)
atrioventricular bundle (bundle
    of His)
Perkinje fibers
systole
diastole
systolic pressure
diastolic pressure
sphygmomanometer
stem cells
erythrocyte (red blood cell, or
    RBC)
leukocyte (white blood cell, or
    WBC)
platelets
bilirubin
phototherapy

phagocytes
lymphocytes
B-cells
helper T-cells
killer T-cells
thymocytes (hematopoietic
    precursors)
AIDS
HIV
clotting factor
fibrinogen
fibrin threads
thrombus
embolus
embolisms
pulmonary embolism
prothrombin
thrombin
hemorrhaging
exsanguinating
coagulopathic
albumin
antigen
transfusion
agglutination
Rh factors
RhoGAM
intercellular clefts
capillary endothelium
edema
adenopathy
neutrophils
monocytes
macrophages
chemotaxis
basophils
eosinophils
mast cells
degranulate
histamine
complement proteins
cytokines
interferons
phagocytosis
innate immunity
febrile
cytotoxic T-cells
cell-mediated response

humoral immunity
long-term immunity
active immunization
artificial active immunization
hepatitis B vaccine
MMR (measles, mumps, and
    rubella)
varicella
passive immunization
pathogens
antibiotic
antiviral drugs
prodrome phase
urine
uric acid
creatinine
filtration
reabsorbtion
secretion
renal cortex
collecting ducts
pyramids (renal papillae)
nephrons
Bowman's capulse
glomerulus
proximal convoluted tubules
distal convoluted tubules
loop of Henle
final collecting duct
ureters
bladder
urethra
urinary meatus
micturation
juxta glomerulosa
erythropoietin
renin
angiotensinogen
angiotensin I
angiotensin II
vasoconstrictor
zona glomerulosa
aldosterone
epithelial tissue
squamous
cuboidal
columnar
simple epithelium

stratified epithelium
pseudostratified epithelium
connective tissue
dense connective
elastic connective
muscle tissue
nervous tissue
stratum corneum
keratin
stratum lucidum
keratohyalin
eleidin
stratum granulosom
stratum spinosum
stratum basale (germinativum)
melanocytes
melanin
cellulitis
lacerations
dehiscence
debridement
revisions
decubidus ulcers (bed sores)
decubidi (plural of decubidus)
turgor
subcutaneously
skin graft
epidermis
dermis
papillary layer
hypodermis
hemopoietic
bone ossification
bones
cartilage
collagen
osteoblasts
osteoclasts
ligaments
tendons
skeletal muscle
voluntary muscle
cardiac muscle
involuntary muscle
smooth muscle
sarcomere
actin
myosin

sarcoplasmic reticulum
sliding filament theory
neuron
cell body (soma)
dendrites
axon
sensory (afferent) neurons
motor (efferent) neurons
interneurons (association)
polarized
action potential
voltage gated sodium channels
depolarization
potassium channels
repolarization
refractory period
sodium-potassium pump
myelin
Schwann cells
myelin sheath
nodes of Ranvier
terminal end
neurotransmitter
acetylcholine
norepinephrine
GABA (gamma-amino-buteric
    acid)
synaptic cleft
myelination
central nervous system (CNS)
peripheral nervous system (PNS)
spinal cord
cranial nerves
cerebrum
cerebellum
midbrain
hypothalamus
medulla
pons
corpus collosum
grey matter
white matter
pincer grasp
hindbrain
pia mater
dura mater
meninges
frontal lobe

parietal lobe
temporal lobe
occipital lobe
coccyx bone (tailbone)
somatic nervous system
autonomic nervous system
sympathetic nervous system
epinephrine
parasympathetic nervous system
pituitary gland
anterior pituitary
posterior pituitary
hypothalamus
growth hormone (GH)
thyroid stimulating hormone
    (TSH)
adrenocorticotropic hormone
    (ACTH)
adrenal cortex
glucocorticoids
mineralcorticoids
follicle stimulating hormone
    (FSH)
gonads
ovaries
mature eggs
estrogen
sperm
luteinizing hormone (LH)
ovum
menstrual cycles
testosterone
prolactin
mammary glands
oxytocin
antidiuretic hormone (ADH)
vasopressin
thyroid gland
thyroxine
calcitonin
parathyroid gland
adrenal glands
adrenal cortex
adrenal medulla
pancreas
insulin
glucagon
islets of Langerhans

gonads
progesterone
secondary sex characteristics
spermatogenesis
cyclic AMP (cAMP)
testes
scrotum (scrotal sac)
seminiferous tubules
spermatogonia
spermatids
epididymis
interstitial cells
androgens
vas deferens
seminal vesicles
prostate gland
semen
vagina
penis
follicles
ova
fertilization
fallopian tube
uterus
thelarche
adrenarche

oogenesis
menstrual cycle
menarche
follicular phase
proliferative phase
ovulation
middleschmertz (intermenstrual
    pain)
corpus luteum
luteal phase
secretory phase
implantation
endometrium
pregnancy
fetus
human chorionic gonadotropin
    (HCG)
early pregnancy factor test
early conception factor test
embryogenesis
zygote
zona pellucida
hyaluronidase
pronucleus
germ-cell division
cleavage

morula
blastocyst
blastula phase
blastocoel
ectoderm
trophoblast
fundus
gastrulation phase
differentiation
ectoderm
endoderm
mesoderm
yolk sac
amnion
amniotic fluid
allantois
chorion
organogenesis
neurula stage (neuralation)
notochord
neural tube
vernix
Braxton hicks
rupture of membranes
effacement
placental afterbirth

Chapter 6
Physics

WHY PHYSICS?

You definitely won't be using physics in your nursing career, unless you go into rehabilitative medicine, specialize in prosthetics and orthotics, or dare to use a Hoyer lift (a pulley system used for lifting heavy patients).

So, no, you do not have to understand the mechanics or physics behind how a Hoyer lift works at the hospital—just know that it does work. But you will have to understand physics if you are planning to take the NLN PAX-RN (with 80 science questions, including some about physics) or the TEAS (with 30 science questions, including some about physics). The NET is the only test that does not focus heavily on the sciences, meaning, no physics either.

Hoyer Lift

Hoyer lifts are often found on medical-surgical units and rehabilitation floors of chronic care facilities. The Hoyer lift uses simple pulleys and physics to do the heavy lifting for you.

Keep in mind that a wise physics move, which will be useful in your nursing career and at home, is proper injury prevention or calisthenics. An example is using the proper procedure for lifting heavy objects—that is, using leg muscles to squat or bend down, not bending over and using back muscles. That squat bend-down movement (as opposed to bending over) can protect you from soft tissue injury and several weeks of unhappy and unnecessary lower back spasms. See? That's good physics and proper thinking. The NLN PAX-RN and TEAS writers will expect you to be familiar with all the laws of physics, including concepts, formulas, and simple machinery mechanics, even though you probably won't ever have to see it again.

Let's begin with a review of the math that goes along with physics. The next pages will be useful in a lot of the problem solving.

SCIENTIFIC NOTATION

It's usually much easier to write very large or very small numbers in scientific notation. For example, the speed of light through empty space is approximately 300,000,000 meters per second. In scientific notation, this number would be written as 3×10^8. Here's another example: In standard units, Newton's universal gravitational constant is about 0.0000000000667; in scientific notation, this number would be written as 6.67×10^{-11}. In general, we say that a number is in **scientific notation** when it's written in the form $a \times 10^n$, where $1 \leq a < 10$ and n is an integer. As the two examples above show, when a very large number is written in scientific notation, the value of n is a large positive integer, and when a very small number is written in scientific notation, n is a negative integer with a large magnitude. To multiply or divide two numbers written in scientific notation, just remember that $10^m \times 10^n = 10^{m+n}$ and $10^m/10^n = 10^{m-n}$. So, for example, $(3 \times 10^8)(2.5 \times 10^{-12}) = 7.5 \times 10^{-4}$ and $(8 \times 10^9)/(2 \times 10^{-5}) = 4 \times 10^{14}$.

BASIC TRIG REVIEW

If you're given a right triangle, there are certain special functions, called **trig functions**, of the angles in the triangle that depend on the lengths of the sides. We'll concentrate on three of these functions: the **sine**, **cosine**, and **tangent** (abbreviated sin, cos, and tan, respectively). Take a look at the following right triangle, *ABC*. The right angle is at *C*, and the lengths of the sides are labeled *a*, *b*, and *c*.

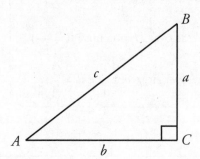

Triangles and Beans?

Pythagoras was actually a cult leader around 500 B.C. Some rules of his number-worshipping group included prohibitions against eating beans and wearing wool.

First, we'll mention one of the most important facts about any right triangle. The **Pythagorean theorem** tells us that the square of the **hypotenuse** (which is the name of the side opposite the right angle, always the longest side) is equal to the sum of the squares of the other two sides (called the **legs**):

$$a^2 + b^2 = c^2$$

Now for the trig functions. Let's consider angle *A* in the right triangle pictured above. The sine, cosine, and tangent of this angle are defined like this:

$$\sin A = \frac{\text{opposite}}{\text{hypotenuse}} = \frac{a}{c} \qquad \cos A = \frac{\text{adjacent}}{\text{hypotenuse}} = \frac{b}{c} \qquad \tan A = \frac{\text{opposite}}{\text{adjacent}} = \frac{a}{b}$$

By *opposite* we mean the length of the side that's opposite the angle, and by *adjacent* we mean the length of the side that's adjacent to the angle. The same definitions, in words, can be used for angle *B* as follows:

$$\sin B = \frac{\text{opposite}}{\text{hypotenuse}} = \frac{b}{c} \qquad \cos B = \frac{\text{adjacent}}{\text{hypotenuse}} = \frac{a}{c} \qquad \tan B = \frac{\text{opposite}}{\text{adjacent}} = \frac{b}{a}$$

Notice that sin *A* = cos *B* and cos *A* = sin *B*.

SOHCAHTOA

Here's a word you should remember on test day so you can keep clear on the definitions of sin θ, cos θ, and tan θ: **SOHCAHTOA**. This isn't some magic word to chant during the test; it simply helps you remember that

$Sine$ = Opposite side over Hypotenuse $(S = \dfrac{O}{H})$

$Cosine$ = Adjacent side over Hypotenuse $(C = \dfrac{A}{H})$

$Tangent$ = Opposite over Adjacent side $(T = \dfrac{O}{A})$

The definitions

$$\sin\theta = \frac{\text{opposite}}{\text{hypotenuse}} \qquad \cos\theta = \frac{\text{adjacent}}{\text{hypotenuse}} \qquad \tan\theta = \frac{\text{opposite}}{\text{adjacent}}$$

can be used for any acute angle θ (theta) in a right triangle.

The values of the sine, cosine, and tangent of the acute angles in a 3-4-5 right triangle are listed in the specific example that follows:

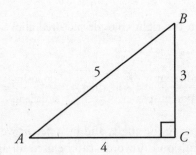

$$\sin A = \frac{3}{5} \qquad \sin B = \frac{4}{5}$$

$$\cos A = \frac{4}{5} \qquad \cos B = \frac{3}{5}$$

$$\tan A = \frac{3}{4} \qquad \tan B = \frac{4}{3}$$

We can also figure out the values of the sine, cosine, and tangent of the acute angles in a couple of special (and common) right triangles: the 30°-60° and the 45°-45° right triangles:

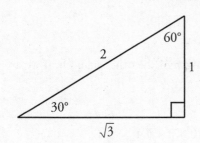

$$\sin 30° = \cos 60° = \frac{1}{2} = 0.50$$

$$\cos 30° = \sin 60° = \frac{\sqrt{3}}{2} \approx 0.87$$

$$\tan 30° = \frac{1}{\sqrt{3}} \approx 0.58, \quad \tan 60° = \sqrt{3} \approx 1.73$$

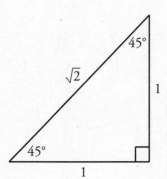

$$\sin 45° = \cos 45° = \frac{1}{\sqrt{2}} \approx 0.71$$

$$\tan 45° = 1$$

Triangle Mnemonics

A 30°-60°-90° triangle has three different angles with sides in proportions 1-$\sqrt{3}$-2. A 45°-45°-90° triangle has three distinct angles with sides in proportions 1-1-$\sqrt{2}$. The number of distinct angles is what goes under the root sign.

If we know the values of these functions for other acute angles, we can use them to figure out the missing sides of a right triangle. This is one of the most common uses of trig for the physics in this book. For example, consider the triangle below, with hypotenuse 5 and containing an acute angle, θ, of measure 30°:

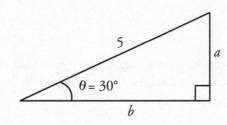

Sin 30° is 0.5, so because $\sin\theta = a/5$, we can figure out that

$$a = 5 \sin\theta = 5 \sin30° \approx 5(0.5) = 2.5$$

We can use the Pythagorean theorem to figure out b, the length of the other side. Or, if we are told that cos 30° is about 0.87, then since $\cos\theta = b/5$, we'd find that

$$b = 5 \cos\theta = 5 \cos30° \approx 5(0.87) = 4.4$$

This gives us

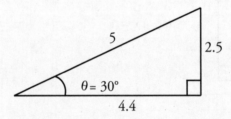

These values can be checked by the Pythagorean theorem, since

$$2.5^2 + 4.4^2 \approx 5^2.$$

This example illustrates this important, general fact: If the hypotenuse of a right triangle is c, then the length of the side opposite one of the acute angles, θ, is $c \sin\theta$, and the length of the side adjacent to this angle is $c \cos\theta$ as follows:

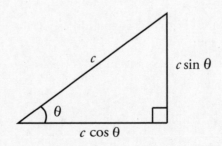

VECTORS

Definition

A **vector** is a quantity that involves both magnitude and direction and obeys the **commutative law for addition,** which we'll explain in a moment. A quantity that does not involve direction is a **scalar**. For example, *55 miles per hour* is a scalar quantity, while *55 miles per hour to the north* is a vector quantity. Speed and distance are scalar quantities. Other examples of scalars include mass, work, energy, power, temperature, and electric charge.

The scalars of distance and speed are paired with the vectors of displacement and velocity, respectively.

Vectors can be denoted in several ways. Here are some examples:

$$\mathbf{A}, A, \vec{\mathrm{A}}, \vec{A}$$

In textbooks, you'll usually see one of the first two, but when it's handwritten, you'll see one of the last two. In this book, we will show all vector quantities in bold. For example, A would be the scalar quantity, and **A** the vector quantity.

Graphically, a vector is represented as an arrow whose length represents the magnitude and whose direction represents, well, the direction.

A ⟋   **A** = 9 m/s northeast

B ⟵   **B** = 4 m/s west

Displacement is the prototypical example of a vector:

$$\underbrace{\mathbf{A}}_{\text{displacement}} = \underbrace{4 \text{ miles}}_{\text{magnitude}} \underbrace{\text{to the north}}_{\text{direction}}$$

Two vectors are equal if they have the same magnitude and the same direction.

MOTION BASICS

The basics of motion are seen in everyday life (sometimes even in nursing school entrance exams). Motion is any physical movement or change in position or place characterized by **position**, **displacement**, **speed**, **velocity**, or **acceleration**.

- Position refers to the location of an object (the object is on the nightstand).
- Displacement refers to the distance that an object has moved (the patient fell 6 feet from the ladder to the ground; an athlete runs exactly once around an oval track).
- Speed is the time-rate of displacement or object movement (the car was struck moving forward while traveling 35 miles per hour).
- Velocity is the direction of speed represented by a vector which has magnitude and direction (for example, going 30 miles per hour north, south, east, west, in a tunnel, or out of a tunnel).
- Acceleration refers to the rate of velocity change, the rate of change per unit time (we were driving at 30 miles per hour and then had to speed up to 40 miles per hour to pass that truck!)

Position, Distance, and Displacement

What's important to know about position is that it refers to an object's relation to a coordinate (x, y) axis system. Distance is a scalar that represents the total amount traveled by the object—it is a physical quantity, a dimension that has no direction. Displacement is an object's change in position. It is the vector that points from the object's initial position to its final position, regardless of the path taken. Displacement, or change in position, is denoted as Δs, where Δ (Greek letter **delta**) denotes change in and s means spatial location or distance. The symbol that resembles the letter p (but is actually the Greek letter **rho**) is not used for position because it's reserved for another quantity: momentum.

In the coordinate axis that we mentioned before, if the displacement is horizontal, then it can be called Δx; if the displacement is vertical, then it's Δy. Since a distance is being measured, the unit for displacement is the meter: $\Delta s = $ m.

Velocity and Speed (Not Starring Keanu Reeves)

When you are in a moving train, subway, or motor vehicle, a speedometer tells the driver (or conductor or Sandra Bullock playing the role of Annie Porter) how fast you are going. In other words, it indicates your speed. But what does it mean to have a specific speed? It means that you are covering a specific distance over a certain period of time. For example, if the speedometer says you are driving at 60 miles per hour, you are covering a distance of 60 miles every 60 minutes (one hour). Or if you are traveling 10 meters per second, you are covering a distance of 10 meters every second.

By definition, the **average speed** is the ratio of the total distance traveled to the time required to cover that distance. Here's that formula:

$$\text{average speed} = \frac{\text{total distance}}{\text{time}}$$

Once again, the speedometer doesn't care in which direction you are traveling (just that the wheels are moving forward). You can be headed north, east, south, or west. We need to include only direction in our descriptions of motion. We already covered displacement (which takes net distance and direction into account), but now let's combine speed and direction. The single concept that embodies both speed and direction is called the velocity. Here's the formula for average velocity:

$$\text{average velocity} = \frac{\text{displacement}}{\text{time}}$$

$$\overline{\mathbf{v}} = \frac{\Delta s}{\Delta t}$$

The bar line above the **v** means average.

Because Δs is a vector, $\overline{\mathbf{v}}$ is also a vector, and because Δt is a positive scalar, the direction of $\overline{\mathbf{v}}$ is the same as the direction of Δs. The magnitude of the velocity vector is called the object's speed, and is expressed in units of meters per second (m/s).

The Distinction Between Speed and Velocity

In everyday language, the terms *speed* and *velocity* are often used interchangeably. However, in physics, speed and velocity are technical terms with two different meanings. Velocity is speed plus direction.

Acceleration

Suppose you speed up to pass a car on the highway, or you begin to hit your breaks and your car slows down quite a bit, or you turn the wheel and go in a different direction. In all three of these scenarios, the velocity changes. To describe a change in velocity, physicists use the word *acceleration*. The same way that velocity measures the rate of change of an object's position, acceleration measures the rate of change in an object's velocity.

Here's the formula for an object's average acceleration:

$$\text{average acceleration} = \frac{\text{change in velocity}}{\text{time}}$$

or

$$\overline{\mathrm{a}} = \frac{\Delta v}{\Delta t}$$

The units of acceleration are meters per second per second: m/s^2.

For example, if a ball is thrown off the top of the Empire State Building, it falls at an acceleration rate of 32 feet per second per second. Because Δv is a vector, $\bar{a}$ is also a vector, and because Δt is a positive scalar, the direction of $\bar{a}$ is the same as the direction of Δv. Furthermore, if we take an object's original direction of motion to be positive, then an increase in speed corresponds to a positive acceleration, while a decrease in speed corresponds to a negative acceleration (deceleration).

Keep this important concept in mind: An object can accelerate even if its speed doesn't change. This is a matter of not allowing common, conversational usage of the word *accelerate* to interfere with its technical, physics usage. Acceleration depends on Δv and the velocity changes if (1) speed changes, (2) the direction changes, or (3) both speed and direction change. An example is a car traveling around in circles, say around a race track. The car is constantly accelerating even if the car's speed is constant, because the direction of the car's velocity vector is constantly changing.

GRAVITY AND FORCE

The value of gravity at Earth's surface (denoted g) is approximately expressed below as the standard average

$$g = 9.81 \text{ m/s}^2 = 32.2 \text{ ft/s}^2 \text{ (32 feet per second per second).}$$

An interaction between two bodies—a push or a pull—is called a **force**. If you lift a book, you exert an upward force (created by your arm muscles) on it. If you pull a rope attached to a huge crate, you create a tension in the rope that pulls the crate. When a sky diver is falling through the air, Earth is exerting a downward pull called **gravitational force** and the air exerts an upward force called **air resistance**.

When you stand on the floor, the floor provides an upward, supporting force called the **normal force**. If you slide a book across a table, the table exerts a **frictional force** against the book so the book slows down and then stops. Static cling provides a directly observable example of **electrostatic force**. Protons and neutrons are held together in the nuclei of atoms by strong nuclear forces and radioactive nuclei decay thru the action of the weak **nuclear forces**.

NEWTON'S LAWS: COLLECT ALL THREE

You need to be familiar with Newton's laws for NSEE test questions. You can remember them easily with the examples we provide.

The First Law

> **Newton's first law** says that an object will continue in its state of motion unless compelled to change by a force impressed upon it.

If an object is at rest, then it will stay at rest, and if it is moving, then it will continue to move at a constant speed in a straight line.

Basically, no force means no change in velocity. This property of objects—their natural resistance to changes in their state of motion—is called **inertia**. In fact, the first law is often referred to as the **law of inertia**.

The Skinny on the First Law

Mass is a measure of inertia; the more mass an object has, the more the object resists changing its velocity. For example, if you hit a bowling ball with a bat, there's not much change in the ball's velocity. But if you hit a baseball with a bat with the same force, there's a bigger change in velocity. Since a bowling ball has more mass, it has more inertia.

The Second Law

Newton's second law predicts what will happen when a force *does* act on an object: The object's velocity will change and it will accelerate. More precisely, it says that its acceleration, **a**, will be directly proportional to the magnitude of the total—or *net*—force ($\mathbf{F}_{net}$) and inversely proportional to the object's mass, *m*.

> $$\mathbf{F}_{net} = m\mathbf{a}$$
>
> This is the most important equation in mechanics!

The mass of an object is directly related to its weight: The heavier an object is, the more mass it has. Two identical boxes, one empty and one full, have different masses. The box that's full has the greater mass, because it contains more stuff; more stuff means more mass. Mass is measured in **kilograms (kg)**. (*Note:* An object whose mass is 1 kg weighs about 2.2 pounds on the surface of Earth, though, as will be discussed later, mass and weight are not the same thing and should not be confused with each other.) It takes twice as much force to produce the same acceleration of a 2 kg object than of a 1 kg object. **Mass** measures an object's inertia—its resistance to acceleration.

The Skinny on the Second Law

Newton's second law defines force. It relates the acceleration that an object of a certain mass experiences when a force is applied to it. The larger the force on the object, the larger its acceleration. It's like the difference between pulling a wagon filled with heavy packages alone and having a friend help you pull. The wagon pulled by your joint force has a greater acceleration.

F_{net} is the sum of all the forces acting on an object. *Beware:* There can be forces acting on an object without causing a net acceleration. This happens when the forces cancel each other out—that is, $F_{net} = 0$ N.

Forces are represented by vectors; they have magnitude and direction. If several different forces act on an object simultaneously, then the **net force**, $\mathbf{F}_{net}$, is the vector sum of all these forces. (The phrase **resultant force** is also used to mean *net force*.)

Since $\mathbf{F}_{net} = m\mathbf{a}$, and m is a *positive* scalar, the direction of $\mathbf{a}$ always matches the direction of $\mathbf{F}_{net}$. Finally, since $F = ma$, the units for F equal the units of m times the units of a.

$$[F] = [m][a]$$
$$= \text{kg·m/s}^2$$

A force of 1 kg·m/s^2 is renamed 1 **newton** (abbreviated N).
A medium-size apple weighs about 1 N.

The relationship between the direction of net force and velocity is the same as the relationship between acceleration and velocity. Forward forces speed up objects, backward forces slow down objects, and forces perpendicular to the velocity are responsible for turning.

speeding up   slowing down   turning

The Third Law

> If object 1 exerts a force on object 2, then object 2 exerts a force back on object 1, equal in strength but in the opposite direction.

Newton's third law was originally stated in the form, "For every action, there is an equal and opposite reaction." Because of this historical phrasing, these two forces, $F_{1\text{-on-}2}$ and $F_{2\text{-on-}1}$, are called an **action/reaction pair**.

The Skinny on the Third Law

Two objects must interact for a force to exist. When both objects interact, each body experiences a force due to the other interacting body. If A and B are the two interacting masses, let F_1 be the force acting on A due to B; F_2 is the force acting on B due to A. F_1 and F_2 are the same magnitude but have opposite directions. $\mathbf{F_1 = -F_2}$.

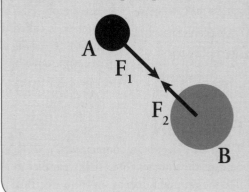

WEIGHT

For your test, remember that although they are used interchangeably in every-day life, mass and weight are not the same thing; there is a clear distinction between them in physics. The **weight** of an object is the gravitational force exerted on it by Earth (or by whatever planet on which it happens to be). Mass, in contrast, is an intrinsic property of an object that measures its inertia: An object's mass does not change with location. If you put a baseball in a rocket and send it to the moon, its weight on the moon would be less than its weight on Earth (because the moon's gravitational pull is weaker than Earth's due to its much smaller mass), but its mass would be the same.

Conversion

In preparing for the nursing exam, you should learn how to convert weight in pounds (lbs) to kilograms (kg). If you are asked to convert lbs to kg, just take that number in lbs and divide it by 2.2 and you will have the correct conversion.

Since weight is a force, we can use $F_{net} = ma$ to compute it. What acceleration would gravitational force impose on an object? The gravitational acceleration, of course! Therefore, setting $a = g$, the equation $F_{net} = ma$ becomes

$$F_w = mg$$

This is the equation for the weight of an object of mass m (weight is often symbolized just by w, rather than F_w). Notice that mass and weight are proportional but not identical. Furthermore, mass is measured in kilograms, while weight is measured in newtons.

Normal Force Notation

The normal force is denoted by F_N, or simply by N. (If you use the latter notation, be careful not to confuse it with N, the abbreviation for the newton.)

THE NORMAL FORCE

When an object is in contact with a surface, the surface exerts a contact force on the object. The component of the contact force that's *perpendicular* to the surface is called the **normal force** on the object. (In physics, the word *normal* means *perpendicular*.) The normal force is what prevents objects from falling through tabletops or you from falling through the floor.

FRICTION

When an object is in contact with a surface, the surface exerts a contact force on the object. The component of the contact force that's parallel to the surface is called the **friction force** on the object. Friction, like the normal force, arises from electrical interactions between atoms that make up the object and those that make up the surface.

We'll look at two main categories of friction: (1) **static friction** and (2) **kinetic (sliding) friction**. If you attempt to push a heavy crate across a floor, at first you meet with resistance, but then you push hard enough to get the crate moving. The force that acted on the crate to cancel out your initial pushes was static friction, and the force that acts on the crate as it slides across the floor is kinetic friction. Static friction occurs when there is no relative motion between the object and the surface (no sliding); kinetic friction occurs when there is relative motion (when there's sliding).

The strength of the friction force depends, in general, on two things: the nature of the surfaces and the strength of the normal force. The nature of the surfaces is represented by the **coefficient of friction**, denoted by μ (*mu*). The greater this number is, the stronger the friction force will be. For example, the coefficient of friction between rubber-soled shoes and a wooden floor is 0.7, but between rubber-soled shoes and ice, it's only 0.1. Also, since kinetic friction is generally weaker than static friction (it's easier to keep an object sliding once it's sliding than it is to start the object sliding in the first place), there are two coefficients of friction: one for static friction (μ_s) and one for kinetic friction (μ_k). For a given pair of surfaces, it's virtually always true that $\mu_k < \mu_s$. The magnitude of these two types of friction forces is given by the following equations:

$$F_{\text{static friction, max}} = \mu_s\, F_N$$
$$F_{\text{kinetic friction}} = \mu_k\, F_N$$

Notice that the equation for the magnitude of the static friction force is for the *maximum* value. This is because static friction can vary, counteracting weaker forces that are less than the minimum force required to move an object. For example, suppose an object feels a normal force of $F_N = 100$ N, and the coefficient of static friction between it and the surface it's on is 0.5. Then, the *maximum* force that static friction can exert is (0.5)(100 N) = 50 N. However, if you push on the object with a force of, say, 20 N, then the static friction force will be 20 N (in the opposite direction), *not* 50 N: The object won't move. The net force on a stationary object must be zero. Static friction can take on all values, up to a certain maximum, and you must overcome the maximum static friction force to get the object to slide.

The direction of $F_{\text{kinetic friction}} = F_{f\,(\text{kinetic})}$ is opposite to that of motion (sliding), and the direction of $F_{\text{static friction}} = F_{f\,(\text{static})}$ is opposite to that of the intended motion.

Kinetic vs. Static

For a person walking, the friction between the person's shoes and the floor is static (no sliding) and is directed forward (in the direction the person is walking). The person pushes on the floor in the backward direction. Static friction prevents it from moving backward, and so therefore must be forward. For similar reasons, objects that are rolling without slipping—rolling normally, not skidding—roll because of static friction.

SIMPLE MACHINES

Simple machines are an important piece in learning about motion and energy. There are six classical simple machines:

1. A **lever** is a rigid object that is used with a **fulcrum** (pivot point) to multiply the mechanical force (**effort**) that can be applied to another object (**load**). This leverage is called **mechanical advantage.** An example of a lever is a teeter-totter.
2. A **wheel and axle** is a modified first-class lever that rotates in a circle around a center point (fulcrum). The larger wheel (or outside wheel) rotates around the smaller wheel (axle). Examples include bicycle wheels, ferris wheels, and gears.
3. A **pulley** is a device that changes the direction of the tension force in the cords that slide over them. These are often seen on ships, where they are called "blocks." We mentioned the Hoyer lift earlier—that is the only type of pulley that you are likely to see in nursing.
4. An **inclined plane** is basically a ramp. If you've ever loaded furniture into and out of a moving truck, you know that placing an inclined plane from the road to the truck bed makes life a lot easier.
5. A **wedge** is a triangular-shaped tool that is really a compound inclined plane. It can be used to separate two objects or portions of an object, lift an object, or hold an object in place. Examples include nails (split and separate the material into which they are driven; the shafts may then hold fast due to friction) and doorstops.
6. A **screw** is a shaft with some type of helical groove or thread formed on its surface. It is basically an inclined plane wrapped around a shaft. Examples include a drill bit, a nut and bolt, and a corkscrew.

A simple machine is a mechanical device that changes the direction or magnitude of force. In general, these simple machines are the building blocks from which more complicated machines are composed. For example, wheels, levers, and pulleys are used together in the mechanism of a bicycle. Simple machines are used to accomplish difficult tasks through manipulating and leveraging small forces.

More on Levers

Earlier we discussed the lever as a type of simple machine. Let's review the three classes for levers.

1. A **first-class lever** is a lever in which the fulcrum is between the applied force and the load. Examples include scissors and a seesaw.
2. A **second-class lever** is a lever in which the load sits between the fulcrum and the force. Examples include a wheelbarrow and a nutracker.
3. A **third-class lever** is a lever in which the effort force (E) is between the fulcrum and the load. An example of a third-class lever is tweezers.

Mechanical advantages reduce the amount of effort on our part. The amount of work done by a person is the same as the amount of work done by the object.

ENERGY

It wasn't until more than one hundred years after Newton's studies that the idea of energy became incorporated into physics. Today it permeates every branch of the subject.

It's difficult to give a precise definition of energy; there are different forms of energy because there are different kinds of forces. The NLN PAX-RN and TEAS focuse on the following forms of energy:

- **Solar energy** is radiant light and heat from the Sun, and it is used along with secondary solar-powered resources such as wind, wave power, and hydroelectricity. One example of solar energy is the use of solar panels to harness energy that can be used even when it's nighttime.
- **Chemical energy** is the interrelation of work and heat with chemical reactions. Natural gas, coal, and petroleum are examples of stored chemical energy.
- **Electrical energy** is associated with conservative Coulomb forces (electrostatic interaction between electrically charged particles). Examples include batteries and lightning.
- **Magnetic energy** and electrical energy are related by Maxwell's equations (the fundamentals of electricity and magnetism). These equations can be combined to show that light is an electromagnetic wave. Magnets align with magnetic fields. One example of magnetic energy in action includes the compass.
- **Nuclear energy** is released by the splitting (**fission**) or merging (**fusion**) of atoms. Examples include nuclear power plants and atomic and hydrogen bombs.
- **Sound energy** is the same thing as sound waves. Sound is a traveling wave that is an oscillation of pressure transmitted through a solid, liquid, or gas. One example is an opera singer hitting a high note and shattering a glass.

- **Energy of light** is also known as **luminous energy.** This is not the same as radiant energy. The human eye can see light only in the visible spectrum and has different sensitivities to light of different wavelengths within the spectrum. Examples include the way in which you process the physical world.
- **Electromagnetic energy** is a phenomenon that takes the form of self-propagating waves in a vacuum or matter. Examples include radio waves, micro waves, X rays, gamma rays, and much more.

All energy can be put into one of two categories:

1. **Potential energy** is energy of position—gravitational energy. Examples include chemical, mechanical, nuclear, gravitational, and electrical energy.
2. **Kinetic energy** is energy of motion—of waves, objects, substances, and molecules. Examples include radiant, thermal, motion, and sound energy.

Energy can come into a system or leave it via various interactions that produce changes. One of the best definitions we know reads as follows:

> Force is the agent of change, energy is the measure of change, and **work** is the way of transferring energy from one system to another.

And one of the most important laws in physics (the **law of conservation of energy,** also known as the **first law of thermodynamics**) says that if you account for all its various forms, the total amount of energy in a given process will stay constant; that is, it will be conserved. For example, electrical energy can be converted into light and heat (this is how a light bulb works), but the amount of electrical energy coming into the light bulb equals the total amount of light and heat given off. Energy cannot be created or destroyed; it can only be transferred (from one system to another) or transformed (from one form to another).

WORK

When you lift a book from the floor, you exert a force on it, over a distance; when you push a crate across a floor, you also exert a force on it, over a distance. The application of force over a distance, and the resulting change in energy of the system that the force acted on, give rise to the concept of work. When you hold a book in your hand, you exert a force on the book (normal force), but since the book is at rest, the force does not act through a distance, so you do no work on the book. Although you did work on the book as you lifted it from the floor, once it's at rest in your hand, you are no longer doing work on it.

> If a force F acts over a distance d, and F is parallel to d, then the work W done by F is the product of force and distance: $W = Fd$.

Notice that, although work depends on two vectors ($\mathbf{F}$ and $\mathbf{d}$), work itself is not a vector. Work is a scalar quanity.

POWER

Simply put, **power** is the rate at which work gets done (or energy gets transferred, which is the same thing). Suppose you and I each do 1,000 J of work, but I do the work in 2 minutes while you do it in 1 minute. We both did the same amount of work, but you did it more quickly; you were more powerful. Here's the definition of power:

$$\text{Power} = \frac{\text{Work}}{\text{time}} \quad \text{(in symbols)} \quad \rightarrow \quad P = \frac{W}{t}$$

The unit of power is the joule per second (J/s), which is renamed the **watt**, and symbolized W (not to be confused with the symbol for work, W). One watt is 1 joule per second: 1 W = 1 J/s.

FORMS OF ENERGY

Heat

Energy can present in the form of **heat**. But **temperature** is best characterized as a measure of the aggregate atomic or molecular activity pertaining to a particular object. Measurements of temperature may be calculated with such devices as thermometers, thermocouples, and optical methods.

When heated to a certain temperature, a mercury or alcohol **thermometer** uses principles of expansion properties. Fluids, when heated, expand or contract to an exact amount, which can then be read by the identifiers on the thermometer.

A **thermocouple** is also a temperature sensor. A small electrical signal is produced by metals that are joined together.

Optical methods may be used for certain solids (such as metals). For example, some metals will begin to glow when heated. Color plays a major role in this with warmer temperatures exhibiting a dull red, which may progress to a yellow/white and at the highest temperatures appear as a blueish white.

Transfer of Heat

Conduction, radiation, and convection are different ways in which the transfer of heat may occur. **Conduction** refers to instances in which heat flows from a hotter object to a cooler one. **Radiation** refers to heat transfer in a vacuum where there is no possibility of conduction. The heat radiates or emits from the heated object into a space area. **Convection** involves the heating and circulation of a substance that changes density when it is heated.

Light Sources

The nursing exams require that you know about light sources including the Sun, light bulbs, and excited atoms. The light given off by the Sun enables photosynthesis (more below and in the biology chapter). We can also produce light, as in light bulbs. The basic idea behind light bulbs is simple. Electricity runs through the filament. Because the filament is so thin, it offers some resistance to the electricity, and this resistance converts electrical energy into heat. The heat is enough to make the filament white hot, and the white part is light. That is how an **incandescent light bulb** works. A fluorescent light bulb works differently. A **fluorescent bulb** has electrodes at both ends of a fluorescent tube, and a gas containing argon and mercury vapor inside the tube. A stream of electrons flows through the gas from one electrode to the other. These electrons bump into the mercury atoms and excite them. As the mercury atoms move from the excited state back to the unexcited state, they give off ultraviolet photons. These photons hit the phosphor that coats the inside of the fluorescent tube. This phosphor creates visible light. Light sources emanate from wavelengths (meaning color). **Polychromatic** refers to a mixture of colors, or a white light source. Single-color sources are known as **monochromatic**.

White light includes the visible spectrum: ROY G. BIV.

ROY G. BIV denotes

> Red
> Orange
> Yellow
> Green
> Blue
> Indigo
> Violet

You know from before that we perceive a red ball as red because the ball absorbs all colors (ROY G. BIV) except for red, and it reradiates (not reflects like a mirror) the color red.

When something is **opaque**, light cannot travel through that item. Therefore, no image or light can be seen through that object (for example, a piece of wood). When something is **translucent**, light travels through that thing, but no clear image can be seen (for example, a foggy shower door). When something is **transparent**, light travels through that item (for example, a window), and clear images can be seen through the item.

Surfaces of materials could be rough, wavy, or smooth. Rough and wavy surfaces cause scattering of light, poor reflection, and poor images. Smooth and parallel surfaces, however, give much clearer images.

In a **convex lens**, the center of the lens is thicker than the edges. Images are reversed with convex lenses. In a **concave lens**, the center of the lens is thinner than the edges. Images in a concave lens disperse the incident parallel rays.

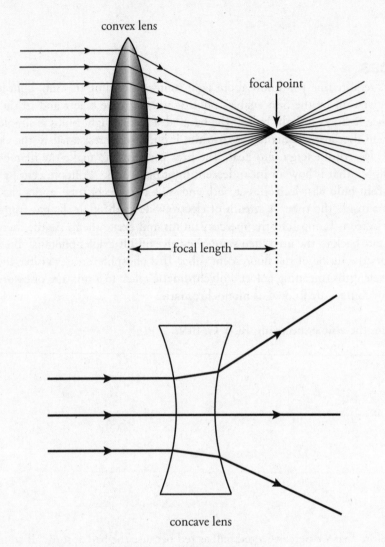

Concave and Convex Lenses

Cataracts

As a nurse, you may hear the medical term *cataracts,* which means clouding or darkening of the lens of the eye, which causes visual abnormality.

Mirror Mirror on the Wall

A **mirror** is an opaque object that reflects light from other objects. There are three types of mirrors: plane, convex, and concave. In **plane mirrors**, the **angle of incidence** equals the **angle of reflection**. A wall mirror is an example of a plane mirror. The smoother the surface of the mirror, the better the reflection. You have probably interacted with concave and concave mirrors and perhaps not realized it. **Concave mirrors** are used in telescopes, and **convex mirrors** are used in supermarkets to see around corners, and in big trucks as side mirrors, for maximum coverage.

Light and Matter Interaction

Vision, photosynthesis, and photoemission are modes of light and matter interaction. **Vision** (light in the visible spectrum) interacts with the human eye, producing electrical signals that the brain is able to read and decipher as color. We perceive color in an object because of the way the object reflects the light reaching it. For example, we see bananas as yellow because bananas absorb all the colors of the spectrum except yellow. **Photosynthesis** is the process by which organisms (plants and bacteria) use energy in the form of light and convert it to chemical form (oxygen and reduced carbon compounds). **Photoemission** refers to the interaction of light with certain types of materials. Electrons are emitted by the lighted material.

Let's try a problem.

Which of the following is an explanation for why we perceive a red apple as red?

A. The apple reflects all the colors of the spectrum except for red, which is absorbed.
B. The apple absorbs all the other colors of the spectrum, but reflects red.
C. The apple reflects green and blue, the other two primary colors, but absorbs red.
D. The apple absorbs green, blue, and red.

Here's How to Crack It

Primary colors have nothing to do with anything here, so immediately scratch out choice C. Choice A gets the information that we know about light and color backward. We see color because that color is reflected back to us, not absorbed. So you can eliminate choice A. Choice B gets the information right exactly—this is the correct answer. Choices C and D maintain that we see colors that are absorbed by the object, rather than reflected by the object, so cross them off.

Waves

Waves are designated as transverse or longitudinal. A **transverse wave** has a wave disturbance, or **amplitude,** perpendicular or transverse to the direction of propagation. However, in a **longitudinal wave**, wave disturbances are parallel to the direction of propagation. One way to think about a wave's energy is simply a disturbance traveling through a medium at speeds that depend on the medium.

Waves are reflected or refracted. **Reflection** occurs when all or part of a wave bounces off a surface and is redirected to another surface. **Refraction** refers to a wave's penetration of a surface.

Frequency is one way to measure sound waves. The frequency is the number of complete cycles of a sound wave within one second. One cycle per second is called **1 hertz**. Human ears can detect sounds from about 20 hertz (the lowest sound) to about 20,000 hertz (the highest sound). Below 20 hertz, humans feel only the vibration of the sound. Above 20,000 hertz, they can't hear the sound at all (but dogs can!). All sound travels at the same speed, regardless of frequency.

MAGNETS

The NLN PAX-RN and TEAS will likely have a few questions about magnetic properties, so let's do a quick review of magnets.

A **magnet** is a material or object that produces a magnetic field. This magnetic field is a force that pulls or repels other magnets, depending on their magnetism. A magnet pulls unlike charges and repels like charges. In short, opposites attract. The magnetic force surrounding a magnet isn't uniform. Each end of a magnet has a great concentration of force, while the center of a magnet has a weak magnetic force. The two ends of a magnet are called the **poles**, much like the poles on Earth.

A **compass** works because its needle is a freely rotating magnet. The painted end, or **needle**, of a compass is drawn to the north (magnetic) pole of Earth to align itself in a northerly direction. It seems confusing, but the needle labeled "N" in a compass is actually a magnet of the opposite charge (S)—it is drawn to north because opposites attract. The area to which the needle points is called the **north magnetic pole**, which is close to the geographic North Pole (but not the exact same place).

Let's tackle a magnetism question of the type you may encounter on the NLN PAX-RN or TEAS.

Magnets are often made of polarized metal bars, especially bars made of iron. Magnets are attracted only to certain types of metal. Typically, metals that make good magnets are also attracted to magnets. Based on this information, which of the following is a magnet most likely attracted to?

A. Copper penny
B. Aluminum can
C. Plastic wrap
D. Iron filings

Here's How to Crack It

Choice C is obviously wrong—plastic is not magnetic, even in the best of science fiction movies. The passage states that magnets are often made of iron and also that the materials used to make magnets are also attracted to magnets. Thus, it can be inferred that magnets and iron attract. Therefore, choice D is correct.

Let's try another practice question.

Which of the following waves can be used for breaking down kidney stones into smaller parts in order to be removed?

A. Gamma rays
B. Infrared radiation
C. Radio waves
D. Ultrasonic waves

Here's How to Crack It

We know the correct answer is not choice A because gamma rays are electromagnetic radiation of high frequency. This is a form of ionizing radiation that, if absorbed by living tissue, can pose a serious health risk. Therefore, the risk of radiation never outweighs the need for breaking down a kidney stone, so choice A is wrong. Gamma radiation or gamma knife surgery is utilized in a process to remove certain tumors or blood clots from the brain. Infrared light is benign, electromagnetic radiation with a long wave length that includes the thermal radiation emitted by objects near room temperature. It has no breakdown capability, so choice B is incorrect. Choice C is not correct because radio waves are electromagnetic waves that use radio frequency waves to generate images of the human body, but they don't break down anything. Ultrasonic waves are cyclic sound pressure waves that are widely used in the medical field. An ultrasound reveals characteristics of a baby in the womb of his or her mother. With regard to kidney stones, the medical term is extracorporeal shock wave lithotripsy (ESWL), which is a common treatment for kidney stones. This treatment uses shock waves outside the body to pass through the skin and break down the stones into smaller pieces that can more easily be eliminated. Again, choice D is correct.

Magnets in Health Care

Magnetic resonance imaging (MRI) is a procedure that uses a large magnet for creating images. The procedure is used in hospitals and out-patient imaging centers. It is a costly test, but well worth the price. The MRI functions to perform a diagnostic test by using a magnetic field and pulses of radio wave energy that create images of various organs and structures inside the human body. This test does not emit any radiation, unlike the CT scan. It is a safe test and can be performed on pregnant woman. MRIs are not fast scans and they are very sensitive to motion. Therefore, the patient must remain completely still. In younger patients, sedation may be required in order to obtain an accurate study. Contraindications would include patients with pacemakers, body piercings, internal defibrillator devices, certain endovascular meshes, and intrathecal pump devices, just to name a few.

BATTERIES AND CURRENTS

Double A (AA) batteries are cells used in objects such as toys and cameras. They are most often placed in these electronic devices in opposite directions—that is, the positive end opposes the negative end of the cells. The end with the bump is positive, and the flatter end is always negative. The appliance that the batteries go into is called the **resistor**, in which all of the resistance of the system is concentrated. Resistors are represented by the following symbol:

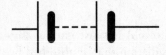

Batteries are denoted by the following symbol:

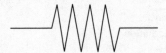

In the preceding symbol, the longer line represents the positive (higher potential) terminal, and the shorter line represents the negative (lower potential) terminal.

A series of connected cells (positive-negative-positive-negative-positive-negative) is called a **battery**. Each cell is about 1.5 volts. The direction of flow for batteries is negative to positive. That is, electrons always travel from the negative pole to the positive pole.

Metal wires (such as copper) are good conductors of electricity. Some materials make better wires than others because they offer less resistance. The longer the wire, the greater the resistance and vice versa. Today, computer manufacturers want to make circuits shorter so that the electric current (electron movement) has a shorter distance to travel, enabling the computers to function more quickly.

Nothing moves unless there is something moving it. With that, electrons are moved along depending upon the voltage (pushing power).

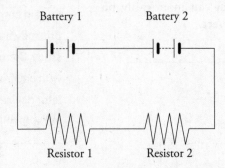

When lights are on (illuminating a room), the circuit is closed, so that the electrons can flow. When a light switch is turned off, the circuit is open, so that electrons don't flow.

SUMMARY

- Scientific notation is used to more easily write very small or very large numbers.

- Right triangles have special functions called trig functions. Three of those functions are sine, cosine, and tangent.

- The Pythagorean theorem for triangles is $a^2 + b^2 = c^2$ for right triangles with legs a and b and a hypotenuse c.

- A vector is a quantity that involves magnitude and direction and is written $A, A, \overline{A}, \overline{A}$.

- Displacement is the prototypical example of a vector.

- Motion is any physical movement or change in position. It is characterized by position, displacement, speed, velocity, and acceleration.

- Average speed = $\dfrac{\text{total distance}}{\text{time}}$.

- Average velocity = $\dfrac{\text{displacement}}{\text{time}}$.

- Average acceleration = $\dfrac{\text{change in velocity}}{\text{time}}$. The units of acceleration are m/s^2.

- Gravity (g) = 9.81 m/s^2 = 32.2 ft/s^2.

- Newton's first law says that an object will continue in its state of motion unless compelled to change by a force impressed upon it.

- Newton's second law predicts what will happen when a force does not act on an object: The object's velocity will change and it will accelerate.

- Newton's third law states that if object 1 exerts a force on object 2, then object 2 exerts a force back on object 1, equal in strength but opposite in direction.

- Weight = gravitational force exerted on an object by Earth.

- Mass = intrinsic property that measures the inertia of an item.

- Two main categories of friction are static friction and kinetic (sliding) friction.

- Simple machines are the lever, wheel and axle, pulley, inclined plane, wedge, and screw.

- Types of energy include solar, chemical, magnetic, nuclear, electrical, sound, luminous, and electromagnetic.

- Work: When a force **F** acts over distance d and **F** is parallel to d, then $W = Fd$.

- Power is the rate at which work gets done. Power $= \dfrac{\text{work}}{\text{time}}$ or $P = \dfrac{W}{t}$ in which the unit of power is the joule per second [J/s], or watt [W].

- Energy can present in the form of heat. Heat can be transferred via conduction, radiation, and convection.

- Light sources include the Sun, lightbulbs, and excited atoms.

- The visible light spectrum is designated as ROY G. BIV.

- A mirror is an opaque object that reflects light from other objects. Three types of mirrors are plane mirrors, convex mirrors, and concave mirrors.

- Waves are transverse or longitudinal.

- Sound waves are measured in hertz [1 cycle/second = 1 hertz].

- A magnet is a material or object that produces a magnetic field. Opposite ends of a magnet attract.

- A series of connected cells is a battery.

KEY TERMS

Hoyer lift

scientific notation

trig functions

sine

cosine

tangent

Pythagorean theorem

hypotenuse

legs

vector

commutative law for addition

scalar

displacement

position

displacement

speed

velocity

acceleration

Δt

Δs

delta

rho

average speed

force

gravitational force

air resistance

normal force

frictional force

electrostatic force

nuclear force

Newton's first law (law of inertia)

inertia

Newton's second law

kilograms (kg)

mass

net force (resultant force)

newton (N)

Newton's third law

action/reaction pair

weight

normal force

friction force

static friction

kinetic (sliding) friction

coefficient of friction

simple machines

lever

fulcrum

effort

load

mechanical advantage

wheel and axle

pulley

inclined plane

wedge

screw

first-class lever

second-class lever

third-class lever

solar energy

chemical energy

electrical energy

magnetic energy

nuclear energy

fission

fusion

sound energy

energy of light (luminous energy)

electromagnetic energy

potential energy

kinetic energy

work (W)

law of conservation of energy (first law of
    thermodynamics)

power

watt (W)

heat

temperature

thermometer

thermocouple

optical methods

conduction

radiation

convection

incandescent light bulb

fluorescent bulb

polychromatic

monochromatic

opaque

translucent

transparent

convex lens

concave lens
cataracts
mirror
plane mirrors
angle of incidence
angle of reflection
concave mirrors
convex mirrors
vison
photosynthesis
photoemission
transverse wave
amplitude

longitudinal wave
reflection
refraction
frequency
hertz
magnet
poles
compass
needle
north magnetic pole
magnetic resonance imaging (MRI)
resistor
battery

Chapter 7
Chemistry

INTRODUCTION TO CHEMISTRY

Chemistry, chemicals, and chemical reactions play an important role in life and life cycles. Especially for those of you who are seriously considering the path to an exciting nursing career, chemistry will be your friend for quite a long time. The NLN PAX-RN and the TEAS have a section of chemistry questions, but the NET has no chemistry at all.

Chemistry (inorganic and organic) is neat because you can learn to make something as simple as toothpaste or write something that appears complicated such as a mass composition conversion into an empirical formula. Don't worry, though. You already learned how to convert glucose into energy from biology review. When you take your first pharmacology class, you will see how elements come together to form compounds and how compounds are made into the very medications that will be administered to your patients on a daily basis. Let's dive in.

MATTER

Objects (things, stuff) that take up space and have mass (weight) are known as **matter**. Matter is made up of **elements**, which are substances that cannot be broken down into simpler substances by chemical means. Everything in the physical world is made up of microscopic matter comprised of **atoms** or **molecules**.

Matter has physical, thermal, electrical, and chemical properties. These specific properties include **color** (the human eye response to light as reflected by matter), **density** (the amount of mass contained in a given substance), **hardness** (the resistance to penetration by a given substance), and **conductivity** (the ability to transmit heat or current).

In **homogeneous matter**, the properties are the same throughout. Coal and glass are examples of homogeneous matter.

In **heterogeneous matter**, the properties may vary in their make-up. Concrete and soil are examples of heterogeneous matter.

Subatomic Particles

If you break down a substance into smaller pieces, you eventually come to the atom—the tiniest unit of an element that retains its characteristic properties. Atoms are the building blocks of the physical world. Within atoms are smaller subatomic particles called **protons**, **neutrons**, and **electrons**.

Here's an illustration of a typical atom:

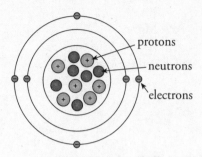

Make-up of an Atom

Protons and neutrons are particles that are packed together in the core of an atom called the **nucleus**. Protons are positively charged particles (+), and neutrons are uncharged particles, which renders them neutral. Electrons are negatively charged particles (–) that orbit the outside of the nucleus. They are in constant motion. Electrons are quite small compared to protons and neutrons. In an electrically neutral atom, the number of electrons is equal to the number of protons: The charges inside and outside the nucleus are balanced.

An example of an electrically neutral atom is hydrogen, which is written as ^{1}H. This atom contains 1 proton and 1 electron, so you may see it written as

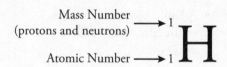

Some atoms have the same number of protons but differ in the number of neutrons in the nucleus. These atoms are called **isotopes**. An example of an isotope is tritium, which has 1 proton, 2 neutrons, and 1 electron. You could see tritium written as ^{3}T or as

Mass Number
(protons and neutrons) $\longrightarrow$ 3
Atomic Number $\longrightarrow$ 1 T

If an atom loses or gains one or more electrons, the number of electrons outside the nucleus is not equal to the number of protons on the inside. Therefore, the atom is not electronically neutral any longer. It has become an **ion**. Na$^+$ (sodium) and Cl$^-$ (chlorine) are examples of ions.

If an atom loses one or more electrons, it has fewer negative charges than positive charges, so it is then a positively charged ion, or **cation**. If the atom gains one or more electrons, it has more negative charges than it does positive. In such a case, it is called an **anion**.

Examples of cations include $(NH_4)^{+1}$, Fe^{+2}, Mg^{+2}.

An example of an anion is $(NO_3)^{-1}$, which is the nitrate ion.

PHYSICAL PROPERTIES OF MATTER

Solids, **liquids**, and **gases** are made up of atoms, molecules, and/or ions, but the behaviors of these particles differ in the three phases.

- In the gas phase, matter has neither definite shape nor definite volume.
- In the liquid phase, matter has a definite volume but an indefinite shape. Liquids take the shape of their containers.
- In the solid phase, matter has both definite shape and definite volume.

Liquids and solids are often referred to as **condensed phases** because the particles are very close together.

Characteristics of Gases, Liquids and Solids		
Properties of a Gas	Properties of a Liquid	Properties of a Solid
• A gas assumes the shape and volume of a closed container. • Gas particles are separated with no regular arrangement, no shape, or volume. • Gas particles vibrate and rotate, and they move freely at high speeds. • Gas particles are compressible, due to the distance between molecules. • Gas flows easily because particles can move past one another.	• A liquid assumes the shape of the container which it occupies. • Liquid particles are close together with no regular arrangement; they have definite volume, but not a definite shape. • Liquid particles are not easily compressible because there is little free space between particles. • Liquid particles flow easily because particles can move/slide past one another.	• A solid retains a definite or fixed volume and shape. • A solid is tightly packed, usually in a regular pattern. A solid is rigid—particles are locked into place. Therefore, it has a definite geometric pattern, crystalline structure. • Solids can vibrate (jiggle) but generally do not move from place to place. • Solids are not easily compressible because there is little free space between particles. • A solid does not flow, because particles cannot move/slide past one another.

Changing Phases

Change of phase occurs because of a change in the potential energy level of molecules. This phase change also occurs at a specific temperature for each substance. Before reading more about phase changes, let's review two important things:

Energy!
Energy is measured in joules and calories.
1 calorie = 4.1856 joules.

1. Heat is a form of energy.
2. Temperature measures the average kinetic energy of particles in a particular system.

With temperature increase or decrease and change in pressure, matter can undergo phase changes. Matter can undergo both physical changes and chemical changes.

Physical changes are changes in state (phase) or form. As temperature is increased under conditions of constant pressure, a substance will move from the solid phase to the liquid phase. As temperature is further increased, the substance will move from the liquid phase to the gas phase. The change in phase that occurs when a solid becomes a liquid is called **melting**. The opposite of melting is **freezing**, or **solidification**. When a liquid becomes a gas, this process is **boiling**, or **vaporization**.

The evaporation of water is an example of a physical change. During vaporization (also called evaporation), water changes from a liquid to a vapor (gas). **Sublimation** occurs when a solid changes directly to a gas without first becoming a liquid. For example, when CO_2, or dry ice, is placed in water, it sublimates to form gas bubbles which show up as smokey fog. **Vapor pressure** is the amount of pressure exerted by the escaping vapor. **Condensation** is the change that occurs when a vapor changes to a liquid. An example of condensation is the formation of water droplets on the outside of a glass of ice water on a humid day.

Interesting points
- Melting and freezing occur at the same temperature.

For example, an ice cube of water will melt at 0 degrees Celsius (32 degrees F). Water will also freeze at 0 degrees Celsius (32 degrees F). The phase change depends on whether temperature is going up or down.

Since energy is always conserved (as we know from Newton), the transition from a phase that contains more energy to a phase that contains less energy must involve the release of energy in the form of heat. These reactions are said to be **exothermic**. Condensation and freezing are exothermic processes. Conversely, a transition from a phase that contains less energy to a phase that contains more energy requires the input of energy in order to take place. These reactions are said to be **endothermic**. Melting, vaporization, and sublimation are all endothermic processes.

The temperature at which the vapor pressure is equal to the atmospheric pressure is called the **boiling point**. The boiling point of water at standard pressure is 100 degrees Celsius (100° C). Temperature is measured in Celsius degrees and Kelvin. To convert Celsius to Kelvin, simply add 273. So if a liquid is 44 degrees Celsius, its equivalent in Kelvin is 44 + 273 = 317 K. To convert Kelvin to Celsius, simply subtract 273. For example, if an item is 354 K, its equivalent in Celsius is 354 − 273 = 81 degrees Celsius.

Ripping open a wrapped gift or shredding a paper document is a physical change. Water freezing and becoming ice is a physical change. Water boiling is a physical change. Crushing a rock is a physical change. Crushing ice cubes to make a snow cone is a physical change.

However, when you sautée sugar in a frying pan and the sugar caramelizes due to the heat, a chemical change occurs. A **chemical change** occurs when bonds are broken and new bonds are formed between different atoms. A change that results in a product that is different from the original substance in both properties and composition is a chemical change. Examples of chemical changes included metal rusting, photosynthesis in plants, and baking a cake.

OTHER PROPERTIES OF MATTER

Thermal Properties of Matter

When heat energy is added to a solid, the temperature of the solid increases up to the melting point of the substance. At the melting point, the temperature stays the same as the substance melts. When all is melted and heat is continued to be added, the temperature will begin to rise to its boiling point. At this time, the temperature will stay the same until the liquid is evaporated into a gaseous state. This process is called the **heating curve**.

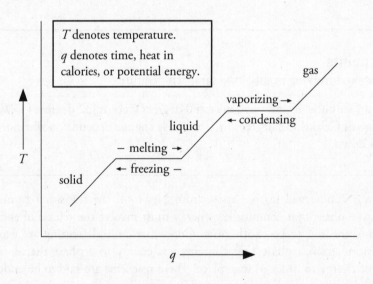

Heating-Cooling Curve

The reverse progression occurs when cooling occurs and a substance changes from a gas to a liquid to a solid.

Electrical Properties of Matter

Matter can be either a **conductor** or a **nonconductor** (very poor conductor). Conductors have a high number of free electrons, while nonconductors do not. Examples of conductors include copper, aluminum, silver, gold, and tap water. Examples of nonconductors include wood, cloth, glass, rubber, and plastic. Nonconductors are also known as insulators.

And There's More

Here are some additional properties of matter that you should review.

- **Density** is the mass (weight) per unit volume of any substance.
- **Specific gravity** is the density of a specific unit of substance compared to an equal volume of water.
- **Solubility** is the ability to dissolve in a solvent (for example, salt is able to dissolve in water).
- **Luster** refers to the shine of a substance.
- **Malleability** is the ability to bend and be shaped into other shapes.
- **Ductility** refers to the ability to be drawn into rods and wires.
- **Tenacity** is the ability to resist being pulled apart.
- **Brittleness** refers to the ability to shatter when struck.
- **Conductivity** is the ability to transfer heat or electricity.

The concept of specific gravity will be important in your nursing career because assessing a person's hydration status may include dipping the urine for the specific gravity. A person who is not well hydrated has dark yellow-orange urine. This individual may have a specific gravity of 1.030. A person who is well hydrated has very clear or pale yellow urine. This person may have a specific gravity of 1.010.

CLASSES OF MATTER

All matter is classified as either **metal, nonmetal, metalloid,** or **noble gas (inert gas)**. All of these elements are found on the periodic table.

Metals
- are ductile
- conduct heat and electricity
- have luster
- are solids (except mercury, which is a liquid at room temperature)
- have a tendency to shed electrons
- form cations and ionic bonds with nonmetals

Examples of metals include iron (Fe), copper (Cu), and sodium (Na).

> Gold, silver, and platinum are considered precious metals because they are rare metallic elements that have a high economic value. It's no wonder that these precious metals are used in long-lasting jewelry such as wedding bands.

Nonmetals
- can be gases or brittle solids while at room temperature
- are *not* ductile or malleable (except bromine, which is a liquid at room temperature)
- do not conduct electricity
- do not have luster
- have a tendency to snag or hog electrons
- have low melting points

Examples of nonmetals include carbon (C), oxygen (O_2), and nitrogen (N_2).

Metalloids have both metal and nonmetal characteristics and may gain or lose electrons. An example of a metalloid is boron (B).

Noble gases are referred to as inert gases because they hardly react with each other or other elements under normal laboratory conditions (meaning temperatures and pressures). They are mono-atomic or single atoms. Examples of noble gases include helium (He) and krypton (Kr).

Which of the followings statements about mercury is true?

A. Mercury is liquid at room temperature.
B. Mercury is the most volatile liquid.
C. Mercury has the lowest electrical conductivity among all metals.
D. Mercury is readily soluble in water.

Here's How to Crack It

You probably know from using a thermometer that choice A is correct—mercury is liquid at room temperature. Choice B is incorrect because mercury is a liquid metal and does not evaporate easily. Therefore, it isn't volatile. Mercury is a good conductor of electricity, so choice C is wrong. If you have ever seen a broken thermometer, you know that mercury beads and is not soluble in water, so eliminate choice D as well.

THE PERIODIC TABLE

The **periodic table** is a visual method of organizing and classifying elements. Elements are classified by their similar and dissimilar properties. The location of a substance on the periodic table determines how it reacts to other substances. Each element is represented by its one- or two-letter chemical symbol and is arranged according to increasing atomic number (the number of protons found in the nucleus of the atom). Below the symbol for each element is its **atomic number**, which gives a numeric value to its number of protons. Above the symbol for each element is its **atomic weight**, or **atomic mass** (found in the upper, left corner). As you move from left to right within a horizontal row, the atoms get smaller.

The horizontal rows of the periodic table are known as **periods**, **rows**, or **series**. The vertical columns are called **groups**, or **families**. Elements in the same period have the same number of electron energy shells. Generally, the larger the atom of a metal, the less firmly it holds its valence electrons, which means that larger metal atoms are more active and more likely to enter into reactions with other atoms. Elements in the same group have the same valence configuration and similar chemical properties. You need not memorize the table for your nursing exam. Just be familiar with how to use it and how it's organized. You may be surprised at how much chemistry is in the home and kitchen too.

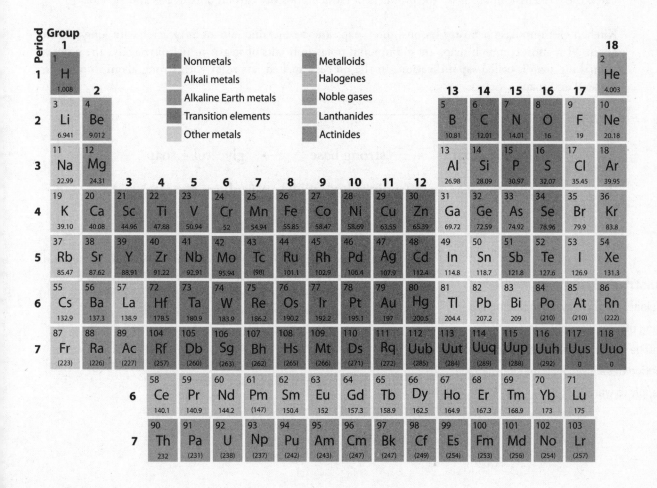

Periodic Table

CHEMISTRY AT HOME

Sodium benzoate is a chemical used to preserve food. It is often found in canned goods. **Monosodium glutamate (MSG)** also acts as a food preservative and a food flavor enhancer. Unfortunately, many people are sensitive or even allergic to MSG and don't even realize it.

Earlier in the biology chapter, we reviewed carbohydrates, simple and complex sugars, starches, proteins, amino acids, lipids, and fatty acids. Remember that the structure of the food and its nutrients can be changed by hydrolysis, oxidation, or coagulation. All of these processes assist in the breakdown of food into smaller more absorbable products for cell life and homeostasis.

Here are some examples of chemistry that you'll find in the kitchen. If you heat up a starch, it will absorb great quantities of liquid. Once it is cooled, a gel is formed. An example of that process is Jell-O. Sodium bicarbonate (baking soda) reacts with acids, such as vinegar or even lactic acid found in sour milk, to form carbon dioxide gas. Baking powder contains sodium bicarbonate and an acid or an acid salt. When water is added, the acid reacts with the baking soda and forms carbon dioxide gas. Steam is used to leaven sponge cake and cream puffs. The gluten chains formed by a large number of egg whites plus the gluten found in flour trap the steam upon heating and the product is leavened. Yeast produces enzymes that cause the fermentation of sugar. The products of fermentation are carbon dioxide gas and alcohol.

Kitchen clean-up has chemistry lessons, too. Soaps are the metallic salts of fatty acids with long carbon chains. The most common soaps are sodium and potassium salts of stearic or palmitic acids. The process of making soap is called **saponification**. In the process, melted fats react with strong alkali to produce glycerol and soap.

$$\text{melted fat} \quad + \quad \text{strong base} \quad \rightarrow \quad \text{glycerol + soap}$$

$$\text{(glycerol stearate)} + \text{(sodium hydroxide)} \rightarrow \text{(sodium stearate)}$$

Chemistry and Home Remedies

Apple cider vinegar may aid in ridding the annoying plantar wart phenomena. Its strength is similar to the prescription application of salicylic acid that dermatologists apply to warts!

Detergents are the sodium salts of long-chain alkyl sulfates. Disinfectants are substances that destroy the cell structure directly oxidizing the disease-causing agent (**pathogen**) or by interfering with the enzymes' reactions essential for the organisms existence.

Chlorine, in the presence of a strong soap such as ammonia or an acid such as vinegar, forms green and fatally toxic chlorine gas. That's why one should never mix cleaning agents.

WHEN THEIR POWERS COMBINE

Compounds

If two or more elements are combined in a fixed ratio, they form a chemical **compound**. Examples of a chemical compound are $KCLO_3$ (potassium chlorate) and CH_4 (methane, or natural gas). Compounds can be broken down by chemical means. An **empirical formula** is the simplest whole number ratio of atoms of each element present in a compound. If you have a compound and you wish to calculate how much of one element is found in the compound (called the **percent composition**), simply add the masses of each element in the compound and divide that number by the molecular mass of the entire molecule. Finally, multiply by 100.

Speaking of math, you should be familiar with a **mole**—not the kind on your skin, but rather the mole that is a unit of measurement used in chemistry to express amounts of a chemical substance (number of particles). A mole is the quantity of anything that has the same number of particles found in 12.000 grams of carbon-12, which is equal to about 6.02×10^{23} particles of that substance (we say particles because they can be ions, electrons, atoms, or molecules). That number of particles is called **Avogadro's number** (roughly 6.02×10^{23}). A mole of carbon atoms is 6.02×10^{23} carbon atoms. Used entertainingly, a mole of nurses is 6.02×10^{23} nurses (there are not that many human beings, but it would certainly prevent any nursing shortages for the next several decades). It's much easier to write the word *mole* than to write out 6.02×10^{23} anytime you want to refer to a large quantity of things.

The mole is used in chemistry to express the amounts of reagents and products of chemical reactions. For example, the chemical equation $2\,H_2 + O_2 \rightarrow 2\,H_2O$ shows that 2 mol of hydrogen molecules and 1 mol of oxygen molecules react to form 2 mol of water.

Bonding

Atoms combine when their valence shells are incomplete. By gaining, losing, or even sharing electrons, the atoms can achieve a complete outermost or valence shell.

Atoms of a compound are held together by chemical bonds. You may recall from the biology review that bonds can be ionic or covalent. **Ionic bonds** are formed between atoms when one or more electrons are transferred from one atom to the other. With this type of reaction, one atom loses electrons and becomes positively charged while the other atom gains electrons and becomes negatively charged. The charged forms of the atoms are called ions—hence, the ionic bond. An example of an ionic bond is table salt, NaCl. All ionic bonds are polar.

Covalent bonds are formed when electrons are shared between atoms. If the electrons are shared equally between the atoms, the bond is called **nonpolar covalent**. An example of a nonpolar covalent bond is good 'ole oxygen, O_2. If the electrons are shared unequally, the bond is called **polar covalent**. When two pairs of electrons are shared, the result is a **double covalent bond**. When three pairs of electrons are shared, the result is a **triple covalent bond**.

As you know from Chapter 4, a hydrogen bond is technically a third kind of bond that occurs when a hydrogen atom weakly interacts with a nearby hydrogen atom that is already part of a covalent bond. The hydrogen atoms in a cup of water are an example of hydrogen bonds.

Organic and Inorganic Compounds

Organic compounds (compounds that contain carbon) are important to know because all living things on Earth are made up of carbon (in addition to a few other elements). Each carbon atom can form up to four bonds with other atoms; this ability enables carbon to form long chains with itself and with certain other atoms, which is what makes it such an important biomolecule. Organic molecules almost always contain nonpolar covalent bonds. Here are some other properties of organic compounds that you should know:

- Organic compounds are much more soluble in nonpolar solvents than in polar solvents. *Remember:* Like dissolves like, so since carbon compounds are generally nonpolar, they will be soluble in nonpolar solvents. That means that organic substances are not very soluble in water, which is a highly polar solvent.
- Organic compounds don't dissociate in solution; since organic compounds do not contain ionic bonds, they will not dissociate into ions. Therefore, organic solutions are poor conductors of electricity, and organic compounds do not behave as electrolytes in solution.

When you think of inorganic compounds, think of fake things like silicon or plastic. An **inorganic compound** is any substance in which two or more chemical elements other than carbon are combined. This combination is almost always in definite proportions and can involve some compounds containing carbon but lacking carbon-carbon bonds.

The simplest organic compounds are **hydrocarbons** (compounds that contain only carbon and hydrogen). Hydrocarbons can be grouped into three categories:

1. **Alkanes**, which contain only single carbon-carbon bonds
2. **Alkenes**, which contain carbon-carbon double bonds
3. **Alkynes**, which contain carbon-carbon triple bonds

Let's take a look at some alkanes, alkenes, and alkynes.

Ethane and propane are examples of alkanes.

Ethane   Propane

Ethene and propene are examples of alkenes.

Ethene   **Propene**

Ethyne and propyne are examples of alkynes.

Ethyne   **Propyne**

Mixtures

A **mixture** is a combination of substances that are mixed together but are not combined chemically. Mixtures have at least two components that vary in property and composition, they can be separated by physical means, and they retain their properties when separated. Mixtures, just like matter, can be homogeneous or heterogeneous.

Mixtures are divided into **suspensions**, **solutions**, and **colloidal suspensions**. Suspensions are cloudy combinations of a solid and liquid, such as sand and water. Solutions consist of **solute** (the substance of which there is less) and **solvent** (the substance of which there is more). **Tinctures** are solutions in which the solvent is a mixture of alcohol and water. Tincture of iodine is still used today in some practices. Colloidal suspensions are made up of **dispersed substances** (insoluble particles) and a **dispersing medium** (the medium containing the substance). They can be solid, liquid, or gas. Examples of a colloidal suspension are homogenized milk, whipped cream, and mayonnaise. In nursing, certain blood products and IV fluids are considered colloids, also known as **volume expanders**. They are often utilized during resuscitation efforts, especially when the patient has experienced trauma or excessive blood loss in the operating room.

ACIDS AND BASES

Acids are compounds in which hydrogen acts as a metal. An example is sulfuric acid (H_2SO_4). Here is a run-down of the properties that you should know for acids.

- Acids release hydrogen ions (H^+) in solution.
- Acids are sour tasting.
- Acids neutralize bases to form water and salt.
- Acids turn litmus paper pink-red.
- All acids react with carbonates to yield CO_2 gas.

Bases are compounds in which the hydroxide radical (OH^-) acts as a nonmetallic radical. An example is potassium hydroxide (KOH). Here is a run-down of the properties of bases that you should know.

- Bases are bitter tasting and caustic.
- Bases neutralize acids to form water and salt.
- Bases emulsify fats and oils.
- Bases turn litmus paper blue.
- Bases are slippery (soap), which makes for easy slippage in the bathtub or freshly-cleaned floors.

Salts form when acids and bases react together in a neutralization reaction. Salts include compounds that have any element except hydrogen and any ion except hydroxide.

acid + base = salt + water

Buffers are solutions of weak acid/base conjugate pairs that resist changes in pH when other acids or bases are added to it.

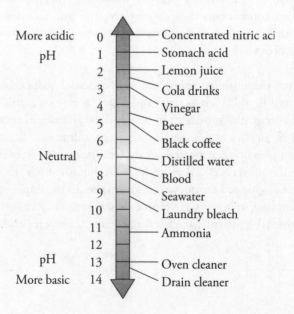

pH Scale

CHEMISTRY AND THERMODYNAMICS

Thermodynamics is the area of chemistry that deals with energy relationships. We touched on this earlier when we discussed phase changes and exothermic versus endothermic reactions. One of the most important things to know about thermodynamics is that low-energy states are more stable than high-energy states. Fundamentally, the universe prefers low-energy states and tends toward disorder. When we talk about disorder, we use the term **entropy**, which is symbolized by S. Everything tends toward maximum entropy and the greater the disorder in or randomness in a system, the larger the entropy. The entropy of a substance always increases as it changes state from solid to liquid to gas. When we talk about a chemical reaction and the difference between entropy of the products and entropy of the reactants, we use the symbol ΔS. If ΔS is negative, the reaction has lost entropy; the products are more orderly than the reactants. If ΔS is positive, the reaction has gained entropy; the products are less orderly than the reactants. When you see the word *entropy*, think "disorder" and just remember

$$\text{higher entropy} + \text{lower energy} \rightarrow \text{more stability}$$

$$\text{lower entropy} + \text{higher energy} \rightarrow \text{less stability}$$

Because the universe tends toward low energy, chemical reactions that release energy are favored in the universe. When we talk about the energy states of reactants or products, we use the term **enthalpy**, which is symbolized by H. High enthalpy means high-energy state, and low enthalpy means low-energy state. So, the universe likes reactions in which enthalpy decreases—reactions in which ΔH (the change in enthalpy that occurs in the course of a reaction) is negative. As we mentioned before, these reactions are said to be exothermic, and they result in the release of energy in the form of heat. If, however, the enthalpy of the products is greater than the enthalpy of the reactants, then ΔH is positive and the reaction is said to be endothermic. Endothermic reactions require the input of energy in order to take place. In layman's terms, here are the basic rules of enthalpy that you might need to know for your nursing exam:

- When bonds are formed, energy is released.
- When bonds are broken, energy is absorbed.

An example of enthalpy is a closed container of helium, which has low entropy and is considered fairly ordered. When you remove the cork, helium expands into the air where it has less entropy and more randomness.

All substances have a tendency to be in the lowest possible energy state with higher energy, which gives them the greatest stability. Therefore, in general, exothermic processes are more likely to occur spontaneously than endothermic processes.

> **Helpful Memorization Trick**
> When in doubt, remember that EnthAlpy **adds** a bit of heat and **Ent**ropy is open (like an entrance) to randomness. (ENTer the room of madness.)

SUMMARY

- Everything in the world is made up of matter comprised of atoms or molecules.

- Atoms contain protons, neutrons, and electrons.

- Matter can be a solid, liquid, or gas.

- Phase change occurs when there is a change in temperature or pressure.

- All matter is classified as either metal, metalloid, or noble gas.

- Energy is measured in joules and calories. 1 calorie = a bit more than 4 joules.

- The periodic table is a useful tool for organizing all elements.

- Every element has an atomic number, which is the number of protons in an atom of the element. This number defines the element within the periodic table.

- The rows of the periodic table are called periods; the columns are called groups.

- Two or more elements combined are referred to as a chemical compound.

- Atoms of a compound are held together by chemical bonds.

- Bonds can be ionic, covalent, or hydrogen.

- Solutions can be acidic, basic, or neutral. The acidity or alkalinity of a solution is measured on the pH scale.

- Most of the chemical compounds in living organisms contain a selection of carbon atoms, also known as organic compounds. Molecules without carbon atoms are inorganic compounds.

- A mole is 6.02×10^{23} particles.

- Hydrocarbons can be alkanes, alkenes, or alkynes.

- Mixtures are divided into suspensions, solutions, and colloid suspensions. They can be homogeneous or heterogeneous.

KEY TERMS

matter
elements
atoms
molecules
color
density
hardness
conductivity
homogeneous matter
heterogeneous matter
protons
neutrons
electrons
nucleus
isotopes
ion
cation
anion
solid
liquid
gas
condensed phases
physical change
melting
freezing (solidification)
boiling (vaporization)
sublimation
vapor pressure
condensation
exothermic
endothermic
boiling point
chemical change
heating-cooling curve
conductor
nonconductor
density
specific gravity
solubility
luster
malleability
ductility
tenacity
brittleness
conductivity
metal
nonmetal

metalloid
noble gas (inert gas)
periodic table
atomic number
atomic weight (atomic mass)
period (row or series)
group (family)
sodium benzoate
monosodium glutamate (MSG)
saponification
pathogen
compound
empirical formula
percent composition
mole
Avogadro's number
ionic bonds
covalent bonds
nonpolar covalent bonds
polar covalent bonds
double covalent bonds
triple covalent bonds
hydrogen bonds
organic compounds
inorganic compounds
hydrocarbons
alkanes
alkenes
alkynes
mixture
suspension
solution
colloidal suspension
solute
solvent
tincture
dispersed substance
dispersing medium
volume expanders
acids
bases
salts
buffers
thermodynamics
entropy
enthalpy

Chapter 8
Earth Science

MOTHER EARTH, SISTER MOON

Here are some of the topics you need to be familiar with for the nursing school entrance exam: Earth, the solar system, and astronomy (not astrology, silly), including weather patterns, water vapor, mineral composition, beach erosion, glaciers, horizontal sorting, water wells, earthquakes, and much more. Someday you may even become an American Red Cross nurse volunteer and be deployed to provide disaster relief services in a region that has been devastated by a tornado or earthquake. In addition to the preceding topics, you should know about pollution, air pollutants (look at those effects on asthmatics), humidity, and much more. You may find questions related to Earth science on the NLN PAX-RN and TEAS, but the NET doesn't test science topics.

Environmental shifts and atmospheric changes affect everyone. A change in our environment and universe creates change in humankind. A change in humans or a trend in a segment of the population can create stress, stimuli, and further changes. This type of snowball effect is called **disease sequela.** Let's get cracking (and beam me up, Scotty).

THE SOLAR SYSTEM AND UNIVERSE (ASTRONOMY)

Our **solar system** consists of the **Sun** and other **celestial objects** bound to it by **gravity.** It includes **planets, moons,** and other smaller bodies. You should recall the planet names in order from the Sun:

> Mercury
> Venus
> Earth
> Mars
> Jupiter
> Saturn
> Uranus
> Neptune
> **Pluto** was considered a planet until 2006, when it was reclassified as a **dwarf planet.**

Earth has only one moon. There are many moons around all the planets in our solar system, and many more are being discovered each year. These many moons are even named. Did you know that Mars has 2 moons, Jupiter 63, Saturn 61, Uranus 27, Neptune 13, and Pluto 4?

Asteroids, Comets, Stars, Meteoroid, and Meteors (Where Is Clark Kent?)

Asteroids are smaller bodies made up of carbonaceous or rocky-metallic materials that orbit the Sun. (*Remember:* If they contain carbon, they are organic). **Comets** contain significant amounts of ice and water, so when they orbit the Sun, they look as if they have a comma, or a tail, about them. Comets leave a trail of debris behind them during their orbits. **Stars** are luminous balls made of plasma held together by their own gravity. They are made up of hydrogen. (The Sun is a star and is the star nearest to Earth). A **meteoroid** is a particle of debris in the solar system, and a **meteor** is the visible path of that meteoroid when it has entered Earth's atmosphere. So a meteor shower is a beautiful display of solar system debris in the sky.

Earth's Rotational Pull

Earth rotates on its own axis once every 24 hours, with the actual time of day varying at different points on its surface. Therefore, at one point on Earth, it may be 3:00 P.M., while at another point on Earth it may be 3:00 A.M., relative to the hemispheric location of the point. For our daily purposes, Earth is viewed as grid with **longitudinal** and **latitudinal lines.**

> Longitudinal lines are designated by linear forms from pole to pole.
> Around Earth are 360 of these longitudinal lines in one-degree increments.
>
> Each hour, a given location on Earth's surface rotates through 15 degrees of longitude.

The Sun's Position, the Milky Way Galaxy, and Other Galaxies

The Sun is in a fixed position and does not move, even though it appears to move across the sky from early morning to afternoon to evening. At dawn, the Sun appears before the eastern horizon where it rises, and it sets below the western horizon at dusk. Earth's constant rotation is what makes our day and nights appear and makes it seem that the Sun is moving.

A **galaxy** is a large collection of hundreds of millions of stars that contains hydrogen and helium, particles of dust, and various gases. Earth is in the **Milky Way galaxy**. There are billions of stars in the Milky Way galaxy and thanks to the Hubble telescope, many galaxies are still being discovered every year. Galaxies are located **light years** away from Earth. (A light year is a unit of distance, indicating the distance that light can travel in one year.) Galaxies are classified according to their appearances.

- An **irregular system** is without form.
- A **spiral system** resembles a pinwheel.
- An **elliptical system** appears round with spiral-like arms.

> ### Big Bang Theory (No, Not the TV Show)
> The **Big Bang Theory** suggests that the universe began billions of years ago, expanded, and continues to expand today. Galaxies are expanding apart from each other at an increasingly rapid pace. Scientists, astrophysicists, and astronomers are trying to establish just how long ago the big bang may have actually happened.

THE MOON

The Moon makes a complete orbit around Earth once every 27.3 days. This time frame is called the **sidereal period**. Meanwhile, Earth orbits the Sun. The period from one full moon to the next full moon (called the **synodic period**) is 29.5 days. What's the story with the difference between 27.3 and 29.5? It takes a little bit longer for the Moon to catch up to the same phase when the interval is observed from Earth.

Scientists believe that during Earth's formation, billions of years ago, a piece of Earth was hit by an object, and the impact caused a large piece to break off and become the Moon. The Moon is thousands of miles away from Earth. It would take about two days to get to the Moon from Earth in a spaceship.

The Moon has no air, no weather, and no atmosphere. Its gravity is 1/6 of Earth's gravity. The Moon also has no organic material. On the Moon are craters; two inches of surface dust, which contains potassium, rare Earth elements, and phosphorous (also referred to as KREEP); sodium; helium; dead volcanoes; and **lunar maria**. Lunar maria (or mare) are large, dark plains that resemble seas on the Moon. The word *mare* comes from Latin for "the sea," because Galileo's telescope revealed objects that resembled seas on the surface of the Moon.

The Moon gets very hot when the Sun is shining upon it. The area receiving the sunlight can reach temperatures as high as 250° Fahrenheit. These high temperatures are why the Moon has no real water—it would evaporate. In any shadow on the Moon, where there is no sunlight, it is extremely cold, with temperatures as low as –250° Fahrenheit. With those temperature swings, life as we know it could not exist in that environment.

As already mentioned, from our perspective it takes the Moon approximately 29.5 days (one lunar cycle) to orbit Earth. The Moon is in **synchronous rotation** with Earth—that is, we always see the same side of the Moon (and this affects tides, as we'll discuss a bit later). The Moon can sometimes be seen during daylight hours because during the last half of a lunar cycle, the Moon sets after sunrise. So for a brief period, you can see the Sun and the Moon at the same time! Every month, the Moon is visible during the second half of the month, during the daytime.

Blue Moon

You may have heard the phrase "once in a blue moon." A **blue moon** is a situation that happens when two full moons occur within one calendar month. Quite a rarity!

The Moon goes through **five lunar phases: new moon, crescent moon, half moon, gibbous moon,** and **full moon**. The **waxing** Moon is the increasing of the lighted portion of the Moon, and the **waning** Moon is the decreasing of the lighted portion of the Moon. Here's a helpful way to remember the term *waxing*: When you dip a wick into melted wax to make a candle, the candle becomes larger each time it's dipped. When the Moon is waxing, it too is getting larger.

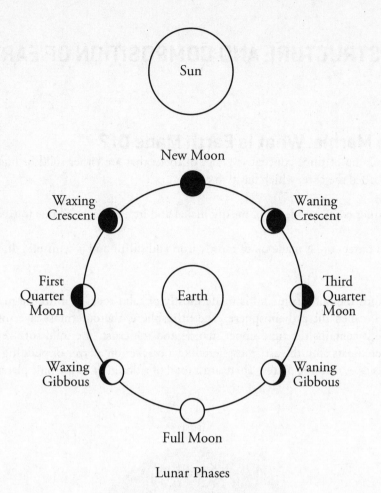

Lunar Phases

What Is a Solar Eclipse? What Is a Lunar Eclipse?

Eclipses can occur only when the Sun, Earth, and Moon are in a straight line. A **solar eclipse** can occur only at the new moon phase—when the Moon is between the Sun and Earth. The Moon is then in the middle, blocking our sunlight.

In contrast, a **lunar eclipse** occurs only at a full moon, when Earth is between the Sun and Moon. With Earth in the middle of this line-up, we see Earth's shadow cast across the Moon, making the Moon appear to be dark. Speaking of shadows, **umbra** and **penumbra** are the two major parts of a shadow.

The Moon causes the **ocean tides,** due to the pull of the Moon's gravity on the oceans. On the side of Earth nearest the Moon, the Moon's gravity is the strongest and it pulls the water slightly upward, which is what we experience as high tide. The high tide is always on the side facing the moon. Every day there are two alternating high tides and two low tides.

On the side of Earth furthest from the Moon, the Moon's gravity is the weakest and the water moves away from the Moon (which is also high tide). The high tide on the far side of Earth is not as high as the one facing the moon. This also affects Earth itself, believe it or not, because as the high tide brings up the water, actual rocks on Earth also move. During high tide, Earth rocks rise by an inch or two—not enough for us to notice.

GEOLOGY: STRUCTURE AND COMPOSITION OF EARTH

The Big Blue Marble: What Is Earth Made Of?

Planet Earth is made up of three concentric zones of rocks that are either solid or liquid (**molten**). The innermost zone is called the **core**, which has two parts:

1. The **solid inner core** is made up of mostly nickel and iron and is solid due to tremendous pressures.
2. The **molten outer core** is made up of mostly iron and sulfur and is semisolid due to lower pressures.

The **mantle** surrounds the outer core and is made mostly of solid rock. Within the mantle is an area of slowly flowing rock called the **asthenosphere**. The **lithosphere**, the outermost layer of Earth, is a thin, rigid layer of rock. It contains the rigid upper mantle and the **crust**, the solid surface of the Earth. Because the lithosphere floats atop the asthenosphere like a cracker on a layer of pudding, it can move and break into large pieces or **tectonic plates**. There are a total of a dozen or so tectonic plates that move about independently.

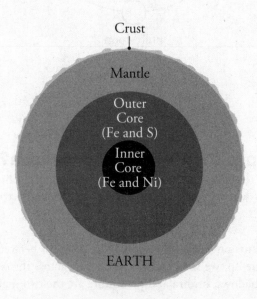

Earth's Zones

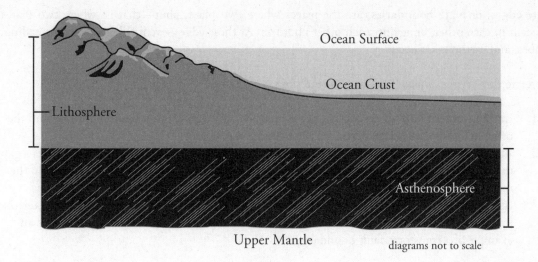

Earth's Outer Layers

When the Earth Moves Under Your Feet and Plates Collide

Earth's tectonic plates (made up of mantle and crust) move about freely. The majority of the land on Earth sits above six big plates, and the remaining plates lie under the ocean floor. Don't worry about memorizing this information. Just use the following diagram to familiarize yourself with Earth's plates:

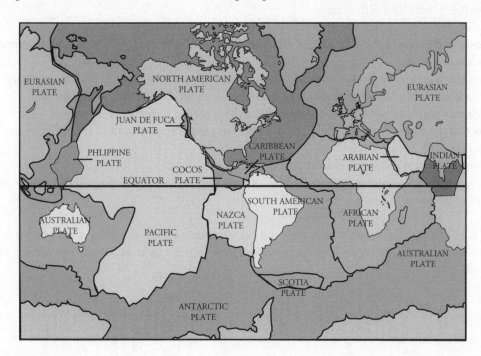

Earth's Plates

Plate edges, or **plate boundaries**, are the places where two plates abut—that is, where two plates are adjacent to each other, or against each other's borders. At these edges, events like sea floor spreading, volcanoes, and earthquakes occur.

There are three types of plate boundary interactions.

1. In a **convergent boundary**, two plates are pushed toward each other (with one above and the other being shoved below, deep into the mantle).
2. In a **divergent boundary**, two plates move away from each other. This movement causes a gap that can be filled with **magma** (molten rock). When magma cools, new crust is formed. The mid-Atlantic ridge is an example of a divergent boundary.
3. In a **transform fault boundary** (**transform boundary**), two plates slide along the fault, relative to each other. This type of boundary is also called a **slip fault**. The San Andreas fault is an example of a transform fault boundary.

Plate **subduction** happens when two plates converge, pushing one plate beneath the other. When neither of the converging plates subducts, both plates are uplifted to form mountains. The Himalaya Mountains are an example of such convergence.

Earthquake prediction is getting better but it is not accurate. Seismologists can tell us where earthquakes are most likely to happen. You may see a question or two about earthquakes on your exam, so be sure you know the following vocabulary associated with earthquakes:

- **Fault**—a break in Earth's crust
- **Epicenter**—the surface of Earth that is directly above the focus
- **Focus**—the exact spot where an earthquake occurs beneath the ground, thousands of meters below the surface
- **Seismic waves**—waves of energy that travel through Earth. This group includes primary waves, secondary waves, and longitudinal waves, which radiate out from the focus.
- **Primary waves (P waves)**—the fastest of the three waves; arrive at a seismograph first
- **Secondary waves (S waves)**—slightly slower than primary waves; arrive at a seismograph second, after the primary waves
- **Longitudinal waves**—travel along Earth's surface
- **Magnitude** or **Richter magnitude scale**—a scale that measures the magnitude of an earthquake based on the energy released

When a large earthquake occurs underneath the ocean, a **tsunami** may result. A tsunami is a series of waves that can travel at speeds of 600 miles per hour. These waves can be extremely destructive when they hit land.

ROCK ON

We are surrounded by rocks—rocks that came from other rocks. The oldest rocks on Earth are over three billion years old, and many other rocks are "only" a few million years old. Time, pressure, and Earth's heat interact to create three basic types of rock in the rock cycle.

1. **Sedimentary rock** is formed as sediment (eroded rocks and the remains of plants and animals) builds up and is compressed. One place this can occur is at a subduction zone where sediments are pushed deep into Earth and compressed by the weight of rock above it. Sandstone is an example of sedimentary rock.

2. **Metamorphic rock** is formed when a great deal of pressure and heat is applied to rock. This can happen as sedimentary rocks sink deeper into Earth, where they are heated by the high temperatures in Earth's mantle. Slate and marble are examples of metamorphic rock.

3. **Igneous rock** results when rock is melted (by heat and pressure below the crust) into a liquid and then resolidifies. The molten rock (magma) comes to the surface of Earth. When it emerges, it is called **lava**. Solid lava is igneous rock. Basalt is an example of an igneous rock.

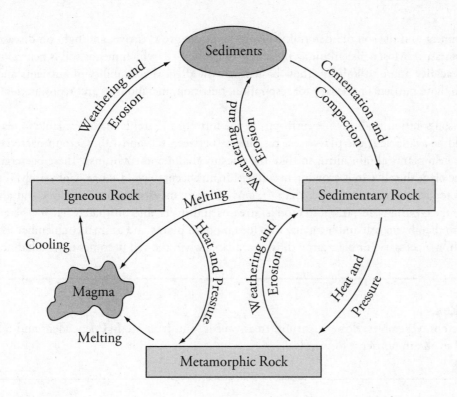

The Rock Cycle

GIVE ME THE DIRT

You don't have to have a green thumb to know the dirt about dirt. Just know that it's complex ancient material teeming with living organisms: protozoa, bacteria, algae, fungi, earthworms, and bugs. Pores between the grains of minerals in soil are filled with air or water—so the pores determine the water-holding capacity of the dirt.

Soil and dirt are made up of organic (living, or **biotic**), dead (**abiotic**), and inorganic matter. The United States Department of Agriculture (USDA) divides soil textures into three large groups: **clay, silt,** and **sand.** Clay is the category with the smallest particles, the next largest is silt, and sand is the coarsest soil.

Soil, loam, and dirt all came from a combination of organic and inorganic material that has been broken down by **physical weathering, chemical weathering,** and **biological weathering.**

Soil pH

Their environment and the soil pH determine plants' ability to grow, thrive, and fight off disease (remind you of homeostasis?). Most soils fall into a pH range of about 4–8, which means soil is neutral to slightly acidic. Soil's **acidity** and/or **alkalinity** (how basic it is) will affect the solubility of nutrients and the way plants absorb those nutrients necessary for respiration, nutrition, metabolism, and reproduction.

If the pH of soil solution is above 5.5, nitrogen (in the form of nitrate) is made available to plants. Phosphorus would be available if the pH were a bit higher (between 6.0 and 7.0). Certain bacteria living in root nodules help plants obtain nitrogen (like the ones in alfalfa and soybeans). These bacteria function best when the plant they live in is growing in soil within an acceptable pH range. Conversely, if the pH of soil becomes too acidic (meaning lower than 4), ions of **heavy metals** (such as **mercury** and **aluminum**) can leak into the ground water; travel to brooks, streams and rivers; and ultimately harm vegetation. That vegetation can then harm fish and humans, who feed on both plants and animals (remember food chains and webs?). Iron, necessary for plant growth is unavailable when the soil becomes more alkaline.

> **pH is Key**
> Many crops, vegetables, flowers, shrubs, trees, weeds, and fruit are pH dependent and rely on the soil to obtain nutrients for survival.

Soil Layers

You may be asked to recall the different **soil layers** for your exam. Here's a quick recap:

- The **O horizon** is the uppermost horizon containing waste from organisms (and decomposing bodies of organisms).
- The **A horizon** lies just below the top O horizon. It is made up of weathered rock and some organic material. The A horizon, often called **topsoil**, is important for plant growth. This layer is called the **zone of leaching**.
- The **B horizon** lies just below the A layer. It receives all minerals that are leached out from the A layer as well as organic material washed down from the topsoil. This is the zone of **illuviation**.
- The **C horizon** is the bottommost layer composed of large pieces of rock that have not undergone much weathering.
- The **R horizon** is the bedrock, which lies below all of the other layers of soil.

> Some things that are damaging to soil:
>
> - Repeated plowing with machinery (overtilling)
> - Monoculture and avoidance of crop rotation
> - Use of pesticides, fossil fuels, and toxic fertilizers
> - Water-logging with salinization, which leads to land degradation
> - Deforesting
> - Soil erosion

THE ATMOSPHERE AND WEATHER PATTERNS

Do you need to be a meteorologist to be a nurse? Of course not. But for your exam, familiarity with certain weather phenomena will be key to gain extra points.

The atmosphere is a layer of gases held close to Earth by the force of gravity. The layer of gases that lies closest to Earth is the **troposphere**, which extends from the surface of Earth to about 10–20 kilometers (5–10 miles) upward. The troposphere is where all the weather happens, and this layer contains the majority of atmospheric water vapor and clouds. This level gradually becomes much colder with an increase in altitude.

The troposphere contains gases called the **greenhouse gases**. The most important of those gases are carbon dioxide and water vapor. As the Sun's rays strike Earth, some of the solar radiation (UV) is reflected back into space; however, greenhouse gases in the troposphere intercept and absorb a lot of this radiation. The environmental movement today comes from the need for humans to stop depleting rain forests and to plant more trees. Green plants absorb carbon dioxide and produce water and oxygen in their living cycle. (So, keep talking to your house plants!)

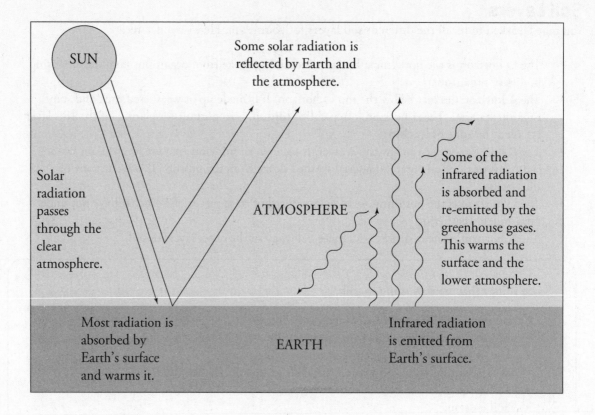

Some solar radiation is reflected by Earth and the atmosphere.

Solar radiation passes through the clear atmosphere.

ATMOSPHERE

Some of the infrared radiation is absorbed and re-emitted by the greenhouse gases. This warms the surface and the lower atmosphere.

Most radiation is absorbed by Earth's surface and warms it.

EARTH

Infrared radiation is emitted from Earth's surface.

The Greenhouse Effect

The Layers of the Atmosphere

The boundary between the troposphere and the stratosphere is called **tropopause**. At this level, the temperature no longer decreases with altitude—rather, it begins to increase with altitude.

Shuttle Mix Up

Poor Clementine spacecraft got lost in outer space in the 1990s due to human error, when its tracking system used the wrong metric.

The **stratosphere** sits on top of the tropopause buffer zone and extends up 20–50 km above the surface of Earth. Unlike the troposphere, its gases are not very well mixed, and like the tropopause, the temperature in the stratosphere increases as the distance from Earth increases. This warming effect occurs due to a thin band of **ozone** (O_3) that exists in this layer. The ozone traps the high-energy radiation of the Sun, holding some of the heat and protecting the troposphere and Earth's surface from this radiation.

Above the stratosphere are two layers called the **mesosphere** and the **thermosphere (ionosphere)**. The mesosphere extends up about 80 kilometers above Earth's surface and is the area where the meteors usually burn up. The thermosphere is the thinnest layer of all the gas layers and is located about 110 km above Earth. In this layer, radio waves are reflected, which enables long-distance radio communication. It's also the site in which **auroras (aurora borealis)** take place. This phenomenon is caused by electrons from the Sun striking oxygen atoms in the thermosphere. The thermosphere is the layer in which the space shuttles orbit. Finally, the thermosphere is also known as the ionosphere because of the ionization that takes place in that layer. This region absorbs most of the **energetic photons** (**solar winds**) from the Sun.

Weather and Climate

The temperamental weather patterns that we experience and their effects on climates are all dependent upon Earth's atmosphere, which has physical features that change from day to day, as well as patterns that are consistent over a period of many years. The day-to-day features like wind speed and direction, temperature, sunlight, pressure, and humidity are what we commonly refer to as the **weather**.

The patterns that are constant over many years are referred to as **climate**. The most important factors in describing climate are the **average temperature** and **average precipitation** amounts. (Wouldn't you want to know the average yearly temperature and amount of rain or snow a region has before you consider relocating there? See, it's not always just about the schools, now is it?) Meteorologists are scientists who study both weather and climate.

> The weather and climate of any given area is the result of the Sun unequally warming Earth (and the gases above it—its atmosphere), as well as the rotation of Earth on its axis.

Air Circulation in the Atmosphere

The motion of air around the big blue marble Earth is the result of unequal solar heating, Earth's rotation, and the physical properties of air, water, and the land. There are three major reasons that Earth is unevenly heated:

1. More of the Sun's rays strike Earth at the equator in each unit of surface area than strike the poles in the same unit area.
2. The tilt of Earth's axis points certain regions toward or away from the Sun.
3. Earth's surface at the equator is moving faster than the surface at the poles. This factor changes the motion of air into major **prevailing winds** (belts of air that distribute heat and moisture unevenly). Winds in the northern hemisphere of the globe are deflected to the right and winds in the southern hemisphere are deflected to the left. This deflection pattern is known as the **Coriolis effect.**

Convection Cells

Solar energy warms Earth's surface and that heat is transferred to the atmosphere by radiation heating. The warmed gases expand, become less dense, and then rise, creating vertical currents called **convection currents**. The warm currents can also hold a lot of moisture compared to the surrounding air. As these large masses of warm, moist air rise, cool air flows along the surface of Earth into the area where the warm air was located. This flowing air, called **horizontal airflow** (or wind), is one way that **surface winds** are created.

As warm moist air rises into the cooler atmosphere, it cools to the **dew point** (the temperature at which water vapor condenses into a liquid form). This **condensation** creates clouds. When condensation continues and the clouds become bigger, they can no longer be held up by gravity. They then fall as precipitation (rain, snow, sleet, or hail). This cold, dry air is now denser than the surrounding air. This air mass then sinks to the surface where it is warmed and can gather more moisture, thus starting the **convection cell** rotation again.

You may be asked to recall the different types of cloud formations. The following is a list of cloud types that you should know:

- **Stratus clouds** are layers of clouds.
- **Nimbostratus clouds** are rain clouds. So when it is raining, you will see a layer of nimbostratus clouds lining the sky.
- **Cumulus clouds** are fluffy and can look like objects (use your imagination); cumulus clouds are fair weather clouds.
- **Cumulonimbus clouds** (big thunder clouds) are large rain clouds that can cause localized thunder storms with rain, wind, lightning, and thunder.
- **Cirrus clouds** are wispy clouds that look like horse tails. They are actually high altitude ice crystals that do not produce rain or any kind of precipitation.

Wind is caused by the unequal heating of Earth's surface. On the local level near the ocean, there are two types of winds: land and sea breezes. A **sea breeze** (wind from the water) occurs when the land is hotter than the large body of water. A **land breeze** occurs when the relative temperature of the water is warmer than that of the land. You can see why kite-flying is very popular at the hot, sunny beach.

The Four Seasons and Wind Types

Seasons occur because of Earth's motion around the Sun and the fact that Earth is tilted on its axis by 23.5 degrees. When Earth is in the part of its orbit in which the northern hemisphere is tilted toward the Sun, the northern half of the planet receives more direct sunlight for a longer period of time each day than does the southern hemisphere. Therefore, when the northern hemisphere is experiencing summer, the southern hemisphere is experiencing winter. Interestingly, because of Earth's tilt, the Sun rises and sets just once a year at the North and South Poles. Approximately six months of the year at the poles is daytime, while the other six months is dark and considered nighttime.

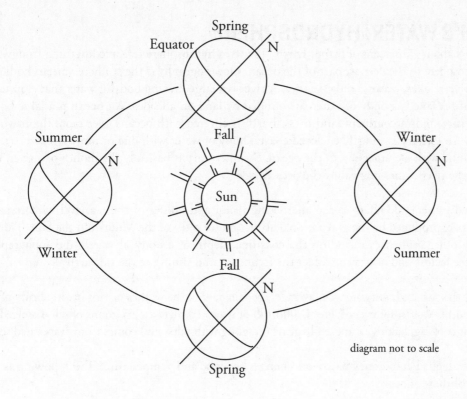

Four Seasons

diagram not to scale

Wind Storms and Weather Events

Trade winds are steady, strong winds named for their ability to quickly propel trading ships across the ocean. These winds can travel 11–13 miles per hour (mph). They occur in somewhat predictable patterns but may cause local disturbances when they blow over very warm ocean water. When this happens, the air warms and forms an isolated, intense low-pressure system, while also picking up more water vapor from the ocean's surface. The wind circles around this isolated low-pressure air (counterclockwise in the northern hemisphere and clockwise in the southern hemisphere). The low pressure system continues to move over warm water, increasing in strength and wind speed which eventually results in a **tropical storm**. When these tropical storms intensify, they are classified as **hurricanes**, with sustained wind speeds starting at a minimum of 74 miles per hour (which is consistent with category one). The rotating winds of a hurricane remove water vapor from the ocean's surface and heat energy is created by the condensing water vapor. This addition of heat energy continues to contribute to the increase in wind speed. Some hurricanes can have winds traveling at speeds up to 155 mph (category five).

Three storm types are **typhoons**, hurricanes, and **cyclones**. The differentiation between each depends upon the location in which the storm forms. Cyclones form in the Indian Ocean or over the Southwest Pacific Ocean. Typhoons form in the Northwest Pacific, and hurricanes form anywhere in the Atlantic Ocean. Generally, tornadoes are smaller than hurricanes and form directly over land (think of the twister from *The Wizard of Oz*).

Monsoon Moment

A **monsoon** is a large-scale version of the type of circulation seen in land and sea breezes. Monsoons occur in southern Asia. A monsoon acts like a large-scale sea breeze in the summer and land breeze in the winter.

EARTH'S WATER: HYDROSPHERE

Water covers about 75 percent of planet Earth. The term **hydrosphere** refers to anything from water vapor in the stratosphere to the deepest part of the ocean. **Oceanography** is the study of various bodies of water including rivers, lakes, oceans, and estuaries. A **river** is a large flowing body of water that empties into the sea or ocean. A **lake** is a body of water surrounded by land on all sides. An **ocean** is a large body of salt-water that surrounds a continent land mass. Earth is covered with oceans over more than two-thirds of the planet. An **estuary** is a partly enclosed coastal body of water with one or more rivers or streams flowing into it, and with a connection to the ocean. So an estuary is basically the mouth of a river, where the current of the river comes up against the ocean's tide.

As discussed earlier, tide refers to the alternating rising and falling of the sea level with respect to the land. Tides are produced by the gravitational attraction (or pull) of the Moon and the Sun. Tides are also affected by other influences including the coastline, depth of a body of water, and topography of the ocean. These factors and others can affect the frequency and timing of the tide arrival.

Most of Earth's surface is saltwater. On average, the saltwater in the world's oceans has a **salinity** of about 3.5 percent. In other words, for every 1 liter (1,000 ml) of seawater, there are 35 grams of salt dissolved in it. **Sea salt** used for cooking, baking, and even hygiene (gargling with saltwater) comes from evaporated seawater.

Oceans are divided into zones based on changes in light and temperature. The following is a helpful review list of those zones:

- The **coastal zone** consists of the ocean water closest to land (the shore).
- The **euphotic zone** is the upper layers of water—that is, the warmest region of the water with the highest levels of dissolved oxygen.
- The **bathyal zone**, or the middle region, receives insufficient light for photosynthesis and is colder than the euphotic zone.
- The **abyssal zone** is the deepest, darkest region marked by extreme cold and very low levels of oxygen, but very high levels of nutrients because of the decaying plant and animal matter that sinks down from the zones above.

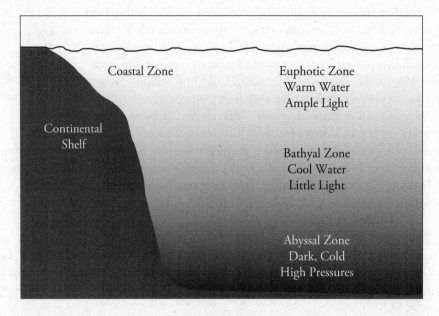

Ocean Zones

Freshwater contains minimal quantities of dissolved salts, especially sodium chloride. Freshwater comes from the precipitation of atmospheric water vapor, which reaches inland lakes, rivers, and groundwater bodies directly or from melting snow or ice. The Great Lakes form the largest collection of freshwater lakes (by surface area) found on Earth.

Red Tide

Occasionally, organisms in the photic regions experience an exponential growth in the population, especially the single-cell algae. This single-cell algae may form blooms of color called algal blooms, the most famous of which is known as **red tide**. These algae can produce toxins that may kill fish and poison the beds of filter feeders such as oysters and mussels. Red tide is caused by a proliferation of **dinoflagellates**.

Ocean Currents and Ocean Circulation

Ocean currents play a major role in modifying conditions around Earth and can affect where certain climates are located. As the Sun warms water in the equatorial regions of the globe, prevailing winds, differences in salinity, and Earth's rotation set ocean water in motion. An example is the **Gulf Stream**, which carries sun-warmed water along the east coast of the United States and as far as Great Britain. This warm water displaces the colder denser water in the polar regions, which can move south to be rewarmed by the equatorial sun. Northern Europe is kept 5–10 degrees Celsius warmer than it would be were the current not present. Oceanographers also study a major current called the **ocean conveyer belt**, which moves cold water in the depths of the Pacific Ocean while creating major upwellings in other areas of the Pacific.

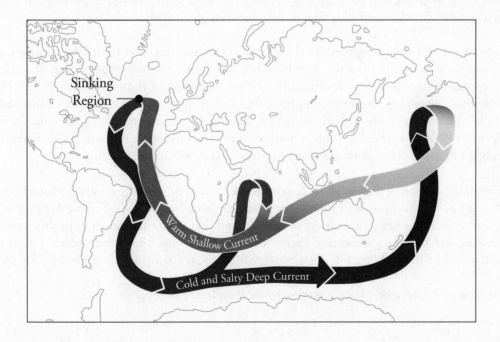

Ocean Circulation

Let's end this review chapter with the cycles that bridge the gap between living and nonliving—water, nitrogen, carbon, and phosphorous—and how they cycle through the environment. We briefly mentioned them at the end of the biology chapter, but let's further review here.

CYCLES IN NATURE

As you may have learned in biology class, nutrients such as carbon, oxygen, nitrogen, phosphorus, sulfur, and water move through the environment in complex cycles known as **biogeochemical cycles.**

As you can probably tell from the collective name of these natural cycles, living organisms, geologic formations, and chemical substances are involved in these cycles. Keep in mind that when we describe the movement of these inorganic compounds, it's important to understand both the destinations of the compounds and how they move toward their destinations. For example, it won't be enough for you to know that water moves from the atmosphere to Earth. You'll need to know the different ways it has of getting there. In other words, you'll need to know that water moves from the atmosphere to Earth's surface through precipitation, either in the form of snow or rainfall.

But, let's talk about a few things that all of these cycles have in common before we go into each one in detail. First of all, the term **reservoir** is used to describe a place where a large quantity of a nutrient sits for a long period of time (in the water cycle, the ocean is an example of a reservoir). The opposite of a reservoir is an **exchange pool**, which is a site where a nutrient sits for only a short period of time (in the water cycle, a cloud is an example of an exchange pool). The amount of time a nutrient spends in a reservoir or an exchange pool is called its **residency time.** In the water cycle, water might exist in the form of a cloud for a few days, but it might exist as part of the ocean for a thousand years! Perhaps surprisingly, living organisms can also serve as exchange pools and reservoirs for certain nutrients.

The energy that drives these biogeochemical cycles in the biosphere comes primarily from two sources: the Sun, and the heat energy from the mantle and core of Earth. The movements of nutrients in all of these cycles may be via abiotic mechanisms, such as wind, or may occur through biotic mechanisms, such as through living organisms. Another important fact to note is that while the **law of conservation of matter** states that matter can be neither created nor destroyed (sounds familiar, right?), nutrients can be rendered unavailable for cycling through certain processes—for example, in some cycles, nutrients may be transported to deep ocean sediments where they are locked away interminably.

Though we won't get into a discussion of trace elements here, you should also know that certain trace elements such as zinc, copper, and iron are necessary in small amounts for living organisms. Trace elements can cycle in conjunction with the major nutrients, but there's still much to be discovered about these elements and their biogeochemical cycles. For this exam, just know that there are certain trace elements required by living things that cycle, along with the major elements, through the biosphere.

Let's start with perhaps the best-known biogeochemical cycle: the water cycle.

The Water Cycle

Water exists in the atmosphere is in a gaseous state. When it condenses from the gaseous state to form a liquid or solid (there's phase change again), it becomes dense enough to fall to Earth because of the pull of gravity. This process is formally known as **precipitation.** When precipitation falls onto Earth, it may travel below ground to become **groundwater**, or it may travel across the land's surface as runoff and enter a drainage system, such as a stream or river, that will eventually deposit it into a body of water such as a lake or an ocean. Lakes and oceans are reservoirs for water. In certain cold regions of Earth, water may also be trapped on the surface as snow or ice; in these areas, the blocks of snow or ice are reservoirs.

Water is also cycled through living systems. For example, plants absorb water (and carbon dioxide) in the process of photosynthesis, in which they produce carbohydrates. Because all living organisms are primarily made up of water, they act as exchange pools for water.

Water is returned to the atmosphere from Earth's surface and from living organisms in a process called **evaporation.** Specifically, animals respire and release water vapor and additional gases to the atmosphere. In plants, the process of **transpiration** releases large amounts of water into the air. Finally, other major contributors to atmospheric water are the vast number of lakes and oceans on Earth's surface. Incredibly large amounts of water continually evaporate from their surfaces.

Take a look at the graphic below, which shows all of the forms that water takes in the biosphere and atmosphere.

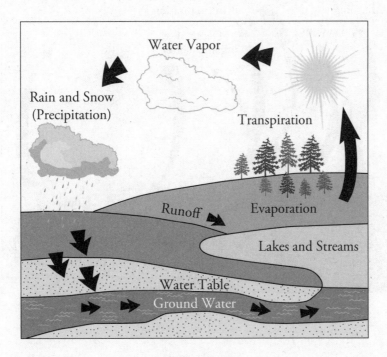

The Water Cycle

The Carbon Cycle

Now let's talk about carbon. The key events in the **carbon cycle** are respiration, in which animals (and plants!) breathe and give off carbon dioxide; and photosynthesis, in which plants take in carbon dioxide, water, and energy from the sun to produce carbohydrates. In other words, living things act as exchange pools for carbon.

When plants are eaten by animal consumers, the carbon locked in the plant carbohydrates passes to other organisms and continues through the food chain. In turn, when organisms—both plants and animals—die, their bodies are decomposed through the actions of bacteria and fungi in the soil; this releases CO_2 back into the atmosphere.

When the bodies of once-living organisms are buried and subjected to conditions of extreme heat and extreme pressure, eventually this organic matter becomes oil, coal, and gas. Oil, coal, and natural gas are collectively known as fossil fuels. When fossil fuels are burned, or **combusted**, carbon is released into the atmosphere. Finally, carbon is also released into the atmosphere through volcanic action.

There are two major reservoirs of carbon. The first is the world's oceans, because CO_2 is very soluble in water. The second large reservoir of CO_2 is Earth's rocks. Many types of rocks—called carbonate rocks—contain carbon, in the form of calcium carbonate.

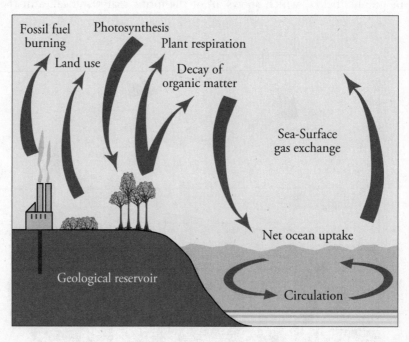

The Carbon Cycle

The Nitrogen Cycle

Earth's atmosphere is made up of approximately 78 percent nitrogen and 21 percent oxygen (the other components of the atmosphere are trace elements); nitrogen is the most abundant element in the atmosphere. For this reason, it might not seem like living organisms would find it difficult to get the nitrogen they need in order to live. But it is! This is because atmospheric N_2 is not in a form that can be used directly by most organisms. In order to keep this rather complicated **nitrogen cycle** straight, let's look at it in steps.

▬ STEP 1:

Nitrogen fixation—In order to be used by most living organisms, nitrogen must be present in the form of ammonia (NH_3) or nitrates (NO_3^-). Atmospheric nitrogen can be converted into these forms, or "fixed," by atmospheric effects such as lightning storms, but most nitrogen fixation is the result of the actions of certain soil bacteria. These nitrogen-fixing bacteria are often associated with the roots of legumes such as beans and clover. In the future we may be able to insert the genes for nitrogen fixation into crop plants, such as corn, and reduce the amount of fertilizer that is used.

▬ STEP 2:

Nitrification—In this process, soil bacteria converts ammonium (NH_4^+) into one of the forms that can be used by plants—nitrate (NO_3).

▬ STEP 3:

Assimilation—In assimilation, plants absorb ammonium (NH_3), ammonia ions (NH_4^+), and nitrate ions (NO_3^-) through their roots. Heterotrophs, or organisms that receive energy by consuming other organisms, then obtain nitrogen when they consume the proteins and nucleic acids in plants.

▬ STEP 4:

Ammonification—In this process, decomposing bacteria convert dead organisms and other waste to ammonia (NH_3) or ammonium ions (NH_4^+), which can be reused by plants.

▬ STEP 5:

Denitrification—In denitrification, specialized bacteria convert ammonia back into nitrites and nitrates and then into nitrogen gas (N_2) and nitrous oxide gas (N_2O). These gases then rise to the atmosphere.

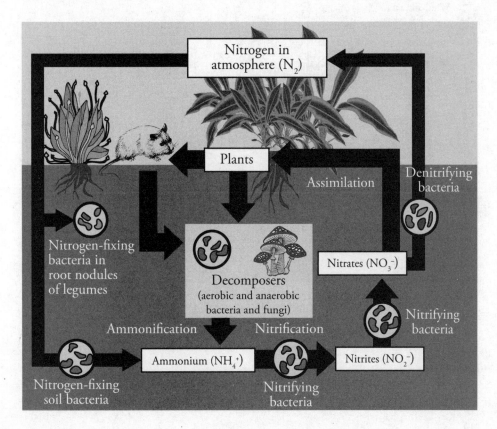

The Nitrogen Cycle

The Phosphorus Cycle

The **phosphorus cycle** is perhaps the simplest biogeochemical cycle, mostly because phosphorus does not exist in the atmosphere outside of dust particles. Phosphorus is necessary for living organisms because it's a major component of nucleic acids and other important biological molecules. One important idea for you to remember about the phosphorus cycle is that phosphorus cycles are more local than those of the other important biological compounds.

For the most part, phosphorus is found in soil, rock, and sediments; it's released from these rock forms through the process of chemical weathering. Phosphorus is usually released in the form of phosphate (PO_4^{3-}), which is very soluble and can be absorbed from the soil by plants. You should know that phosphorus is also often a limiting factor for plant growth, so plants that have little phosphorus are stunted.

Phosphates that enter the water table and travel to the oceans can eventually be incorporated into rocks in the ocean floor. Through geologic processes, ocean mixing, and upwelling, these rocks from the seafloor may rise up so that their components once again enter the **terrestrial cycle**. Take a look at the phosphorus cycle shown in the diagram below.

Humans have affected the phosphorus cycle by mining phosphorus-rich rocks in order to produce fertilizers. The fertilizers placed on fields can easily leach into the groundwater and find their way into aquatic ecosystems where they can cause **eutrophication**. Eutrophication occurs when a body of water receives excess nutrients. The adundance of nutrients can cause an overgrowth of algae and deplete the water of oxygen.

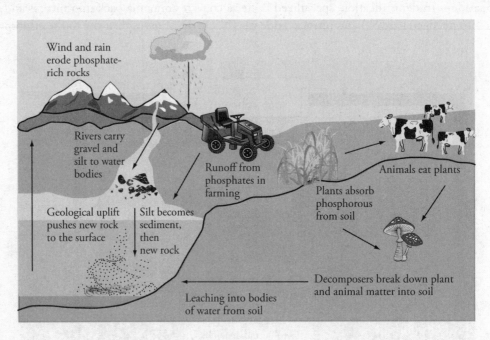

The Phosphorous Cycle

Sulfur

The last biogeochemical cycle we'll talk about is the sulfur cycle. Sulfur is one of the components that make up proteins and vitamins, so both plants and animals need sulfur in their diets. Plants absorb sulfur when it is dissolved in water, so they can take it up through their roots when it's dissolved in groundwater. Animals obtain sulfur by consuming plants.

Most of Earth's sulfur is tied up in rocks and salts or buried deep in the ocean in oceanic sediments, but some sulfur can be found in the atmosphere. The natural ways that sulfur enters the atmosphere are through volcanic eruptions, certain bacterial functions, and the decay of once-living organisms. When sulfur enters the atmosphere through human activity, it's mainly via industrial processes that produce sulfur dioxide (SO_2) and hydrogen sulfide (H_2S) gases.

SUMMARY

- Our solar system consists of the Sun and other celestial objects bound to it by gravity that includes planets, moons, and other smaller bodies.

- We live in the Milky Way galaxy, which includes many planets: Mercury, Venus, Earth, Mars, Jupiter, Saturn, Uranus, and Neptune.

- Earth rotates on its own axis every 24 hours.

- From full moon to full moon is the synodic period (29.5 days).

- The Moon makes a complete orbit around Earth once every 27.3 days (called the sidereal period).

- The lunar phases of the moon are new moon, crescent moon, half moon, gibbous moon, and full moon.

- Earth is made up of three concentric zones of rocks: the solid inner core, the molten outer core, and the mantle.

- There are three plate boundary interactions: convergent, divergent, and transform fault boundary.

- There are three types of rocks in the rock cycle: sedimentary rock, metamorphic rock, and igneous rock.

- Soil, loam, and dirt all came from a combination of organic and inorganic material and rock that was broken down by physical weathering, chemical weathering, and biological weathering.

- The atmosphere has many layers: troposphere, stratosphere, mesosphere, and thermosphere.

- Day-to-day features such as wind speed, temperature, and sunlight make up weather. Patterns of weather over many years are known as climate.

- The different kinds of cloud formations include stratus clouds, nimbostratus clouds, cumulus clouds, cumulonimbus clouds, and cirrus clouds.

- Oceanography is the study of various bodies of water including rivers, lakes, oceans, and estuaries.

- Water covers about 75% of Earth and most of Earth's surface is saltwater.

- There are a number of cycles in nature: the water cycle, the carbon cycle, the nitrogen cycle, and the phosphorus cycle.

KEY TERMS

disease sequela
solar system
Sun
celestial objects
gravity
planets
moons
Mercury
Venus
Earth
Mars
Jupiter
Saturn
Uranus
Neptune
Pluto
dwarf planet
asteroid
comets
star
meteoroid
meteor
longitudinal lines
latitudinal lines
galaxy
Milky Way galaxy
light year
irregular system
spiral system
elliptical system
Big Bang Theory
sidereal period
synodic period
lunar maria
synchronous rotation
lunar phases
new moon
crescent moon
half moon
gibbous moon
full moon
waxing
waning
blue moon
eclipse
solar eclipse

lunar eclipse
umbra
penumbra
ocean tides
molten
core
solid inner core
molten outer core
mantle
asthenosphere
lithosphere
crust
tectonic plates
plate edges (plate boundaries)
convergent boundary
divergent boundary
magma
transform fault boundary (slip fault)
subduction
fault
epicenter
focus
seismic waves
primary waves (P waves)
secondary waves (S waves)
longitudinal waves
Richter magnitude scale
tsunami
sedimentary rock
metamorphic rock
igneous rock
lava
biotic
abiotic
clay
silt
sand
physical weathering
chemical weathering
biological weathering
acidity
alkalinity
heavy metals
mercury
aluminum

soil layers
O horizon
A horizon
topsoil
zone of leaching
B horizon
illuviation
C horizon
R horizon
troposphere
greenhouse gases
tropopause
stratosphere
ozone
mesosphere
thermosphere (ionosphere)
auroras (aurora borealis)
energetic photons (solar winds)
weather
climate
average temperature
average precipitation
prevailing winds
Coriolis Effect
convection currents
horizontal airflow
surface winds
dew point
condensation
convection cell
stratus clouds
nimbo stratus clouds
cumulous clouds
cumulonimbus clouds
cirrus clouds
wind
sea breeze
land breeze
trade winds
tropical storm
hurricane
monsoon
typhoon
cyclone
hydrosphere
oceanography

river
lake
ocean
estuary
salinity
sea salt
coastal zone
euphotic zone
bathyal zone
abyssal zone
freshwater
red tide
dinoflagellates
Gulf Stream
ocean conveyer belt
biogeochemical cycles
reservoir
exchange pool

residency time
law of conservation of matter
water cycle
precipitation
groundwater
evaporation
transpiration
carbon cycle
combusted
nitrogen cycle
nitrogen fixation
nitrification
assimilation
ammonification
dentrification
phosphorous cycle
terrestrial cycle
eutrophication

Chapter 9
Arithmetic

In this chapter, we will review basic math concepts. When it comes to math, there are no tricks, no easy cramming methods—just the basics that come with memorization and application over and over. Not every student feels super comfortable with parts of math tested, so we have compiled a bunch of principles that you should know. It's okay if you feel confident about a science subject, but feel uncertain about math, or vice versa. You will need to be familiar with basic math principles and skills for your nursing school entrance exam preparation, as well as in your nursing career. Medication dosages and concentrations are almost never "ready to administer." You will undoubtedly have to do step-by-step calculations prior to medicating one of your patients.

Let's start by reviewing common definitions. There are a number of mathematical terms that can appear on the math section of the NET, TEAS, and NLN PAX-RN, and you should understand them so that you can be confident and comfortable.

Integers	Positive and negative whole numbers, and zero; NOT fractions or decimals.
Prime Number	An integer that has exactly two distinct factors: itself and 1. All prime numbers are positive; the smallest prime number is 2. Two is also the only even prime number. One is not prime.
Rational Numbers	All positive and negative integers, fractions, and decimal numbers; technically, any number that can be expressed as a fraction of two integers—which means everything except numbers containing weird radicals (such as $\sqrt{2}$), π, or e.
Irrational Numbers	Any number that does not end or repeat (in other words, any number that isn't rational). This includes all numbers with radicals that can't be simplified, such as $\sqrt{2}$ (perfect squares with radicals, such as $\sqrt{16}$, don't count because they can be simplified to integers, such as 4). Also, all numbers containing π or e. Note that repeating decimals like $.33333$ are rational (they're equivalent to fractions, such as $\frac{1}{3}$).
Real Numbers	Any number on the number line; everything except imaginary numbers (see below).
Imaginary Numbers	The square roots of negative numbers, that is, any numbers containing i, which represents $\sqrt{-1}$.
Consecutive Numbers	The members of a set listed in order, without skipping any; examples of consecutive integers are –3, –2, –1, 0, 1, 2; examples of consecutive positive multiples of 3 are 3, 6, 9, 12.
Distinct Numbers	Numbers that are different from each other.
Sum	The result of adding numbers.
Difference	The result of subtracting numbers.
Product	The result of multiplying numbers.
Quotient	The result of dividing numbers.
Remainder	The integer left over after dividing two numbers. For example, when 17 is divided by 2, the remainder is 1.

Reciprocal	The result when 1 is divided by a number. For example, the reciprocal of 2 is $\frac{1}{2}$, the reciprocal of $\frac{3}{4}$ is $\frac{4}{3}$, and the reciprocal of $\frac{1}{16}$ is 16.
Positive Difference	Just what it sounds like—the number that results when the smaller of two numbers is subtracted from the larger one. You can also think of it as the distance between two numbers on the number line.
Absolute Value	The positive version of a number. You just strike the negative sign if there is one. You can also think of it as the distance on the number line between a number and zero.
Arithmetic Mean	The average of a list of values; also simply referred to as the "mean."
Median	The middle value in a list when arranged in increasing order; in a list with an even number of members, the average of the *two* middle values.
Mode	The value that occurs most often in a list. If no value appears more often than all the others in a list, then that list has no mode.

INTEGERS

Integers are the numbers that most of us are accustomed to thinking of simply as "numbers." Integers are numbers that have no fractional or decimal part. They can be either positive or negative.

The **positive integers** are

1, 2, 3, 4, 5, 6, 7, 8, 9, 10, and so on.

Zero (0) is an integer also, but it is neither positive nor negative.

The **negative integers** are

–1, –2, –3, –4, –5, –6, –7, –8, –9, –10, and so on.

Basically, integers are numbers that have no fractions or decimals. For example, the following numbers are not integers:

–3.4
0.625
17.2
–9.9
2/5
–3/4

Number Line

Integers are often illustrated on a **number line**.

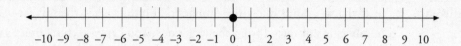

The number line is a two dimensional way of looking at positive and sometimes negative numbers in relation to one another. Positive numbers are to the right of the zero on the number line. Negative numbers are to the left of zero on the number line.

Even and Odd Numbers

Even numbers are integers that can be divided by 2 and leave no remainder. Here are some examples of even numbers:

–4, –2, 0, 2, 4, 6, 8, 10, and so on

You can always tell at a glance whether a number is even—how? It is even if its final digit is an even number (meaning divisible by 2). Consider the following number. Is it even?

333,333,333,338

Yes, you know that it is an even number because 8, the final digit, is an even number.

Odd numbers are integers that have a remainder when divided by 2. Here are some examples of odd numbers:

–5, –3, –1, 1, 3, 5, 7, 9, and so on

You can always tell at a glance whether a number is odd—how? It is odd if its final digit is an odd number. Consider this number:

222,222,222,227

It is an odd number because 7, the final digit, is an odd number.

Addition

Addition is putting integers together to get their sum. The **sum** is the result of addition.

Subtraction

Subtraction is the reverse of addition. The answer to a subtraction problem is called the **difference**.

Rules of Addition and Subtraction

Even and odd numbers are governed by the following important rules that you should know:

1. Even number + even number = even number
$$2 + 2 = 4$$
2. Even number – even number = even number
$$6 - 2 = 4$$
3. Odd number + odd number = even number
$$3 + 3 = 6$$
4. Odd number – odd number = even number
$$5 - 3 = 2$$
5. Even number + odd number = odd number
$$4 + 3 = 7$$
6. Even number – odd number = odd number
$$10 - 7 = 3$$

Multiplication

Multiplication is an outgrowth of addition, only faster. See?

For example, $4 + 4 + 4 + 4 + 4 = 20$. However, you can also say that $5 \times 4 = 20$.

The result of multiplying is called the **product**.

Rules of Multiplication

1. Even number × even number = even number
$$4 \times 4 = 16$$
2. Odd number × odd number = odd number
$$3 \times 3 = 9$$
3. Even number × odd number = even number
$$4 \times 3 = 12$$

Distributive and Commutative Laws Regarding Multiplication

Distributive law, or **distributive property**, says if you are multiplying the sum of two numbers, you can multiply each number in your sum individually. In other words, $a(b + c) = a(b) + a(c)$, which is the same as $a \times b + a \times c$. Here's an example:

$$6(5) + 6(2) = 6(5 + 2) = 42$$

See? $6 \times 5 = 30 + 6 \times 2 = 12 = 42$

The answers to both are the same.

Commutative law, or **commutative property**, says that $a \times b = b \times a$.

Example: $4 \times 2 = 2 \times 4$

Both answers are 8.

Positive and Negative Numbers

Positive numbers are numbers that are larger than zero (0).

Negative numbers are numbers smaller than zero (0).

You can add negative and positive numbers:

$$8 + {-3} = 5 \qquad\qquad 8 + 3 = 11$$

You can subtract negative and positive numbers:

$$-8 - (-5) = -3 \qquad\qquad -8 - 5 = -13$$

There are three rules regarding the multiplication of positive and negative numbers.

1. Positive number × positive number = positive number
$$2 \times 5 = 10$$
2. Negative number × negative number = positive number
$$-3 \times -3 = 9$$
3. Positive number × negative number = negative number
$$4 \times -3 = -12$$

Division is the opposite of multiplication. The result of division is called a **quotient**. Here are the rules for dividing positive and negative numbers:

1. Positive number ÷ positive number = positive number

$4 \div 2 = 2$, which can be written as $2\overline{)4}$ with quotient 2

2. Negative number ÷ negative number = positive number

$-6 \div -2 = 3$, which can be written as $-2\overline{)-6}$ with quotient 3

3. Positive number ÷ negative number = negative number

$6 \div -2 = -3$, which can be written as $-2\overline{)\,6}$ with quotient -3

Zero: What's the Zip About Zero?

Any number × 0 = 0 (no matter what).

$$0 \times 4 = 0 \text{ and } 0 \times 658 = 0$$

Any number ÷ 0 = undefined.

What About 1?

The number 1 is a **multiplicative identity**. In other words, any number multiplied by 1 = itself.

7, one time, is 7.

That is, $7 \times 1 = 7$

Distinct Numbers

Distinct numbers are nothing more than different numbers—that is, a group of numbers in which no number appears more than once. Here's an example of a group of distinct numbers:

2, 3, 5, 8, 9

The following set of numbers cannot be called distinct because the number 7 appears twice:

2, 7, 5, 9, 7

Digits

A **digit** is one of the integers (0, 1, 2, 3, 4, 5, 6, 7, 8, 9) especially when it's part of a larger number. All integers (all numbers, that is) are made up of digits.

The number 2,346 has four digits: 2, 3, 4, 6. Therefore, it is a four-digit number representing two thousand, three hundred forty-six. Each of its digits has a different value that's based on its place in the number. In the number 2,346, the

2 is in the **thousands place**

3 is in the **hundreds place**

4 is in the **tens place**

6 is in the **unit place**, or the **ones place**

If we make that same number bigger by adding a decimal and numbers such as 2,346.782, the

7 is in the **tenths place**

8 is in the **hundredths place**

2 is in the **thousandths place**

The dot separating the decimal places from the whole number is called a **decimal point**. We'll discuss decimals more later in the chapter. Is the suspense killing you?

Rounding a Number to the Nearest "Whatever"

You will often see a number, either as money, a large number, or perhaps a number with a decimal, and you'll be asked to **round** it up or down. A rounded number is almost the same as the original number, just less exact. Rounding can be useful when you're working with large numbers especially, but it can be used on any type of number, really.

The "places" that we just discussed are about to come in handy. Suppose you wish to round the number 2,346 to the nearest tens place. This is where it gets tricky, because you aren't going to look at the digit in the tens place, but rather, the digit to the right of it (in the ones, or unit, place). In this case, that digit is 6.

Generally, if the number to the right is 0, 1, 2, 3, or 4, you would round down; if the number to the right is 5, 6, 7, 8, or 9, you would round up. In 2,346, the number 6 is to the right of the tens place. Therefore, you should round up. The number 2,346 rounded to the nearest tens place becomes 2,350.

Let's look at a few more examples to be sure we get this rounding stuff.

5,003 rounded to the nearest hundreds place is 5,000 (because you look at the tens place and see a 0, so you round down). (*Note:* The numbers to the right of the rounded number become zeroes.)

204,800 rounded to the nearest thousands place is 205,000.

7 rounded to the nearest tens place is 10 (because there is technically a zero in the tens place—07—and then you look at the units place and see 7, which rounds up).

You can also round to places that are found to the right of the decimal point (tenths, hundredths, as we discussed before). For example, if you were asked to round $53.29 to the nearest tenths place, the result would be $53.30 because you should look at the digit to the right of the tenths place, which is 9. Since 9 rounds up, the result is $53.30.

Factors

The **factors** of an integer are all of the integers that divide *evenly* into that number. For example, the factors of 30 are

1, 2, 3, 5, 6, 10, 15, and 30

Multiples

A **multiple** of a number is any product of an integer and the given number. For example, 10, 20, 50, 180, and 370 are multiples of 10.

Make sure you know the difference between a factor and a multiple. Factors are Few; Multiples are Many.

Remember This:

Every positive integer is its own greatest factor and least multiple.

Remainders

If an integer cannot be divided evenly by another number, the integer left over at the end of the division is called the **remainder**. Decimals cannot be remainders.

The best way to figure out a reminder is to actually do the long division. For example if you want to find the remainder when 25 is divided by 3, set up and start solving a long division problem.

$$\begin{array}{r} 8 \\ 3{\overline{\smash{\big)}\,25}} \\ \underline{24} \\ 1 \end{array}$$

As you can see in this long division problem, 3 goes into 25 a total of 8 times, as $8 \times 3 = 24$. Subtract 24 from 25 and you get 1. The 1 that is left over is called the remainder.

Consecutive Integers

Consecutive integers are integers listed in increasing order of size without any integers missing in between them.

For example, −1, 0, 1, 2, 3, 4, 5 are consecutive integers.

The integers 2, 4, 5, 7, and 8 are not consecutive integers because they skip 3 and 6.

The integers −1, −2, −3, −4 are not consecutive integers because they are decreasing in size, not increasing in size. If these numbers were reversed to read −4, −3, −2, −1, then they would be consecutive integers because they are increasing in size.

Prime Numbers

A **prime number** is a positive integer that is divisible only by itself and by 1. For example, 5 is a prime number because it is divisible only by itself (5) and by 1. There are a few important facts about prime numbers that you should know:

- 0 and 1 are not prime numbers.
- 2 is the smallest prime number.
- 2 is the only even prime number.
- Not all odd numbers are prime: 1, 9, 15, 21, and many others are *not* prime.

STANDARD SYMBOLS

Symbol	Meaning
=	is equal to
≠	is not equal to
<	is less than
>	is greater than
≤	is less than or equal to
≥	is greater than or equal to

BIG SIX: THE SIX ARITHMETIC OPERATIONS

1. Addition (3 + 3)
2. Subtraction (3 − 3)
3. Multiplication (3 × 3 or 3 • 3)
4. Division (3 ÷ 3)
5. Raising to a **power** (3^3)
6. Finding a **square root** ($\sqrt{3}$)

Quick Review: What Do You Get?

- The result of addition is a sum or a total.
- The result of subtraction is a difference.
- The result of multiplication is a product.
- The result of division is a quotient.
- In the expression 4^3, the 3 is called an **exponent**.

ORDER OF OPERATIONS

To solve problems involving different operations, you must be sure to perform the operations in the proper order. In general, the problems are written in such a way that you won't have trouble deciding what comes first. In cases in which you are uncertain, you need to remember the following sentence:

Please Excuse My Dear Aunt Sally; she limps from *left* to *right* (**PEMDAS** for short).

This sentence reminds you to perform operations in the following order: **Parentheses, exponents and roots, multiplication** and **division**, and **addition** and **subtraction**.

First clear the parentheses; then take care of any exponents; finally, perform all multiplication and division at the same time from left to right, followed by addition and subtraction from left to right.

FRACTIONS

A **fraction** is a number that names a part of a whole or a part of a group. Fractions are most easily recognized when they use the **fraction bar.** The fraction bar, that line between the two numbers, shows that division is taking place.

$$\frac{6}{3}$$

In some cases, the numbers divide evenly, like $\frac{6}{3}$. In other cases, however, these numbers don't divide evenly, like $\frac{5}{2}$ or $\frac{2}{3}$. They leave remainders.

All of these types of numbers are called fractions, whether they express division or part over whole. Fractions are actually pretty great.

A fraction is made up of two parts: the top, also called the **numerator,** and the bottom, also called the **denominator.** In the fraction $\frac{5}{2}$, 5 is the numerator, and 2 is the denominator. The numerator represents the part, and the denominator represents the whole.

For positive numbers, when the numerator (top) of the fraction is a number larger than the denominator (bottom), like $\frac{5}{2}$, the value of the fraction is greater than 1. You already know that because you know that $\frac{5}{2} = 5 \div 2 = 2$ with a remainder of 1, or r1. People in math call this an **improper fraction.** The part is 5 and the whole is 2. Think of it as cutting up apples into 2 pieces, and having 5 of these pieces. Five halves is more than 1 apple.

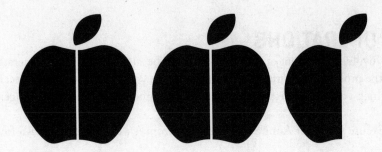

For positive numbers, when the numerator of the fraction is smaller than the denominator, like $\frac{2}{3}$, the value of the fraction is less than 1. This is because 3 can't fit into 2 even one time. This is called a **proper fraction.** It's like cutting up an apple into 3 pieces, and having only 2 of these parts.

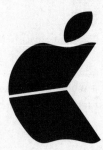

And remember dividing a number by itself? What if you cut an apple into 3 pieces and you had all 3 of them? You would have the whole apple, wouldn't you?

When the numerator and the denominator have the same value, like $\frac{3}{3}$, the fraction is exactly equal to 1.

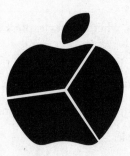

What about when your fraction has a denominator of 1? Any number over 1 is equal to that number. For instance, $\frac{3}{1}$ equals 3. Think about if you had an apple divided into 1 piece—in other words, a whole apple. What if you had three of them? Exactly as it seems; you would have 3 apples.

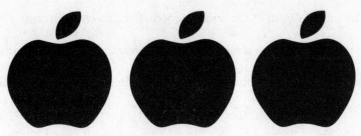

Remember: You can never divide 0 into any number, so the denominator of a fraction can never be 0.

What about when you divide 0 by something else? Well a fraction with the numerator 0 is always equal to 0, no matter what number it has for a denominator. If you had 0 apples cut up into 3 pieces, you would have 0 sets of pieces.

Fractions Smaller Than 1

Lots of math deals with fractions that are smaller than 1. We could think back to the apple and figure that you took a small bite, and maybe the apple consisted of 5 more bites exactly that size, or 6 bites total. So the bite you took was $\frac{1}{6}$, or 1 bite out of a possible 6. The 1 bite represents the part of the apple, and the 6 bites represent the whole. It's back to what we said before—fractions represent part over whole. You say, "one sixth." This number is less than 1, because it is less than the whole of the apple.

Reducing Fractions

Reducing a fraction means dividing *both* the numerator and the denominator by the same number to get a simpler fraction. Use the fraction $\frac{20}{100}$. Look at both the numerator and the denominator. What is a factor of both these numbers? They are both even, so 2 will divide evenly into both of them.

Divide the 20 by 2, and the 100 by 2, and get $\frac{10}{50}$

$$\frac{20 \div 2}{100 \div 2} = \frac{10}{50}$$

Since both 10 and 50 still have a common factor, you can reduce again.

$$\frac{10 \div 10}{50 \div 10} = \frac{1}{5}$$

This fraction, $\frac{1}{5}$, is the simplest form of the same fraction. You know this because 1 has no other factors, so you couldn't divide it again. Equal fractions can look entirely different. For instance, $\frac{20}{100}$ and $\frac{1}{5}$ and $\frac{4}{20}$ and $\frac{3}{15}$ still represent the same number. All the fractions in the last sentence are equal.

Adding Fractions

Think for a minute about what it is you are adding when you add fractions. Let's say you have a box of 100 pencils and you give Julie 3 pencils, or $\frac{3}{100}$ of the box, and you give Sam 1 pencil, or $\frac{1}{100}$ of the box. How many pencils have you given away total? 4. Out of how many pencils? 100. So, you've given away $\frac{4}{100}$ of the box of pencils.

$$\frac{3}{100} + \frac{1}{100} = \frac{4}{100}$$

You add the numerators, but not the denominators. The denominator, or the whole, does not change. You are still talking about 100 pencils. Only the number given away has been altered.

But what happens when the denominators of the fractions are different? If, for example, you want to combine $\frac{1}{2}$ of one apple with $\frac{2}{5}$ of another apple, you need to add the fraction $\frac{1}{2}$ to the fraction $\frac{2}{5}$.

$$\frac{1}{2} + \frac{2}{5}$$

How do you add $\frac{2}{5}$ and $\frac{1}{2}$? By changing the denominators so they are the same. This process is called finding a **common denominator.**

A common denominator is a number that is divisible by both denominators of the fractions you are adding. In this case, since the denominators of the two fractions you are working with are 2 and 5, you can choose the number 10: 10 is divisible by both 2 and 5. The best common denominators are the numbers that are easiest to work with. For instance, 50 is a common denominator because it is also divisible by 5 and 2, but 10 is a smaller number, so it is easier to use.

To change the fraction $\frac{1}{2}$ into a fraction with a denominator of 10, multiply the fraction by $\frac{5}{5}$. *Remember:* Any number over itself is equal to 1, and you can multiply any number by 1 without changing the number. Since $\frac{5}{5}$ is equal to 1, you don't change the value of the fraction. It's like reducing in the opposite direction.

$$\frac{1}{2} \times \frac{5}{5} = \frac{5}{10}$$

To make $\frac{2}{5}$ into a fraction with a denominator of 10, multiply by $\frac{2}{2}$.

$$\frac{2}{5} \times \frac{2}{2} = \frac{4}{10}$$

Now you can add $\frac{4}{10}$ and $\frac{5}{10}$ the same way you added the fractions in which the denominators started out the same.

$$\frac{4}{10} + \frac{5}{10} = \frac{9}{10}$$

You've got $\frac{9}{10}$ of an apple when you combine them.

Finding a common denominator works for fractions larger than 1 in exactly the same way. Try adding $\frac{5}{2}$ and $\frac{4}{3}$.

$$\frac{5}{2} + \frac{4}{3}$$

The easiest to use common denominator of 2 and 3 is 6.

$$\frac{5}{2} \times \frac{3}{3} = \frac{15}{6} \text{ and } \frac{4}{3} \times \frac{2}{2} = \frac{8}{6}$$

You have $\frac{15}{6} + \frac{8}{6} = \frac{23}{6}$.

One way to find a common denominator is to multiply the denominators of a fraction addition problem together. This way, you can be sure that your common denominator is divisible by both.

Sometimes in math, people use the **lowest common denominator.** Look at it this way: You have $\frac{3}{4}$ of a box of erasers and your co-teacher has $\frac{1}{6}$ of a box of erasers. You're trying to figure out if together you have 1 whole box of erasers to give to your students as a class prize. So you want to add the two fractions, $\frac{3}{4}$ of a box and $\frac{1}{6}$ of a box.

$$\frac{3}{4} + \frac{1}{6}$$

As you know, you want to find a common denominator to solve this problem. Of course, one way to find the common denominator would be to multiply the two original denominators together: $4 \times 6 = 24$.

$$\frac{18}{24} + \frac{4}{24} = \frac{22}{24}$$

Reduce $\frac{22}{24}$ and you get $\frac{11}{12}$. You and your co-teacher don't quite have 1 whole box. You are a little bit short.

Here's another way to figure out the same problem. Your denominators, 4 and 6, are factors of 24, but they are also factors of a smaller number: 12. How would you know to look for 12? Try fooling around with the larger denominator. First see if 6 could serve as the denominator. It can't, because 4 is not a factor of 6. Try multiplying 6 by 2. You get 12. Well, what about 12? Sure, because both 4 and 6 are factors of 12.

Multiply $\frac{3}{4}$ by $\frac{3}{3}$ to get 12 as your denominator.

$$\frac{3}{4} \times \frac{3}{3} = \frac{9}{12}$$

Multiply $\frac{1}{6}$ by $\frac{2}{2}$ to get 12 as your denominator.

$$\frac{1}{6} \times \frac{2}{2} = \frac{2}{12}$$

Now add.

$$\frac{9}{12} + \frac{2}{12} = \frac{11}{12}$$

Because fractions can look different and mean the same thing, this is the same addition problem as $\frac{18}{24} + \frac{4}{24} = \frac{22}{24} = \frac{11}{12}$. Same answer, smaller denominator to start, and you skip the step of reducing.

Which is the better way to do it, lowest common denominator or regular old common denominator?

Whichever one you feel more comfortable using.

Let's try a fraction problem.

Of the following fractions, which is smallest?

A. $\frac{3}{5}$

B. $\frac{4}{9}$

C. $\frac{7}{13}$

D. $\frac{2}{9}$

Here's How to Crack It

The trick here is approximation. Choice A is greater than $\frac{1}{2}$, and choices B and C are just under $\frac{1}{2}$. To be around $\frac{1}{2}$, the numerator in choice D would have to be 4 or 5 ($\frac{4}{9}$ or $\frac{5}{9}$) and 2 is far below that. So choice D, $\frac{2}{9}$, is the smallest fraction.

Mixed Numbers

Some fractions are presented as **mixed numbers**. A mixed number is a number that contains both an integer and a fraction, like $4\frac{2}{3}$. You can look at $4\frac{2}{3}$ as representing 4 cans of peas with an additional $\frac{2}{3}$ of a can of peas.

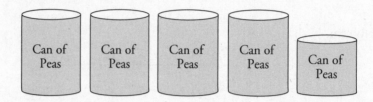

One of the easier ways to work with a number like this is to treat it as an addition problem.

First turn the integer 4 into a fraction, $\frac{4}{1}$. Then $4\frac{2}{3}$ looks like $\frac{4}{1} + \frac{2}{3}$.

Since $4\frac{2}{3}$ has turned into an addition problem, you need to find a common denominator. Since $\frac{4}{1}$ has a denominator of 1, the denominator of $\frac{2}{3}$, which is 3, will work as a common denominator since it is a multiple of 1. Now, just like in any other fraction addition problem, multiply the fraction $\frac{4}{1}$ by $\frac{3}{3}$.

$$\frac{4}{1} \times \frac{3}{3} = \frac{12}{3}$$

Now you can add.

$$\frac{12}{3} + \frac{2}{3} = \frac{14}{3}$$

So you see, $\frac{14}{3}$ is the same number as $4\frac{2}{3}$. You have converted a mixed number into a regular fraction.

Earlier in this chapter, we spoke about ordering integers. You should also understand how to order mixed numbers, factions, decimals, and percents. The exact same rules apply and you just follow the logic that whatever number is farthest down the number line (negative) is the least, and the highest up the number line (positive) is the greatest.

Let's try a problem.

---○---

$$4.5, \frac{50}{100}, 88\%, -26.2$$

Arrange the numbers listed above in the correct order from least to greatest.

A. $4.5, \frac{50}{100}, 88\%, -26.2$

B. $4.5, 88\%, \frac{50}{100}, -26.2$

C. $-26.2, \frac{50}{100}, 88\%, 4.5$

D. $-25.2, 4.5, 88\%, \frac{50}{100}$

Here's How to Crack It

This should be old hat by now. You can eliminate choices A and B immediately, because both choices list

4.5 as the least integer, which cannot be correct since one of the choices is a negative number. Both $\frac{50}{100}$

and 88% $\left(\frac{88}{100}\right)$ are less than 1, so choice D can't be correct. So the correct answer is choice C, –26.2,

$\frac{50}{100}$, 88%, 4.5.

---○---

DECIMALS

As you know from earlier in this chapter, **decimals** are just a way to express fractional parts. The thing to understand about decimals is that they are fractions over powers of ten (10; 100; 1,000; 10,000; and so on).

Adding Decimals

You're saying, "What's so great about decimals?"

One of the great things about decimals is that since they are fractions with powers of ten, you don't have to do anything fancy when you add them. Think about it; their denominators are so similar. All you have to do is make sure that you line the decimal places up evenly so you are adding tenths to tenths, hundredths to hundredths, and all that sort of thing.

Just like with fractions, you wouldn't want to combine decimals with different denominators without thinking about it. And adding decimals will be no problem for you.

Just think about money. A dollar is 100 pennies, so a penny is $\frac{1}{100}$ of a dollar, or 0.01. So you can think about adding money if you ever get confused as to how things should add up.

To add decimals, line them up along the decimal point and add as you would integers.

$$\begin{array}{r} 0.45 \\ + \ 0.1 \\ \hline \end{array}$$

If, as in the problem above, the numbers don't look as if they're the same length—don't worry about it. Just write in a 0 for any missing place and add.

$$\begin{array}{r} 0.45 \\ + \ 0.10 \\ \hline 0.55 \end{array}$$

Subtracting Decimals

Subtracting decimals works much the same way as adding them. Think of fractions again: You need to add and subtract common denominators, so make sure your decimal places are lined up. When one looks shorter, just throw a few 0s onto the end to make it line up.

$$0.01 - 0.002$$

becomes

$$\begin{array}{r} 0.010 \\ - \ 0.002 \\ \hline 0.008 \end{array}$$

You know from working with fractions that numbers can look different and have the same value, like $1 = \dfrac{2}{2} = \dfrac{7}{7}$. The same thing is true of decimals. You can add 0s to the end of a decimal without changing the value of the number, since you are not moving any of the digits with respect to the decimal point.

Adding 0s to a whole number *will* change it.

$$12 \quad \text{to} \quad 120$$

In that case, you move the digits farther to the left of the decimal point, which changes the value of the number. This is just something to keep in mind. If you ever get tempted to start throwing 0s onto the ends of numbers to the left of the decimal point, resist.

Multiplying Decimals

Since you know how to multiply regular numbers, you are eminently qualified to begin multiplication of decimals. If you had four stacks of 50 cents, how much money would you have?

$$4 \times 0.50 =$$

First, multiply the numbers as though they were integers.

$$4 \times 50 = 200$$

Then, count the total number of decimal places, counting from right to left, you had in your *first* setup. You had two places, the tenths place and the hundredths place, so you make sure you put two decimal places in your product, starting from the right.

$$4 \times .50 = 2.00$$

You would have $2.00 if you had four stacks of $0.50 each.

To figure out where the decimal point goes, just count up the total number of decimal places in the numbers you are multiplying and put them in your product, starting from the right.

$$3.5 \times 1.7 =$$

First, multiply the numbers as though they had no decimals at all.

$$
\begin{array}{r}
35 \\
\times\ 17 \\
\hline
245 \\
350 \\
\hline
595
\end{array}
$$

Then, count the number of decimal places you have in the numbers you are multiplying, and add them together. You have one place in 3.5, and one place in 1.7. Together, that gives a total of two places. Count off two decimal places starting at the right.

$$5.95$$

Another way to make sure you have put the right number of decimal places in your answer is to approximate. If you rounded 3.5 and 1.7, what would you have? 4×2. So you know your product will be somewhere near 8. Not 80 or 800.

Dividing Decimals

One of the clearest ways to look at decimal division is to keep this guideline in your head: The divisor should always be in the form of an integer.

$$.3\overline{).45}$$

Since the divisor must be an integer, you don't want to look at it as .3, but rather 3. You may be thinking, "How do I do that?" Just move your decimal place to the right until you have a whole number. In this case, that means you have to move it to the right only once. Once you have transformed your divisor, give the same treatment to your dividend.

$$3.\overline{)4.5}$$

In the dividend, write the decimal point above the place it sits in the dividend. Then divide as you would normally.

$$
\begin{array}{r}
1.5 \\
3\overline{)4.5}
\end{array}
$$

To check your work, you can multiply your quotient by your divisor to see if you get your dividend. And you should always practice approximating to see if your answer looks about right. Are there about 1.5 groups of .3 each in .45? Or how many groups of 30 cents are there in 45 cents? About $1\frac{1}{2}$.

PERCENTAGES

Now we get to **percentages**. And guess what. You know how you feel about decimals after looking at fractions? That whole why-they're-just-fractions-over-powers-of-10,-I'm-not-sure-why-they-seemed-so-terrible feeling? Well it's the same thing with percentages. The only difference is that percentages are an even smaller part of fractions. Percentages are fractions over 100. Percent, when you break it down, becomes per and cent. Per as in "there are 3 hats per every 5 children," which means you have $\frac{3}{5}$ of the hats you need. *Per* means for each.

Cent means 100. Cent is like *cent*ury or *cent*s as in 100 per (there it is again) dollar; so percent means for each 100.

More Practice!

Check out your online companion tools at PrincetonReview.com/cracking to brush up on your math skills with a practice test.

50% means 50 for each 100. It can also look like .5, or $\frac{50}{100}$, or $\frac{1}{2}$ (just reduce the fraction).

100% means 100 for each 100 or $\frac{100}{100}$, which means 1. The whole. If you have 100 percent of something you have the whole thing.

Converting Fractions to Percentages

If a fraction is already over 100, just drop the denominator and add the percent sign.

$$\frac{99}{100} = 99\%$$

If the fraction is over a power of 10, try to convert the denominator to 100 by multiplying by $\frac{10}{10}$, or $\frac{100}{100}$, or reducing to a power of 10 (just move the decimal point on the numerator).

$$\frac{6}{10} = \frac{6}{10} \times \frac{10}{10} = \frac{60}{100} = 60\%$$

$$\frac{5}{1,000} = \frac{5 \div 10}{1,000 \div 10} = \frac{0.5}{100} = 0.5\%$$

And if you are starting from a decimal, translating to a percentage is even easier. The number .68 is 68%, because it is already over 100.

When you want to convert a fraction to a percentage and that fraction is not already over a power of 10, you need to convert the fraction to a decimal. To do this, divide the numerator by the denominator, and then move the decimal place two spaces to the right and add a percent sign.

$$\frac{3}{8} = 8\overline{)3}$$

$$\begin{array}{r} 0.375 \\ 8\overline{)3.000} \\ \underline{2\ 4} \\ 60 \\ \underline{56} \\ 40 \\ \underline{40} \end{array}$$

Put the decimal point two places to the right, and there is your percent: 37.5%. You can also write it as $37\frac{1}{2}\%$. As a fraction, it is $\frac{375}{1,000}$ or back to your original friend, $\frac{3}{8}$. It's all the same number. Isn't that amazing? See how to work it in the other direction now.

Converting Percentages to Standard Fractions

To convert percentages to fractions, put the percentage over 100 and drop the % sign; then reduce.

$$60\% = \frac{60}{100} = \frac{3}{5}$$

Sometimes percentages have fractions in them, like $66\frac{2}{3}\%$. This means it is $66\frac{2}{3}$ over 100, or $66\frac{2}{3}$ divided by 100 (same thing, remember?). To work with this number more easily, try converting $66\frac{2}{3}$ from a mixed number. Once it is converted, you can divide by 100.

Here's another way to convert from a mixed number to a fraction: $66\frac{2}{3} = 3 \times 66 = 198 + 2 = 200; \frac{200}{3}$.

$$66\frac{2}{3} \text{ becomes } \frac{200}{3}$$

$$\frac{200}{3} \div 100 = \frac{200}{3} \times \frac{1}{100} = \frac{200}{300} = \frac{2}{3}$$

Converting Percentages to Decimals

To convert percentages to decimals, move the decimal point two spaces to the left and drop the % sign.

$$75\% = 0.75 \text{ and } 2\% = 0.02$$

Since calculators are not allowed in the NET, the TEAS, or the NLN PAX-RN, you may want to use estimation and time-saving strategies to get through the questions. Problems that concern percentages are a great place to use these shortcuts. Let's take a look at one.

A DVD player is on sale for 20% off its normal price of $400.
If the sales tax is 5%, what is the cost of the VCR?

A. $300
B. $320
C. $336
D. $350

Here's How to Crack It

This question requires two separate operations. First, let's find the sale price of the DVD player.

What is 20% of $400?

By moving the decimal, we can easily deduce that 10% of $400 is $40. Therefore,

20% of 400 = 2 × 40 = $80

So if the DVD player has been marked down by $80, the sale price is $320. Notice that in case you were in too much of a hurry and thought you were already done, $320 was included among the answer choices. Don't fall for it!

Now let's calculate the sales tax.

What's 5% of $320?

Again, by moving the decimal, you can determine that 10% of $320 = $32. Therefore,

$$5\% \text{ of } \$320 = \frac{1}{2} \times 32 = \$16$$

So what is the final price?

$320 + $16 = $336, choice C.

Percent Increase or Decrease

You may have to find the percent that something changes either by increasing or decreasing. Here's the formula to use:

$$\text{Percent increase or percent decrease} = \frac{\text{change}}{\text{original amount}} \times 100$$

Here's an example: Suppose an $80 item is reduced to $60 during a sale. What is the percent decrease? To solve the problem, substitute what you know into the formula above:

$$\text{Percent decrease} = \frac{\text{change}}{\text{original amount}} \times 100$$

$$\text{Percent decrease} = \frac{\$20}{\$80} \times 100$$

$$= .25 \times 100 = 25\%$$

EXPONENTS AND ROOTS

Exponents are a shorthand way of expressing a number multiplied by itself. For instance, 4^3 is 4 times itself three times.

$$4^3 = 4 \times 4 \times 4 = 64$$

The way to express 4^3 aloud is to say either "four to the third power" or "four cubed."

When a fraction is raised to an exponential power, both the numerator and the denominator get raised to that power. For instance, $\left(\dfrac{3}{4}\right)^2 = \dfrac{3 \times 3}{4 \times 4} = \dfrac{9}{16}$.

Multiplying Exponents

What if you wanted to multiply 4^3 by 4^2? How would you express that in exponents? Take a look at what each of those exponents means.

$$4^3 = 4 \times 4 \times 4, \text{ and } 4^2 = 4 \times 4, \text{ so } 4^3 \times 4^2 = 4 \times 4 \times 4 \times 4 \times 4$$

There are 5 fours, so you have 4^5. Since you see how it works, and now it makes perfect sense, from here on in you can just remember this rule: When multiplying exponents with the same **base**, just add the exponents. And what the heck is the base, you say? It is the number that is being raised to a power. In this particular case, the base is 4.

Dividing Exponents

What about when you are trying—you are getting very ambitious here—to divide exponents? For instance, $\dfrac{3^5}{3^2}$.

Again, proceed just as you did with multiplying exponents. Arrange them as multiplication and see what happens.

$$\frac{3 \times 3 \times 3 \times 3 \times 3}{3 \times 3}$$

Two of the threes cancel out, correct? Both $\dfrac{3}{3}$ and $\dfrac{3}{3}$ get counted as 1, because any number over itself is equal to 1 and they both disappear. You are left with $3 \times 3 \times 3$. Or, 3^3. So the rule here is that when you divide exponents with the same base, subtract the exponents.

"But," you ask, "what would have happened if the smaller exponent had been on top, and the larger exponent had been on the bottom?" Well, generally you would leave the larger where it is.

$$\frac{2^4}{2^7} = \frac{2 \times 2 \times 2 \times 2}{2 \times 2 \times 2 \times 2 \times 2 \times 2 \times 2}$$

Cancel where the $\frac{2}{2}$ appears, and you are left with $\frac{1}{2 \times 2 \times 2}$ or $\frac{1}{2^3}$. So you subtract smaller from larger.

But can you subtract and get 2^{-3}? Read on.

Negative Exponents

What happens when you raise 2 to the negative third power (2^{-3})? It is the same as if you had left it $\frac{1}{2^3}$. It becomes $\frac{1}{2 \times 2 \times 2}$, or $\frac{1}{8}$.

Any number raised to a negative power becomes 1 over that number to its exponent's positive power. It all connects.

Adding and Subtracting Exponents

One of the sad things in this world is that there is no real way to add or subtract exponents. Think about it. If you have $2^3 + 2^4$ it is equal to $(2 \times 2 \times 2) + (2 \times 2 \times 2 \times 2) = 8 + 16 = 24$. Unfortunately, you can see that there is no special exponential shortcut, since 24 is not any power of 2, $2^4 = 16$, and $2^5 = 32$.

If you have $2^3 + 2^3$ you can say it is $2(2^3)$, but that is regular old multiplication. Two groups of 2^3 is the same as two times 2^3. Which is 16, by the way. But other than that, there is no way to add exponents with the same base.

Scientific Notation

Numbers can get really huge. Really, really huge. A way to get around it is by using **scientific notation**. Scientific notation uses exponential powers of 10 as a way of expressing numbers. You saw this a few chapters back in the discussion of moles, remember?

$$56.7 \times 10^2$$

Here is an example of scientific notation. Again, to figure out what is going on, expand it. What is 10^2? 100. So you have 56.7×100. To multiply by 100, move the decimal point two spaces to the right, so $56.7 \times 100 = 5,670$.

That is how scientific notation works. Now that you understand it, here is a simpler way to translate the pieces.

Check the exponent of the 10; then move the decimal point that many places to the *right* if the exponent is *positive*.

$$56.7 \times 10^2 = 56.70$$

The exponent here is 2, so you move the decimal point two spaces to the right to get 5,670.

If you get a scientific notation expression in which the exponent is negative, remember what a negative exponent means. $10^{-2} = \dfrac{1}{100}$. Find the exponent of the ten, and move the decimal point that many places to the *left*.

$$56.7 \times 10^{-2} = 0.567$$

Roots

You know that if you square 3, you get 9.

$$3^2 = 3 \times 3 = 9$$

And you know that if you square –3, you also get 9.

$$-3^2 = -3 \times -3 = 9$$

But what about the famed **square roots**? A square root of a particular number is a number that, when squared, will equal that particular number. For example, a square root of 9 is 3. But –3 is also a square root of 9.

The positive square root of a positive number is called the **principal square root.** The sign for square root, called a **radical sign,** looks like this: $\sqrt{}$.

$\sqrt{25}$ = the square root of 25. You need to ask yourself, "What times itself equals 25?" And the answer is 5.

The numbers 9 and 25 are known as **perfect squares.** That is, they are the squares of integers. There are other numbers you will come across that are not perfect squares. For instance, $\sqrt{8}$ is not equal to an integer. In other words, 8 is not a perfect square. You can approximate, of course, and you should, so you feel comfortable with it. Is $\sqrt{8}$ bigger than 2? Well yes, if it were 2, 2^2 is equal to 4, and 8 is bigger than 4, so $\sqrt{8}$ is bigger than 2. Is it bigger than 3? Well, 3^2 is equal to 9, and 9 is bigger than 8, so $\sqrt{8}$ is smaller than 3. In fact, $\sqrt{8}$ is between 2 and 3.

Another way to handle square roots of numbers that are not perfect squares is to factor them out. To do this, find the factors of the number you are taking the square root of, and see if you can take a square root of any of these factors.

$$\sqrt{8} = \sqrt{4 \times 2}$$

Well, 4 is a perfect square, and the square root of 4 is 2. So, you put the 2 outside the square root sign, and leave what remains that cannot be factored to a perfect square, inside. It looks like this:

$$\sqrt{8} = \sqrt{4 \times 2} = 2\sqrt{2}$$

This also shows you that you can multiply square roots by each other. $\sqrt{4} \times \sqrt{2} = \sqrt{8}$.

Other Roots

Square roots are not the only type of roots; there are as many other kinds of roots as there are numbers. Yikes.

To figure out what kind of root a number is, take a look at the number floating high on the left of the radical sign.

$\sqrt[4]{16}$ = the fourth root of 16. This means some number to the fourth power is equal to 16. Here, the number is 2, because $2 \times 2 \times 2 \times 2 = 2^4 = 16$.

Don't worry though; the ones you will come across most frequently are square roots and **cube roots.** A cube root looks like this: $\sqrt[3]{}$.

The cube root of a particular number is a number that, when cubed, equals the particular number. Whew. For instance, what is the cube root of 8?

$$\sqrt[3]{8} = 2, \text{ because } 2 \times 2 \times 2 = 2^3 = 8.$$

Just like with square roots, cube roots are only positive numbers. And just like square roots, and in fact, everything in the world, you should always try to approximate cube roots so you feel comfortable with them as numbers of a certain type.

$$\sqrt[3]{9}$$

Is it bigger than 2? Well, $2^3 = 8$, and 9 is bigger than 8, so yes, $\sqrt[3]{9}$ is bigger than 2.

Is it bigger than 3? Well, $3^3 = 27$, and 9 is not bigger than 27, so no, $\sqrt[3]{9}$ is a lot smaller than 3. It is some number between 2 and 3, that is closer to 2.

Another way to express roots is as fractional exponents. $27^{\frac{1}{3}}$ is just another way of expressing $\sqrt[3]{27}$, or the cube root of 27, which equals 3. And $36^{\frac{1}{2}}$ is another way of expressing $\sqrt{36}$, or the square root of 36, which equals 6.

THE AVERAGE PIE

You probably remember the average formula from math class, which says **average (arithmetic mean)** = $\frac{\text{total}}{\text{\# of things}}$. However, the NLN PAX-RN, NET, and TEAS rarely ask you to take a simple average. Of the three parts of an average problem—the average, the total, and the number of things—you're usually given two of these parts, but often in tricky combinations.

Therefore, the most reliable way to solve average problems is always to use the **average pie**:

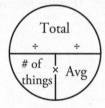

What the pie shows you is that if you know any two of these parts, you can always solve for the third. Once you fill in two of the elements, the pie shows you how to solve for the third part. If you know the total and the number, you can solve the average (total divided by number); if you know the total and the average, you can solve for the number (total divided by average); if you know the number and average, you can solve for the total (number times average).

Let's try this example.

The average (arithmetic mean) of three numbers is 22 and the smallest of these numbers is 2. If the remaining two numbers are equal, what are their values?

A. 22
B. 32
C. 40
D. 64

Here's How to Crack It

Let's start by filling in the average pie. We know that three numbers have an average of 22. So we can fill in the pie, which shows that the sum total of these numbers must be 22 × 3, or 66.

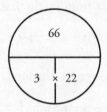

We know that one of the numbers is 2, so we can subtract it from the total we've just found, which leaves 64. What else do we know from the question? That the remaining two numbers are equal, so 64/2 = 32. So the answer is choice B.

MEDIAN AND MODE

There are two more terms you should know: median and mode.

Finding a Median

To find the median of a set containing an even number of items, arrange the numbers in ascending order and then take the average of the two middle numbers.

The **median** of a group of numbers is the number in the middle, just as the "median" is the large divider in the middle of a road. To find the median, here's what you do:

- First, put the elements in the group in numerical order from lowest to highest.
- If the number of elements in your group is *odd*, find the number in the middle. That's the median.
- If you have an *even* number of elements in the group, find the two numbers in the middle and calculate their average (arithmetic mean).

Try this on the following problem:

If the five students in Ms. Jaffray's math class scored 91, 83, 84, 90, and 85 on their final exams, what is the median score for her class on the final exam?

A. 84
B. 85
C. 86
D. 88

Here's How to Crack It

First, place these numbers in order from lowest to highest: 83, 84, 85, 90, 91. The number in the middle is 85, so the median of this group is 85 and the answer is choice B.

The **mode** of a group of numbers is the number that appears the most. (*Remember:* The word *mode* sounds like *most*.) To find the mode of a group of numbers, simply determine which element appears the greatest number of times.

If the seven students in Ms. Holoway's math class scored 91, 83, 92, 83, 91, 85, and 91 on their final exams, what is the mode of her students' scores?

A. 83
B. 85
C. 91
D. 92

Here's How to Crack It

Since the number 91 is the one that appears most often in the list, the mode of these numbers is 91, choice C. Pretty simple!

RATIOS AND PROPORTIONS

Ratios

Ratios vs. Fractions

$$\text{Fraction} = \frac{\text{part}}{\text{whole}}$$

$$\text{Ratio} = \frac{\text{part}}{\text{part}}$$

Ratios are about relationships between numbers. Whereas a fraction is a relationship between a part and whole, a ratio is about the relationship between parts. So, for example, if there were 3 boys and 7 girls in a room, the fraction of boys in the room would be $\frac{3}{10}$. But the ratio of boys to girls would be 3 : 7. Notice that if you add up the parts, you get the whole. 7 + 3 = 10.

Ratio problems usually aren't difficult to identify: The problem will tell you that there is a "ratio" of one thing to another, such as a 2 : 3 ratio of boys to girls in a club. When you see a ratio problem, drawing a **ratio box** will help you organize the information in the problem and figure out the correct answer.

For instance, suppose a problem tells you that there is a ratio of 2 boys to 3 girls in the physics club, which has 40 members total. Here's how you would put that information in a ratio box so that you can answer the question being asked:

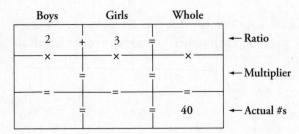

The first line of a ratio box is where you put the *ratio* from the problem. These are parts of the whole; they're not actual numbers of people, animals, books, or anything else. By themselves, they don't tell you *how many* of anything you have.

The second line of a ratio box is for the **multiplier**. The multiplier tells you how much you have to multiply the ratio by to get an actual number of something. The multiplier is the same all the way across; it doesn't change from column to column. And usually, the multiplier isn't in the problem; you have to figure it out yourself.

The third line is for **actual numbers,** so when the problem gives you a number of people (or animals, books, or whatever), that information goes in the third line.

Finally, notice the column labeled "Whole." In the column, you add the numbers in the ratio row and actual numbers row. Don't forget to add a column for the whole—it's usually key in figuring out the problem.

Now that you know some information from the problem and you know how the ratio box works, you can fill in the rest of the box.

	Boys		Girls		Whole	
	2	+	3	=	5	← Ratio
	×		×		×	
	8	=	8	=	8	← Multiplier
	=		=		=	
	16	+	24	=	40	← Actual #s

The first step is adding the ratio columns to find the whole, which is 5. Then you can find the multiplier by figuring out what you need to multiply 5 by to get 40. Once you fill in 8 for the multiplier all the way across the middle row, finding the actual number of boys and girls in the club is a snap.

Now you can answer all kinds of questions about the membership of the physics club. There are 16 boys and 24 girls. Take the $\frac{\text{part}}{\text{whole}}$ from the ratio row to figure out that $\frac{3}{5}$ of the members are girls. That means $\frac{2}{5}$, or 40%, of the members are boys.

Direct Proportion/Variation

Direct proportion problems generally ask you to make a conversion (such as from ounces to pounds) or to compare two sets of information and find a missing piece. For example, a proportion problem may ask you to figure out the amount of time it will take to travel 300 miles at a rate of 50 miles per hour.

> To solve proportion problems, just set up two equal fractions.
> One will have all the information you know, and the other will
> have a missing piece that you're trying to figure out.

$$\frac{50 \text{ miles}}{1 \text{ hour}} = \frac{300 \text{ miles}}{x \text{ hours}}$$

Be sure to label the parts of your proportion so you'll know you have things in the right place; the same units should be in the numerator on both sides of the equal sign and the same units should be in the denominator on both sides of the equal sign. Notice how using a setup like this helps us keep track of the information we have and to find the information we're looking for, so we can use bite-sized pieces to work through the question.

Now we can cross-multiply and then solve for x: $50x = 300$, so $x = 6$ hours.

Let's try the following problem.

John receives $2.50 for every 4 pounds of berries he picks. How much money will he receive if he picks 90 pounds of berries?

A. $36.00
B. $42.25
C. $48.50
D. $56.25

Here's How to Crack It

To solve this, set up a proportion.

$$\frac{\$2.50}{4\,\text{pounds}} = \frac{x}{90\,\text{pounds}}$$

Now we can cross-multiply. $4x = 2.50 \times 90$, so $4x = 225$, and $x = 56.25$. The answer is choice D.

RATE PROBLEMS

You might see one or two questions on the NLN PAX-RN, NET, or TEAS that ask you about rates, so let's do a quick review. **Rate** problems are usually about cars, boats, or trains, and they are often expressed in terms of miles per hour or kilometers per hour.

The formula for rate looks like this:

$$\text{rate} \times \text{time} = \text{distance}$$

For example, if you drive your car for two hours at 50 miles per hour, you will have traveled 100 miles. Fifty miles per hour is the rate at which you traveled, 2 hours is the time it took you to travel, and 100 miles is the distance you traveled.

Let's tackle a rate problem before we close out this thrilling ride through arithmetic.

———————————○———————————

> A train traveled at a speed of 120 kilometers per hour for 2½ hours. How many kilometers did the train travel?
>
> **A.** 300
> **B.** 280
> **C.** 240
> **D.** 200

Here's How to Crack It

As soon as you see the word train and travel, you should immediately be thinking rate $\times$ time = distance. Now all you have to do is plug in the numbers they gave you.

$$\text{rate} \times \text{time} = \text{distance}$$

$$120 \times 2\frac{1}{2} = ?$$

Multiply 120 by $2\frac{1}{2}$ (2.5) to get 300, which is choice A.

———————————○———————————

SUMMARY

- An integer is a number that is not a fraction or a decimal. 0 is an integer.

- A number line is a visual representation of positive and negative numbers.

- The absolute value of a number is its distance from zero on the number line.

- Digits are the integers 0 through 9. The digits in a number have names based on location. To the left of the decimal point are the ones (units) place, the tens place, the hundreds place, the thousands place, and so on. To the right of the decimal are the tenths place, the hundredths place, the thousandths place, and so on.

- Distributive law: If you are multiplying one number by the sum of two numbers, you can multiply each number in your sum individually. With variables, this law is shown as $a(b + c) = a(b) + a(c)$.

- Decimals are a way to express fractions. The numbers to the right of the decimal point are called decimal places.

- A factor is a number that divides evenly into another number. It is smaller than or equal to the original number.

- A multiple of a number is the product of that number and any integer. It is larger than or equal to the original number.

- For the order of operations, remember PEMDAS; she limps from left to right (Parenthesis, Exponents, Multiplication, Division, Addition, Subtraction).

- A fraction is a numerical way of expressing part to whole. The top number in a fraction is called the numerator; the bottom number is called the denominator. Reducing and finding the common denominator are helpful tools for working with fractions.

- A decimal is another way to express a fraction.

- A percentage is a fraction over 100.

- Exponents are a shorthand way of expressing a number multiplied by itself.

- A square root of a particular number is the number that, when squared, will equal that number.

- The average pie is useful when you know two out of three pieces of a puzzle. You can use the two pieces to solve for the third. The average (arithmetic mean) is $\frac{\text{total}}{\text{number of things}}$.

- The median of a group of numbers is the number in the middle when the numbers are arranged in ascending or descending order.

- The mode of a group of numbers is the number that appears most frequently.

- A ratio shows the relationship between two numbers. Use the ratio box to organize information in a ratio question.

- For proportion problems, set up two equal fractions—one with the information you know and another with the information you don't know.

- Rate $\times$ time = distance.

- The formula for percent change is

$$\% \text{ change} = \frac{\text{amount change}}{\text{original}} \times 100$$

KEY TERMS

integers

positive integers

negative integers

number line

even numbers

odd numbers

addition

sum

subtraction

difference

multiplication

product

distributive law (distributive property)

commutative law (commutative property)

positive numbers

negative numbers

division

quotient

multiplicative identity

distinct numbers

digit

thousands place

hundreds place

tens place

unit place (ones place)

tenths place

hundredths place

thousandths place

decimal point

round up or down

factors

multiple

remainder

consecutive integers

prime numbers

power

square root

exponent

PEMDAS

fraction

fraction bar

numerator

denominator

improper fraction

proper fraction

reducing fractions

common denominator

lowest common denominator

mixed number

decimal

percentages

exponent

base

scientific notation

square root

principal square root

radical sign

perfect square

cube root

average (arithmetic mean)

average pie

median

mode

ratio

ratio box

multiplier

actual numbers

direct proportion

rate

Chapter 10
Algebra

ALGEBRA IN NURSING

This section of the review is important not only for your nursing school entrance exam, but also for the foundation of the mathematics you'll need to calculate dosages for medications and the day-to-day drug conversions that are necessary before considering administration to a patient. Most dosage calculations are in the algebraic ratio and proportion type format as derived from the following sample:

Medication order: 5 mg diphenhydramine orally now × one dose.

You have a bottle that reads 12.5 mg diphenhydramine per 1tsp (5 ml).

Calculate 12.5 mg is to 5 ml as 5 mg is to x (how many ml)?

Written as $\dfrac{12.5 \text{ mg}}{5 \text{ ml}} = \dfrac{5 \text{ mg}}{x \text{ ml}}$

$12.5x = 5 \times 5$

$12.5x = 25$

$x = 2$

Answer: 2ml

How did we get there? A few steps:

1. Put what you have on hand on the left side of the equation.
2. Put what you need or want on the right side of the equation.
3. Multiply the two inside numbers.
4. Multiply the two outside numbers.

The equation now looks like this $12.5x = 25$.

x is on the left side and your job is to get x alone.

Then x is the answer.

Units of Measure

The United States health care system uses the **metric system** of measurement. This system of measurement is used on a day-to-day basis in most of the world, except the United States. The United States uses the U.S. system. You're probably quite familiar with this system already, if you have ever talked about losing 5 pounds or drinking a bunch of 8-ounce glasses of water each day, or driving a few miles.

First, let's review each system and then cover conversion of units from one system to another. You will definitely see at least one question about conversion on your nursing school entrance exam.

U.S. System of Measurement

Mass/Weight
16 ounces = 1 pound
2,000 pounds = 1 ton

Fluid/Volume
8 ounces = 1 cup
2 cups = 1 pint
2 pints = 1 quart
4 quarts = 1 gallon

Length
12 inches = 1 foot
3 feet = 1 yard
5,280 feet = 1 mile

Metric System of Measurement

Mass/Weight
1 gram = 1,000 milligrams
1 gram = 100 centigrams
10 grams = 1 dekagram
100 grams = 1 hectogram
1,000 grams = 1 kilogram
1,000 kilograms = 1 metric ton

Fluid/Volume
1 liter = 1,000 milliliters
1,000 liters = 1 kiloliter
1 milliliter = 1 cubic centimeter (known as cc)

Length
1,000 millimeters = 100 centimeters
100 centimeters = 10 decimeters
10 decimeters = 1 meter
1,000 meters = 1 kilometer

The metric system is a **decimal system**. That is, its base is 10. To convert a large metric unit (grams) to a smaller unit (milligrams), simply multiply by 1,000 or move the decimal point 3 places (because 1,000 has 3 zeros) to the right. So, if you need to convert 2 grams to milligrams, the answer is 2,000. To convert milligrams (small unit) to grams (large unit), just do the opposite: Either divide by 1,000 or move the decimal point 3 places to the left. So if you need to convert 40 mg to grams, the answer is 0.040 grams.

In your nursing work, you might see dosages in drops (gtt). This measurement is used for eyedrops, eardrops, and oral drops. For the NCLEX-RN exam you'll take years from now, you'll have to be familiar with IV maintenance. For example, you'll need to know how many gtts are in a ml or an IV machine or drip set that administers 10 gtts per minute or 110 cc per hour.

U.S./Metric Conversions

On your exam, you will definitely see at least one question that will ask you to convert metric units to U.S. units, or vice versa. So let's do a quick review.

U.S. Measurement	Metric Measurement
1.09 yards	1 meter
1 inch	2.54 centimeters
2.2 pounds	1 kilogram
1 ounce	28 grams
1.06 quarts	1 liter
14 pounds	1 stone
1 ounce	30 mL
1 tablespoon	15 mL
About ½ an ounce	15 cc

Let's look at a sample question that requires you to convert from one metric unit to another.

Complete the following conversion: 628 milligrams = _____ grams.

A. .628
B. 6.28
C. 62,800
D. 628,000

Here's How to Crack It

Since 1 gram = 1,000 milligrams, you're converting from a small unit to a larger unit. Therefore, you must divide by 1,000 (that is, move the decimal point three places to the left). If you move the decimal point in 628 three places to the left, the result is .628. Choice A is the correct answer. Notice that choice D is 628 multiplied by 1,000. Make sure you choose the correct function.

Now, let's try a question that requires conversion from the U.S. system of measurement to the metric system.

Approximately how many quarts are in 16 liters?

A. 14.94
B. 15.09
C. 16.96
D. 17.06

Here's How to Crack It

Since 1.06 quarts = 1 liter, you're converting from a large unit to a smaller unit. Therefore, you must multiply. 16 liters × 1.06 = 16.96. Choice C is correct. *Note:* Since you're going from a larger unit to a smaller unit, your answer must be larger than the original number (16). Therefore, you should be able to immediately eliminate choices A and B, since they are smaller than 16.

Finally, here's a question that illustrates real application to the world of nursing.

A patient is receiving solution from an IV of DSW (Dextrose 5% Water)—that is, the bag of solution contains 5 g dextrose per 100 ml of water in it. How much sugar is patient x receiving from this IV, per 1 ml of solution?

Here's How To Crack It

Since you know that 5 g = 5,000 mg, you can rewrite the ingredients to be 5,000 mg per 100 ml. You can further break down that math just as you would simple fractions (as discussed in Chapter 9: Arithmetic) to be 50 mg dextrose per 1 ml, by just removing the two zeros from 5,000 and 100 or by simple long division to give 50/1. Therefore, the answer is 50 mg dextrose per 1 ml solution.

When you get into your nursing career, you will learn that normal saline (NS) is also written as 0.9% saline solution. It is isotonic due to the fact that the osmolarity of normal saline is a close approximation to the osmolarity of NaCl (sodium chloride) found in our cells and blood. In time, you will be familiar with hypotonic solutions (less than 0.9%), hypertonic solutions (more than 0.9%), and other isotonic solutions frequently used in the hospital setting. Let's start reviewing general algebraic equations so you can apply the concepts to nursing situations later on.

PLUGGING IN

One of the most powerful problem-solving skills that you can use on the NLN PAX-RN, NET, or TEAS is a technique we call Plugging In. This technique will turn nasty algebra problems into simple arithmetic and help you through the particularly twisted problems that you'll often see on your exam. There are several varieties of Plugging In, each suited to a different kind of question.

Plugging In Your Own Numbers

The problem with doing algebra is that it's just too easy to make a mistake.

> Whenever you see a problem with variables in the answer choices, PLUG IN.

Start by picking a number for the variable in the problem (or for more than one variable, if necessary), solve the problem using your number, and then see which answer choice gives you the correct answer.

Take a look at the following problem:

_____

When to Plug In
- Phrases like "in terms of k" in the question
- Varables in the answers

If x is a positive integer, then 20% of $5x$ equals

A. x
B. $2x$
C. $5x$
D. $15x$

Here's How to Crack It

Let's start by picking a number for x. Let's plug in a nice round number such as 10. When we plug in 10 for x, we change every x in the whole problem into a 10. Now the problem reads as follows:

If 10 is a positive integer, then 20% of 5(10) equals

A. 10
B. 2(10)
C. 5(10)
D. 15(10)

Look how easy the problem becomes! Now we can solve: 20 percent of 50 is 10. Which answer says 10? Choice A does.

Let's try it again on a harder question.

If $-1 < x < 0$, then which of the following has the greatest value?

A. x
B. x^2
C. x^3
D. $\dfrac{1}{x}$

Here's How to Crack It

This time when we pick a number for x, we have to make sure that it is between -1 and 0, because that's what the problem states. So let's try $-\dfrac{1}{2}$. If we make every x in the problem equal to $-\dfrac{1}{2}$, the problem now reads as follows:

If $-1 < -\dfrac{1}{2} < 0$, then which of the following has the greatest value?

A. $-\dfrac{1}{2}$

B. $\left(-\dfrac{1}{2}\right)^2$

C. $\left(-\dfrac{1}{2}\right)^3$

D. $\dfrac{1}{-\dfrac{1}{2}}$

Plugging In Quick Reference

- When you see *in terms of* and variables in the answers choices, you can plug in.
- Pick your own number for an unknown in the problem.
- Do the necessary math to find the answer you're shooting for, or the target. Circle the target.
- Use POE to eliminate every answer that doesn't equal the target.

Now we can solve the problem. Which has the greatest value? Choice A is $-\frac{1}{2}$, choice B equals $\frac{1}{4}$, choice C equals $-\frac{1}{8}$, and choice D equals -2. So choice B has the greatest value.

Plugging In is such a great technique because it turns hard algebra problems into medium and sometimes easy arithmetic questions. Remember this technique when you see variables in the answers.

Don't worry too much about what numbers you choose to plug in; just plug in easy numbers (small numbers like 2, 5, or 10 or numbers that make the arithmetic easy like 100 if you're looking for a percent). Also, be sure your numbers fit the conditions of the questions (if they say $x \leq 11$, don't plug in 12).

What If There's No Variable?

Sometimes you'll see a problem that doesn't contain an x, y, or z, but which contains a hidden variable. If your answers are percents or fractional parts of some unknown quantity (total number of marbles in a jar, total miles to travel in a trip), try using Plugging In.

Take a look at this problem:

In a certain high school, the number of seniors is twice the number of juniors. If 60% of the senior class and 40% of the junior class attend the last football game of the season, approximately what percent of the combined junior and senior class attends the game?

A. 60%
B. 53%
C. 50%
D. 47%

Here's How to Crack It

What number, if we knew it, would make the math work on this problem incredibly easy? The number of students. So let's plug in a number and work the problem. Suppose that the number of seniors is 200 and the number of juniors is 100.

If 60% of the 200 seniors and 40% of the 100 juniors go to the game, that makes 120 seniors and 40 juniors, or 160 students. What fraction of the combined class went to the game? $\frac{160}{300}$, or about 53%. So the answer is choice B.

———————◯———————

Let's try a problem in which you don't need to solve for the variable, but just place the variable correctly.

———————◯———————

At a state fair, Martha was charged $5.00 for entry, $4.00 for parking, and $1.50 for each game she played. If she played p games, how much did she spend in all?

A. $\dfrac{1.5}{p} + 9$

B. $1.5p + 9$

C. $9p + 1.5$

D. $(1.5 + 9)p$

Here's How to Crack It

This question is an easy one, and it's about placing the variable correctly. Each game costs $1.50 and Martha played p games, so you know that $1.50 and p need to be next to each other because they are going to be multiplied. That makes choice B a pretty obvious answer, but double-check the other part of the equation to be sure. $5.00 + $4.00 = $9.00, so choice B is the only correct answer.

———————◯———————

Plugging In the Answers (PITA)

You can also plug in when the answers to a problem are actual values, such as 2, 4, 10, or 20. Why would you want to do a lot of complicated algebra to solve a problem, when the answer is right there on the page? All you have to do is figure out *which* choice it is.

How can you tell which is the correct answer? Try every choice *until you find the one that works*. Even if this means you have to try all four choices, PITA is still a fast and reliable means of getting the right answer.

But if you use your head, you almost never have to try all four choices. When you plug in the answer choices, begin with the value that's in the middle. If that value works, you're done. If the value is too small, you know the correct answer must be a larger number. If it doesn't work because it's too big, then go in the other direction and try one of the smaller numbers. You can save time by finding the answer in two or three tries.

Let's try PITA on the following problem.

―――――――――○―――――――――

PITA = Plugging In the Answers

Don't try to solve problems like this by writing equations and solving for x or y. Plugging In the Answers lets you use arithmetic instead of algebra, so you're less likely to make errors.

If the average (arithmetic mean) of 8 and x is equal to the average of 5, 9, and x, what is the value of x ?

A. 1
B. 2
C. 4
D. 8

Here's How to Crack It

Let's start with choice C and plug in 4 for x. The problem now reads as follows:

If the average (arithmetic mean) of 8 and 4 is equal to the average of 5, 9, and 4 . . .

Does this work? The average of 8 and 4 is 6, and the average of 5, 9, and 4 is also 6. Therefore, choice C is the answer.

―――――――――○―――――――――

Neat, huh? Let's try one more.

―――――――――○―――――――――

If $(x - 2)^2 = 2x - 1$, which of the following is a possible value of x ?

A. 1
B. 2
C. 3
D. 6

Here's How to Crack It

If we try plugging in choice C, 3, for *x*, the equation becomes 1 = 5, which is false. So choice C can't be right. If you're not sure which way to go next, just pick a direction. It won't take very long to figure out the correct answer. If we try plugging in choice B, 2, for *x*, the equation becomes 0 = 3, which is false. If we try plugging in choice A, 1, for *x*, the equation becomes 1 = 1, which is true. There's no need to try other answers, because there are no variables; only one answer choice can work. So the answer is choice A.

Sets

Sets are basically lists of distinct numbers. The numbers in a set are called **elements,** or **members**.

For example, if a problem asks for the set of even integers greater than 0 but less than 12, the set would be {2, 4, 6, 8, 10}.

Let's try one.

If set *X* = {2, 3, 5, 7} and set *Y* = {3, 6, 8}, then which of the following represents the union of *X* and *Y* ?

A. {3}
B. {2, 3}
C. {2, 3, 5, 7}
D. {2, 3, 5, 6, 7, 8}

Here's How to Crack It

The question asks for the union of the two sets, so you need to combine the elements into one big set, as in choice D. Watch out for choice A, which is the tricky answer; it's the intersection of sets *X* and *Y*, not the union.

EXPANDING, FACTORING, AND SOLVING QUADRATIC EQUATIONS

You're likely to see at least one problem that asks you to work with **quadratic equations**. It may have been a little while since you've done this, so let's review.

Expanding

Most often you'll be asked to **expand an expression** simply by multiplying it out. When working with an expression of the form $(x + 3)(x + 4)$, multiply it using the following rule:

> FOIL = First Outer Inner Last

Multiply the *first* figure in each set of parentheses: $x \times x = x^2$

Now multiply the two *outer* figures: $x \times 4 = 4x$

Next, multiply the two *inner* figures: $3 \times x = 3x$

Finally, multiply the *last* figure in each set of parentheses: $3 \times 4 = 12$

Add them all together to get $x^2 + 4x + 3x + 12$, or $x^2 + 7x + 12$

Factoring

If you ever see an expression of the form $x^2 + 7x + 12$, there is a good chance that **factoring** it will be the key to cracking it.

The key to factoring is figuring out what pair of numbers will multiply to give you the constant term (12, in this case) and add up to the coefficient of the x term (7, in this question).

Let's try an example.

Factor the following expression:

$$x^2 + 7x + 12$$

▬ STEP 1:

Draw two sets of parentheses next to each other and fill an x into the left side of each. That's what gives us our x^2 term.

$$(x \quad)(x \quad)$$

▬ STEP 2:

12 can be factored a number of ways: 1×12, 2×6, and 3×4. Which of these adds up to 7? 3 and 4, so place a 3 on the right side of one parenthesis and a 4 in the other.

$$(x \quad 3)(x \quad 4)$$

▬ STEP 3:

Now we need to figure out what the correct signs should be. Both should be positive in this case, because that will sum to 7 and multiply to 12, so fill plus signs into each parenthesis.

$$(x + 3)(x + 4)$$

If you want to double-check your work, try expanding $(x + 3)(x + 4)$ using FOIL. If your work is correct, you should get the original expression.

Now try the following problem.

───────────○───────────

If $\dfrac{x^2 + 5x - 6}{x - 1} = 2$, then what is the value of x ?

A. -4
B. -1
C. 5
D. 6

Here's How to Crack It

Since we know we can factor $x^2 + 5x - 6$, we should do so. When we factor it, we get $\dfrac{(x-1)(x+6)}{(x-1)} = 2$.

Now we can cancel the $(x - 1)$ and we're left with $x + 6 = 2$. If we solve for x, we find $x = -4$ and our answer is choice A.

Don't forget that we can also just Plug In the Answers!

───────────○───────────

Solving Quadratic Equations

The following test sample question is clearly the most difficult type in the land of algebraic sample questions. It is very unlikely that you will ever see a test question written that has two possible values for x. However, we have broken down the process step by step to demonstrate the ease in finding the most effective method to answer the question (should you feel daring). We guarantee you will *never* see a medication calculation that has more than one value for x. It is one medication per calculation in real life and one variable for x for NLN PAX-RN or NSEE test-taking purposes. Tylenol and Aspirin are Tylenol and Aspirin. You can and must calculate drug dosages one at a time. (*Note:* If you are taking the NET, which is primarily math, there may be a complicated algebraic question that gives more than one value for x. NET test takers be warned.) Either way, it's a good practice question to check your math skills. Let's take a look.

Sometimes you'll need to factor to solve an equation. In this case, there will be two possible values for x, called the **roots** of the equation. To solve for x, use the following steps:

■ STEP 1:

Make sure that the equation is set equal to zero.

■ STEP 2:

Factor the equation.

■ STEP 3:

Set each parenthetical expression equal to zero. So if you have $(x + 2)(x - 7) = 0$, you get $(x + 2) = 0$ and $(x - 7) = 0$. When you solve for each, you get $x = -2$ and $x = 7$. Therefore, -2 and 7 are the solutions or roots of the equation.

Try the following problem.

If $x^2 + 2x - 15 = 0$, then the possible values of x are

A. 2 and 4
B. −13 and −4
C. 5 and −4
D. −5 and 3

Here's How to Crack It

Let's try the steps:

■ STEP 1:

The equation is already set equal to zero.

■ STEP 2:

Factor the left side of the equation to get $(x + 5)(x - 3) = 0$.

■ STEP 3:

Set each parenthetical expression equal to zero to get $x = -5$ and $x = 3$. Therefore, the answer is choice D.

Now that you have a solid foundation of arithmetic and algebra, let's keep moving in our math review. Up next is geometry. We're getting there.

SUMMARY

- The U.S. health care system uses the metric system of measurement. You should know units of measure in both the metric system of measurement and the U.S. system of measurement. You also need to know how to convert from one system to the other.

- Plugging In is a fantastic strategy to turn complex algebra problems into simple arithmetic problems. Try out a few sub-strategies of Plugging In: Plug in your own numbers, plug in even when you don't see an obvious variable, and plug in the answer choices that you are given.

- Tackle quadratic equations by either expanding or factoring.

- When you expand an equation, multiply it using FOIL (first, outer, inner, then last).

- When you factor a quadratic equation, you are trying to figure out what pair of numbers will multiply to give you the constant term that you need.

KEY TERMS

metric system
decimal system
sets
elements (members)
quadratic equations
expand an expression
factoring
roots

Chapter 11
Geometry

LINES, ANGLES, AND TRIANGLES—OH MY!

You won't be using the rule of 180 or the Pythagorean theorem to run any cardiac arrests or calculate IV drips for your patients, that's for sure. As a nurse, you may find yourself moving beds and medication carts, shuffling patients, monitoring visitors and equipment, but that sounds more like physics. There are not any nursing notes or charting tasks that will include geometry in your nursing career. However, in order to be considered a nursing school candidate, you must refresh your geometry knowledge and skills that will be tested on the nursing school entrance exam. Should you decide to take the NET, you must have stellar math skills, as the NET is mostly math. For those of you preparing for the NLN PAX-RN or TEAS, you will encounter around 45–54 math questions, which will definitely cover geometry. So let's get into it.

GEOMETRY DEFINITIONS

Lines and Angles

Common sense might tell you what a line is, but let's review the particulars of a line, a ray, and a line segment.

A **line** continues on in each direction forever. You need only two points to form a line, but that line does not end at those points. A straight line has 180 degrees on each side.

A **ray** is a line with one distinct endpoint. Again, you need only two points to designate a ray, but one of those points is where it stops—it continues on forever in the other direction. A ray has 180 degrees as well.

A **line segment** is a line with two distinct endpoints. It requires two points, and its length is the distance from one point to the other. A line segment has 180 degrees.

Whenever you have **angles** on a line, remember the **rule of 180**: The angles on any line must add up to 180. In the figure below, what is the value of x? We know that $2x + x$ must add up to 180, so we know that $3x = 180$. This makes $x = 60$.

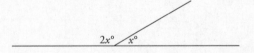

Vertical angles are angles that are opposite each other when two lines cross. These angles have the same measure. In the figure below, angles x and z are vertical angles and y and 130° are vertical angles. Angle z must equal 50, since $130 + z$ must equal 180. Angle y is 130, since it is across from the angle 130. Angle x is 50, since it is across from z.

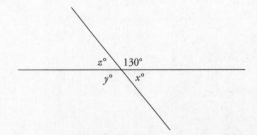

When two lines are crossed by a third line (called a **transversal**), eight angles are formed. In the figure below, the angles formed are *a, b, c, d, e, f, g,* and *h.* Within this configuration are specific pairs of angles called **corresponding angles**, which are angles on the same side of the transversal (either left or right) and the same side of the lines (either top or bottom). In the figure below, the following pairs of angles are corresponding angles: *a* and *e, c* and *g, b* and *f,* and *d* and *h.* When the two lines crossed by a transversal are parallel, all pairs of corresponding angles are equal. Since *l*1 is parallel to *l*2, angle *a* is equal to angle *e,* angle *c* is equal to angle *g,* angle *b* is equal to angle *f,* and angle *d* is equal to angle *h.*

Now, you also just learned that vertical angles are equal. In the figure below, the following angles are vertical angles: *a* and *d, c* and *b, e* and *h,* and *g* and *f.*

If you put corresponding angles and vertical angles together, you can determine that angles *a, e, d,* and *h* are equal; and angles *c, g, b,* and *f* are equal.

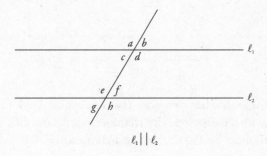

$\ell_1 \| \ell_2$

Four-Sided Figures

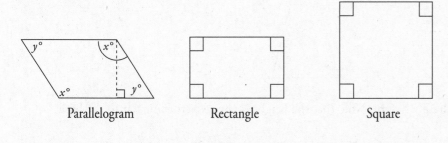

Parallelogram   Rectangle   Square

A figure with two sets of parallel sides is a **parallelogram**. In a parallelogram, the opposite angles are equal, and any adjacent angles add up to 180 degrees. (In the figure above, *x* + *y* = 180 degrees.) Opposite sides are also equal.

If all of the angles are also right angles, then the figure is a **rectangle**. And if all of the sides are the same length, then the figure is a **square**.

The **area** of a square, rectangle, or parallelogram is **length × width**. (In the parallelogram above, the length is shown by the dotted line.) The area of a square, specifically, is sometimes written as $A = s^2$. Since the sides of a square are the same length, the area can be expressed as *s* × *s*, which is the same as s^2. Therefore, the area of a square can be correctly written as $A = s^2$.

Thinking Inside the Box

Here's a progression of quadrilaterals from least specific to most specific:

quadrilateral = 4-sided figure

↓

parallelogram =
a quadrilateral in which opposite sides are parallel

↓

rectangle =
a parallelogram in which all angles equal 90°

↓

square =
a rectangle in which all sides are equal

The **perimeter** of any figure is the sum of the lengths of its sides. Again, because the sides of a square are equal, its perimeter can be expressed as 4*s*.

Triangles

The sum of the angles inside a **triangle** equals 180 degrees. This means that if you know two of the angles in a triangle, you can always solve for the third. Since we know that two of the angles in the following figure are 90 and 60 degrees, we can solve for the third angle, which must be 30 degrees.

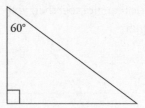

An **isosceles triangle** is a triangle that has two sides that are equal. Angles that are opposite equal sides are equal. In the figure below, we have an isosceles triangle. Since $AB = BC$, we know that angles x and y are equal. And since their sum must be 150 degrees (to make a total of 180 degrees when we add the last angle), they must be 75 degrees each.

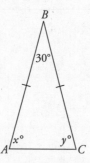

The area of a triangle is $\frac{1}{2}$ **base × height**. Note that the height is always perpendicular to the base.

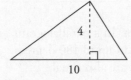 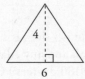

$$\text{Area} = \frac{1}{2} \times 10 \times 4 = 20 \qquad \text{Area} = \frac{1}{2} \times 6 \times 4 = 12$$

An **equilateral triangle** has all three sides equal and all of its angles equal to 60 degrees.

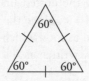

Here's a typical example of a question that you might see on your exam.

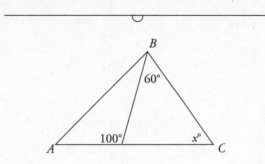

In triangle *ABC* above, *x* =

A. 30°
B. 40°
C. 50°
D. 60°

Here's How to Crack It

We know that the angle adjacent to the 100-degree angle equals 80 degrees since we know that a straight line is 180 degrees. Fill it in on your diagram. Now, since we know that the sum of the angles contained in a triangle equals 180 degrees, we know that 80 + 60 + *x* = 180, so *x* = 40. That's choice B.

Plugging In on Geometry

You can also plug in on geometry questions, just as you did back in the algebra chapter. Anytime you have variables in the answer choices, or hidden variables, plug in! As long as you follow all the rules of geometry while you solve, you'll get the answer.

Take a look at this problem.

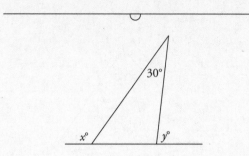

In the figure above, what is the value of $x + y$?

A. 140°
B. 180°
C. 190°
D. 210°

Here's How to Crack It

We can plug in whatever numbers we want for the other angles inside the triangle—as long as we make sure that all the angles in the triangle add up to 180 degrees. So let's plug in 60 and 90 for the other angles inside that triangle. Now we can solve for x and y: If the angle next to x is 60 degrees, then x will be equal to 120. If the angle next to y is equal to 90 degrees, then y will be equal to 90. This makes the sum $x + y$ equal to 120 + 90, or 210. No matter what numbers we pick for the angles inside the triangle, we'll always get the same answer, choice D.

Plugging In is a great tool, but what if you hate it? Let's walk through a problem that combines geometry and algebra and solve it the old-fashioned way.

The perimeter of a regular hexagon is $7x + 10$ cm and one side of the hexagon is $x + 3$ cm. What is the actual length of each side of the hexagon?

A. 5 cm
B. 8 cm
C. 11 cm
D. 12 cm

Here's How to Crack It

The question tells us that one side of the hexagon is $x + 3$, so the perimeter of the entire hexagon must be $6(x + 3)$, which is the same value as $7x + 10$, as the question says. Therefore, $6(x + 3) = 7x + 10$. To solve this equation, first distribute the 6 across the items in parenthesis:

$$6x + 18 = 7x + 10$$

Subtract $6x$ from both sides of the equation and 10 from both sides of the equation. The result is $x = 8$. But you're not done yet, so don't fall for the trick answer choice B. To find the value of one side, you must plug 8 into the equation for one side $(x + 3)$. Since $8 + 3 = 11$, the correct answer is choice C.

─────────○─────────

Let's take a look at another triangle question that you might see on the NLN PAX-RN.

─────────○─────────

In the figure below, $\triangle ABC$ is isosceles, $\triangle ADE$ is equilateral, and $m\angle BAD = 25°$.

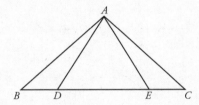

What is the measure of $\angle ABC$?

A. 30°
B. 35°
C. 60°
D. 70°

Here's How to Crack It

Use the given information and your knowledge of triangles to gather more information. We know that angle BAD is 25 degrees and since triangle ADE is equilateral, each of its three angles must be 60 degrees (to total 180). Since angle ADE is 60 degrees, angle ADB must be 120 degrees (to total 180 across the line BC). Since the angles of all triangles total 180 degrees, simply add $120 + 25 = 145$, but we're not done yet. The entire triangle must be 180, so take $180 - 145 = 35$. Choice B is the correct answer.

─────────○─────────

THE PYTHAGOREAN THEOREM

Whenever you have a right triangle, you can use the **Pythagorean theorem**, which says that the sum of the squares of the **legs** of a right triangle (the sides that form the right angle) equals the square of the **hypotenuse** (the side opposite the right angle).

Pythagorean Theorem

$a^2 + b^2 = c^2$, where c is the hypotenuse of a right triangle. Learn it, love it.

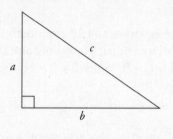

$$a^2 + b^2 = c^2$$

Two of the most common ratios of sides that fit the Pythagorean theorem are 3 : 4 : 5 and 5 : 12 : 13. Since these are ratios, any multiples of these numbers will also work, such as 6 : 8 : 10, and 30 : 40 : 50.

Try the following example.

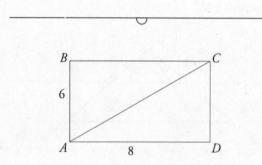

If *ABCD* is a rectangle, what is the perimeter of triangle *ABC* ?

A. 6
B. 8
C. 10
D. 24

Here's How to Crack It

We can use the Pythagorean theorem to figure out the length of the diagonal of the rectangle, which is the hypotenuse of triangle *ABC*. The legs of this triangle are 6 and 8. Therefore, the hypotenuse (diagonal) is 10. (If you remembered that this is one of those well-known Pythagorean ratios, you didn't actually have to do the calculations.) Therefore, the perimeter of the triangle is 6 + 8 + 10, or 24, choice D.

SPECIAL RIGHT TRIANGLES

There are two specific right triangles, the properties of which may play a role in some harder math problems. They are the right triangles with angles 45-45-90 and 30-60-90.

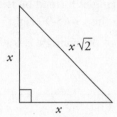

An **isosceles right triangle** has angles that measure 45, 45, and 90 degrees. Whenever you have a 45-45-90 triangle with sides (legs) of x, the hypotenuse will always be $x\sqrt{2}$. This means that if one of the legs of the triangle measures 3, then the hypotenuse will be $3\sqrt{2}$.

This isosceles right triangle is important because it is half of a square. Understanding the 45-45-90 triangle will allow you to easily find the diagonal of a square from its side, or find the side of a square from its diagonal.

Here's an example.

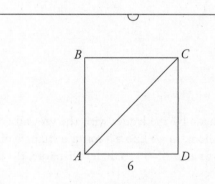

In square *ABCD* above, what is the perimeter of triangle *ABC* ?

A. $6\sqrt{2}$
B. 8
C. $12 + \sqrt{2}$
D. $12 + 6\sqrt{2}$

Here's How to Crack It

This question looks like a question about a square, and it certainly is in part, but it's really more about the two triangles formed by the diagonal of a square.

In this square, we know that each of the triangles formed by the diagonal AC is a 45-45-90 right triangle. Since the square has a side of 6, you can use the 45-45-90 right triangle rule. Each of the sides is 6 and the diagonal is $6\sqrt{2}$. Therefore, the perimeter of the triangle is $6 + 6 + 6\sqrt{2}$, or $12 + 6\sqrt{2}$ and the answer is choice D.

Let's take a look at a question that you might see on the NLN PAX-RN:

A ladder is placed with one end at the top of a bookshelf such that it makes an angle of 45° with the floor. The bookshelf is 5 m tall. How far is the bottom of the ladder from the shelf?

A. 5 m

B. $5\sqrt{2}$ m

C. 10 m

D. $10\sqrt{2}$ m

Here's How To Crack It

The question tells us that the angle made by the ladder with the ground is 45° and the bookshelf must make an angle of 90 degrees with the floor, so we know it forms a triangle of the type we just discussed—an isosceles right triangle, also known as a 45-45-90 triangle. Therefore, the distance from the shelf to the bottom of the ladder is 5 meters, choice A.

The other important right triangle to understand is the 30-60-90 right triangle.

In a 30-60-90 triangle, the side opposite the 30° angle is 1/2 the hypotenuse.

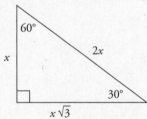

A 30-60-90 triangle with a short leg of x has a hypotenuse of $2x$ and a long leg of $x\sqrt{3}$. If the smaller leg (the x side) of the triangle is 5, then the sides measure 5, $5\sqrt{3}$, and 10. This triangle is important because it is half of an equilateral triangle, and it allows us to find the height of an equilateral triangle.

Third Side Rule

Suppose you don't know anything about a triangle except the lengths of two of its sides. You can also then figure out that the third side must be between certain values; that is, the length of the third side must be less than the sum of the other two and greater than the difference.

> The third side of a triangle is always less than the sum of the other two sides and greater than the difference between them.

Why? Consider a triangle that looks like this:

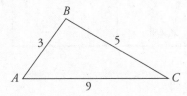

The shortest distance between two points is a straight line, right? And yet in this figure, the straight-line distance from A to C is 9, yet the scenic route from A to B to C is…8? That can't be right! And it isn't. The crooked path must be longer than the straight path, and thus any two sides of a triangle added together must be longer than the third side. In this example, $2 < AC < 8$.

Which of the following is a possible perimeter of a triangle with sides 5 and 8 ?

A. 15
B. 16
C. 17
D. 26

No Figures?
Draw one before you do anything else.

Here's How to Crack It

To find the perimeter of a triangle, you just need to add up the sides of the triangle, so let's see what we know about the sides. We know that the two given sides add up to 13, so the perimeter will be 13 + the third side. The third side will be between the sum and difference of those other two sides. $8 + 5 = 13$ and $8 - 5 = 3$, so the third side will be greater than 3 and less than 13. Add these to the sum of the sides we already know (13), and the perimeter must be greater than 16 (13 + 3) and less than 26 (13 + 13). The only answer choice that fits the bill is choice C.

Let's combine what we learned in the last chapter about isosceles right triangles with what we just covered about perimeters.

What is the perimeter of the polygon *ABCD*?

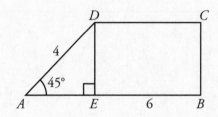

A. $12 + 4\sqrt{2}$

B. $16 + 2\sqrt{2}$

C. $16 + 4\sqrt{2}$

D. $20 + 2\sqrt{2}$

Here's How to Crack It

First, take a look at triangle *ADE* and notice that it is an isosceles right triangle, so we know that the sides are in the ratio for $1 : 1 : \sqrt{2}$ for $45° : 45° : 90°$. Use the Pythagorean theorem to derive that $AE = 2\sqrt{2}$. Because the triangle is isosceles, you also know that *DE* is $2\sqrt{2}$. Because *DE* is opposite *BC*, we know that *BC* is $2\sqrt{2}$ as well. Now simply add $6 + 6 + 4 + 2\sqrt{2} + 2\sqrt{2}$, which then equals $16 + 4\sqrt{2}$. So choice C is correct.

Circles

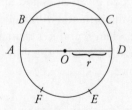

The **radius** of a circle is the distance from the center to the edge of the circle. In the figure above, *OD* is a radius. So is *OA*.

The **diameter** is the distance from one edge, through the center, to the other edge of the circle. The diameter will always be twice the measure of the radius and will always be the longest line you can draw through a circle. In the figure above, *AD* is a diameter.

A **chord** is any line drawn from one point on the edge of the circle to the other. In the figure above, *BC* is a chord. A diameter is also a chord.

An **arc** is any section of the circumference (the edge) of the circle. *EF* is an arc in the figure above.

The **area** of a circle with radius *r* is πr^2. A circle with a radius of 5 has an area of 25π.

The **circumference** is the distance around the outside edge of the circle. The circumference of a circle with radius *r* is $2\pi r$. A circle with a radius of 5 has a circumference of 10π.

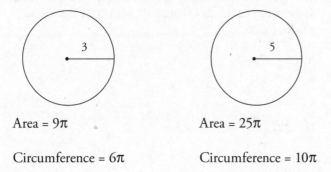

Area = 9π Area = 25π

Circumference = 6π Circumference = 10π

Before we go any further, let's also talk pi (π) for a moment. You probably know that its value is around 3.14. As discussed in Chapter 3, for ballparking purposes, it's useful to think of pi as being around 3. So if you're looking at the circle above with radius 5, the area (25π) is around 75 and the circumference (10π) is about 30. Another useful pi shorthand is $\dfrac{22}{7}$, which is a fraction version of pi.

Let's work out a question that looks confusing, but is a perfect opportunity to break out your ballparking and estimation skills with circles.

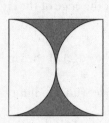

The figure above shows two semicircles inscribed in a square. If the square has a side of length 10, what is the area of the shaded region?

A. $50 - 75\pi$

B. $50 - 25\pi$

C. $100 - 25\pi$

D. $\dfrac{100 - 25\pi}{2}$

Here's How to Crack It

First, let's do some ballparking. Since the square has a side of length 10, the area of the square is 100. The shaded region is pretty small in comparison—maybe about 10 or 12. Only choice D comes close to that approximation: Choices A and B are negative! (*Remember:* π is about 3.) If we want to check our ballparking with math, we would again start with 100 as the area of the square. Now let's remove the area of the circle to get the size of the remaining area (which includes the shaded region and the identically shaped area just below it). Since each of these is a semicircle, together they will make one complete circle with radius of 5. (We know the radius is 5 because it's half of one side of the square.) This means that the area of the circle will be 25π. So once we remove the area of the circle, what is left is 100 − 25π. Now the shaded region is only half of this, so we need to divide by two, and the area of the shaded region will be

$\dfrac{100 - 25\pi}{2}$, choice D.

OVERLAPPING FIGURES

Very often on a harder geometry problem you'll see two figures that overlap: a triangle and a square, a triangle and a circle, or a square and a circle.

> The key to solving overlapping figure problems is figuring out what the two figures have in common. This may be something you have to draw in yourself.

Take a look at the following problem.

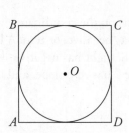

In the figure above, the circle with center O is drawn in square $ABCD$. If the area of square $ABCD$ is 36, what is the area of circle O ?

A. 18
B. 24
C. 9π
D. 12π

Here's How to Crack It

Go ahead and draw a diameter in the figure through point O and parallel to the base. We mentioned earlier that we want to write down things we know about the figure, so let's write the formulas for both of the figures we've been given. The question mentions the area of the square and the area of the circle, so write $A = s^2$ for the square and $A = \pi r^2$ for the circle.

Now let's take the information we've been given and take bite-sized pieces to crack it. Since we know that the area of the square is 36, we can solve the first equation and to get $s = 6$, so $d = 6$ as well. Let's take that information to the other formula, that of the circle, which is what we're being asked to find. The radius is half of the diameter, so $A = \pi 3^2 = 9\pi$, so that's our answer, choice (C).

THE COORDINATE PLANE

You might see one or two questions on your exam that involve the **coordinate plane**. The biggest mistake that people make on these questions is getting the *x*- and *y*-axes reversed. So let's just review:

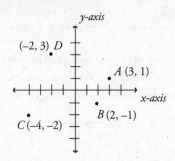

The *x*-**axis** is the horizontal axis, and the *y*-**axis** is the vertical axis. Points are given on the coordinate plane with the *x*-coordinate first. Positive *x*-values go to the right, and negative ones go to the left; positive *y*-values go up, and negative ones go down. So point A (3, 1) is 3 points to the right on the *x*-axis and 1 point up from there. Point B (2, –1) is two points to the right on the *x*-axis and 1 point down from there.

Slope is a measure of the steepness of a line on the coordinate plane. On most slope problems you need to recognize only whether the slope is positive, negative, or zero. A line that goes up and to the right has positive slope; a line that goes down and to the right has negative slope, and a flat line has zero slope. In the figure below, line 1 has positive slope, line 2 has zero slope, and line 3 has negative slope.

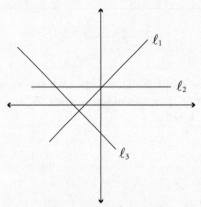

Suppose you need to calculate the slope of a line determined by two points (x_1, y_1) and (x_2, y_2). To find this slope, simply count the distance up (**rise**) and over (**run**) from one point on the line to the other. The formula you would then use is slope = $\dfrac{\text{rise}}{\text{run}}$. Written out with the aforementioned points x_1, y_1, x_2, and y_2, the formula is slope = $\dfrac{y_2 - y_1}{x_2 - x_1}$.

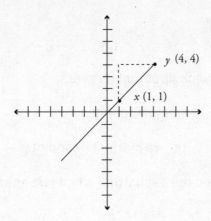

In the graph above, to get from point x to point y, we count up (rise) 3 units, and count over (run) 3 units. Therefore, the slope is $\dfrac{\text{rise}}{\text{run}} = \dfrac{3}{3} = 1$. Always remember to check whether the slope is positive or negative when you use $= \dfrac{\text{rise}}{\text{run}}$.

If you're not given a figure and you can't draw one easily using the points given, you can find the slope by plugging the coordinates you know into the slope formula. So far the line in the above figure, you would set up the formula as slope $= \dfrac{4-1}{4-1} = \dfrac{3}{3} = 1$. You get the same result no matter which way you calculate the slope.

SUMMARY

- A line continues on in each direction forever.

- A ray is a line with one distinct endpoint.

- A line segment is a line with two distinct endpoints.

- Vertical angles are opposite each other when two lines cross. They have the same measure.

- Corresponding angles are pairs of angles on the same side of a transversal and the same side of the lines crossed by the transversal.

- If two parallel lines are cut by a third line, the corresponding angles are equal.

- The rule of 180: the angles on any line must add up to 180.

- A figure with two sets of parallel sides is a parallelogram. In a parallelogram, the opposite angles are equal and any adjacent angles add up to 180 degrees. Also, opposite sides are equal.

- The area of a square, rectangle, or parallelogram is the length $\times$ height.

- The area of a square is $A = s^2$.

- The perimeter of any figure is the sum of the lengths of its sides.

- The sum of the two acute angles in a right triangle is 90 degrees.

- The sum of the angles inside a triangle equals 180.

- Isosceles triangles have two sides that are equal, and the angles opposite these two sides are equal.

- The area of a triangle is ½ the base $\times$ height. Remember that the height is always perpendicular to the base.

- An equilateral triangle has all three sides equal and all of its angles are equal to 60 degrees.

- The Pythagorean theorem ($a^2 + b^2 = c^2$) states that the square of the hypotenuse (c^2) of a right triangle is equal to the sum of the squares of the other two sides ($a^2 + b^2$).

- There are two types of special right triangles with angles measuring 45-45-90 and 30-60-90.

- The third side of a triangle is always less than the sum of the other two sides and greater than the difference between them.

- The radius of a circle is the distance from the center to the edge of the circle.

- The area of a circle with radius r is πr^2.

- The diameter of a circle in the distance from one edge through the center and to the other edge. It is two times the radius.

- 22/7 [3.14] is shorthand for π, which is the pi symbol.

- The x-axis is the horizontal axis on the coordinate plane, and the y-axis is the vertical axis.

- The key to overlapping figure problems is to determine what the figures have in common.

- To find the slope of a line that includes points $[x_1, y_1]$ and $[x_2, y_2]$, use the formula $\dfrac{y_2 - y_1}{x_2 - x_1}$. This formula represents $\dfrac{\text{rise}}{\text{run}}$.

KEY TERMS

lines
ray
line segment
angles
rule of 180
vertical angles
transversal
corresponding angles
four sided figures
parallelogram
rectangle
square
area
length
width
perimeter
triangle
isosceles triangle
base
height

equilateral triangle
Pythagorean theorem
legs
hypotenuse
isosceles right triangle
third side rule
circles
radius
diameter
chord
arc
area of circle
circumference
coordinate plane
x-axis (horizontal axis)
y-axis (vertical axis)
slope
rise
run

Chapter 12 Graphs and Diagrams

GRAPHS, DATA INTERPRETATION, AND DIAGRAMS

Many math questions on the NET, NLN PAX-RN, and TEAS are presented as word problems and number problems. However, you will likely see at least a few questions that will ask you to solve the problem by using a graph or a chart. Graphs can appear in many formats, such as those shown and described below.

A **table** is a tool used to organize information in rows and columns. Here's an example:

Favorite Cereals		
Cereal	Boys	Girls
Cheerios	2	5
Banana Nut Crunch	6	3
Honey Smacks	10	8
Kashi	5	4

Tables have many uses. For example, in the table above, four types of cereal are broken down according the preferences of boys and girls.

A **bar chart** is a visual representation in which rectangular bars are plotted in proportion to the values they represent. A bar chart may be arranged with the bars either vertical or horizontal. Here's an example:

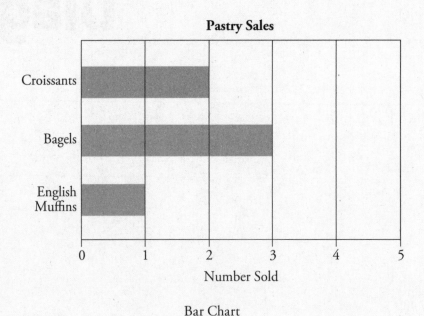

Bar Chart

In the bar chart above, different pastries are shown by the rate at which they sell. As you can see, for this data set, bagels are the most popular pastry. A bar chart can be used, for example, by nursing management to show an increase in infection rate due to poor hygiene techniques over several years. Or a bar chart can be used to applaud a goal, such as the completion of mandatory training by all staff members. You have probably seen bar charts used with fundraising efforts.

In a **line chart,** or **line graph**, information is plotted as dots on a grid. The dots are then connected by line segments. Here's an example:

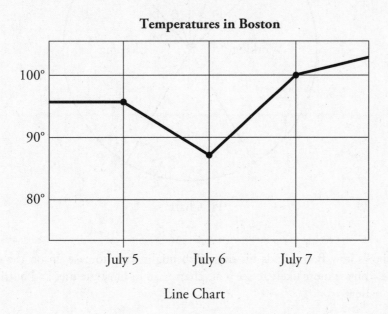

Temperatures in Boston

Line Chart

The line chart above tracks the temperatures in Boston over three days in July. In nursing, a line chart might be used with a patient who has suffered an injury. The patient can record the events that took place and write them on a time line. Attorneys often use line charts when obtaining detailed history prior to litigation.

A **pie chart** is a circle that's divided into sections. Each section proportionally represents an element that makes up the whole circle. Here's an example:

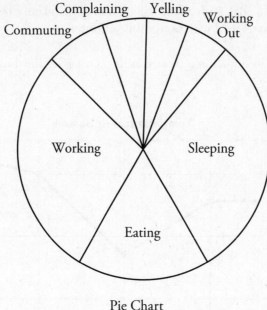

Pie Chart

The chart above shows how Bob spends his day. (Bob might want to ease up on the complaining and yelling.) As a nurse, you are more likely to see a pie chart used to illustrate diet and nutrient recommendations for a specific patient.

Occasionally you will see a **box-and-whisker plot**, which is used to display a data set. Here's an example:

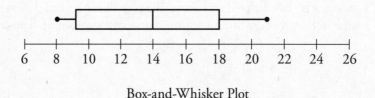

Box-and-Whisker Plot

This chart breaks down the data set that is the ages of people at a church outing. A box-and-whisker plot is a good way to break down data into median, upper median, lower median, and more. In nursing school, your professor might break down an assortment of test scores in this way.

A **stem-and-leaf plot** is also used to display a data set. Here's an example:

Quiz Scores	
Stem	Leaf
5	0, 9
6	1, 2
7	6, 8, 9
8	3, 4
9	1, 7

Stem-and-Leaf Plot

A steam-and-leaf plot is mostly used to present data in statistics. It's very unlikely you will see this type of chart, but it's still useful to know. In the chart above, the quiz scores are organized in a stem-and-leaf plot. The stem is the first digit and the leaf is the second digit. So the chart above is a visual representation of the data set: 50, 59, 61, 62, 76, 78, 79, 83, 84, 91, 97.

Here's a question like one you might see on the TEAS:

The table below shows the height that a mountaineer has climbed over a period of 4 hours.

Time (hours)	Height (ft)
After 2 hours	300
After 4 hours	600

What is the average rate at which the mountaineer is climbing?

A. 50 feet per hour
B. 150 feet per hour
C. 300 feet per hour
D. 450 feet per hour

Here's How to Crack It

You know that the average rate at which the mountaineer is climbing can be found with the formula

$$\frac{\text{total distance covered}}{\text{total time}}$$

So just plug in what you know

$$\frac{\text{total distance covered}}{\text{total time}} = \frac{600}{4}$$

$$= 150 \text{ feet per hour}$$

The correct answer is choice B.

_____

Here's a graph that you will definitely see in your nursing career—a **PQRST wave** of a heartbeat, which shows the electrical conductivity of one beat.

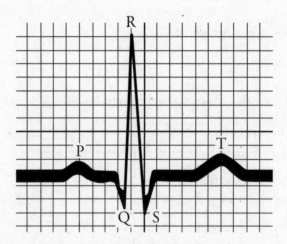

PQRST Wave

GRAPHS IN NURSING

You are probably wondering when you'll use a graph when you become a nurse. Well, quite often, actually. Graphs are used to map the electrical waves from your brain in the form of an EEG. Seizure activity is evident on this graph. Another diagram that you might see as a nurse is an EKG, which shows the electrical activity of the heart over a period of time.

Bone density results (in the form of a graph) map who is at risk for a bone fracture, compared to other people of different ages. If you go into pediatrics, you will undoubtedly work with growth charts. Based on their height and weight, patients are placed in a percentile that compares them to other children of the same age over a period of time. You can follow and compare measurements to see where someone is perhaps overeating or losing too much weight. Growth charts are also useful to monitor a child's growth spurt, or note if he is not growing at all and needs a bone age X ray or a workup for Celiac disease. So yes, you will be using graphs and charts in your career, as well as for your nursing school entrance exam preparation.

Many test takers find graphs and charts intimidating. They are not. Don't let the data tables or figures intimidate you—some can actually be fun. All you have to do is weed out the "too much information" from the "I need to know that" information and answer the question. Keep it simple and don't get thrown off by superfluous data. Find out what the question is asking. Read the chart and look at each element represented. Carefully read the labels on the *x*- and *y*-axis—that is, the vertical and horizontal lines (the ups and downs). Look for the answer on the graph or chart—it will be there. Take only the information you need to answer the question, do the math equation, and move to the next question.

Graph coordinate questions are often more prevalent in the geometry section of the NET, as opposed to the TEAS and NLN PAX-RN. You may be asked to find the mean price of gas from a bar chart that visually represents five years of gas hikes. You may be asked to find the rate of change in the amount of gas left in a tank after a road trip. The next few pages illustrate the types of questions and answers you should review in preparation for your test.

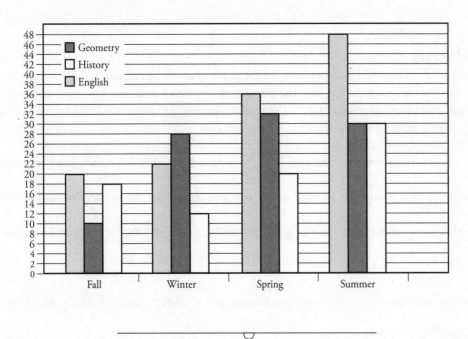

According to the preceding graph, how many more students took geometry in the winter than history in the fall?

A. 3
B. 10
C. 18
D. 28

Here's How to Crack It

In this graph question, you are asked to find the difference between two different values on the graph. First, locate the value of each group: 28 students took geometry in the winter, and 18 students took history in the fall. After you find these two pieces of information, the problem is simple. Subtract 18 from 28 to get 10, or choice B, as the correct answer. *Note:* Partial answer choices will often appear on problems that use graphs (in this case, choices C and D), so be careful.

In the preceding graph, the percentage of geometry students who took geometry in the spring is how much greater than the percentage of history students who took history in the spring?

A. 7%
B. 20%
C. 25%
D. 32%

Here's How to Crack It

This question asks us to compare two percents. In the graph above, no percentages are given, so we'll need to calculate the percentages first. To find the percent of geometry students who took geometry in the spring, we need two pieces of information—the total number of geometry students for the year, and the number of geometry students in the spring.

First, add the geometry students for the year (10 + 28 + 32 + 30 = 100). Nice and round number. In the spring, 32 students took geometry. To express this as a percentage, put the number of students who took geometry in the spring in the numerator of a fraction and the total number of students in the denominator: $\frac{32}{100} = 32\%$.

If you follow the same procedure to determine the percent of history students who took history in the spring, you get $\frac{20}{80} = \frac{1}{4} = 25\%$.

The difference between these two values is 32% − 25%, or 7%. Choice A is the correct answer. Again, watch out for partial answer choices.

Relating Data Found in Graphs

In the previous two examples, you had to take information from a graph and perform certain operations on the numbers. On some math questions, you will be asked to compare numbers to each other. Here are some sample questions:

- What was the percent increase from year x to year y?
- In order to equal the amount of sales of Company x, Company y needs to increase its sales by what percent?
- What year saw the greatest increase in production for Company x?

The formula for finding **percent change** is

$$\% \text{ change} = \frac{\text{difference}}{\text{original amount}}$$

This formula is often helpful when you are asked to compare data within a graph. Using the graph from before, let's examine one of these types of questions.

───────────────────

Which class saw the largest percentage change in enrollment from spring to summer?

A. English
B. Geometry
C. History
D. English and history have the same percentage increase.

Here's How to Crack It

We need to find the largest percent change from the spring term to the summer term. In order to find a percent change, use the percent change formula that we just discussed:

$$\% \text{ change} = \frac{\text{difference}}{\text{original amount}}$$

For English class, the percent change is

$$\frac{(48 - 36)}{36} = \frac{12}{36} = \frac{1}{3} = 33\frac{1}{3}\%$$

For geometry class, the percent change is

$$\frac{(32 - 30)}{30} = \frac{2}{30} = \text{less than } 10\%$$

For history class, the percent change is

$$\frac{(30-20)}{20} = \frac{10}{20} = \frac{1}{2} = 50\%$$

From these calculations, you can see that the correct answer is choice C, history.

Linear Equations

A **linear equation** is an algebraic equation in which each term is either a constant or the product of a constant and (the first power of) a single variable.

A common form of a linear equation in the two variables x and y is

$$y = mx + b$$

This equation is often called the **slope-intercept form** because m is the slope and b gives the y-intercept (where the line crosses the y-axis). Linear equations graph as straight lines, and have simple variable expressions with no exponents on them.

It's very likely that any nursing school entrace exam will throw at least one or two line slope questions at you, so let's take a look at a few sample problems.

What is the equation of the straight line that has slope $m = 4$ and passes through the point $(-1, -6)$?

    A. $y = 4x - 2$
    B. $y = 2x - 4$
    C. $y = -6x - 2$
    D. $y = -1x - 2$

Here's How to Crack It

Remember the slope-intercept form, $y = mx + b$. In this case, they've provided the value of the slope ($m = 4$). Also, in giving you a point on the line, they have given you an x-value and a y-value for this line: $x = -1$ and $y = -6$.

So far, the only thing that you don't have a value for is b (which gives you the y-intercept). Then all you need to do is plug in for the slope and then solve for b:

$$y = mx + b$$
$$(-6) = (4)(-1) + b$$
$$-6 = -4 + b$$
$$-2 = b$$

So the line equation must be $y = 4x - 2$

Slope

As discussed in Chapter 11, **slope** is the measure of the steepness of a line; mathematically it's represented by the letter m. To calculate the slope of a line, put the difference between two y-coordinates over the difference between two corresponding x-coordinates:

$$m = \frac{y_2 - y_1}{x_2 - x_1}$$

The slope of the line we just graphed, $y = 3x + 2$, can be calculated by the coordinates we identified, $(0, 2)$ and $(1, 5)$. The expression of these coordinate pairs in the formula for slope is $\frac{5-2}{1-0}$, or 3. Thus, the slope of the line is 3.

The linear equation we've been working with here is $y = 3x + 2$, which is in the form $y = mx + b$. What is m again? Why, it's the slope.

What is the slope of the line that is represented by the equation $y + 5 = x$?

A. 1
B. 2
C. −1
D. 3

Here's How to Crack It

There are two ways to find the slope here: You could use the slope formula, or you could put the equation into the slope-intercept form $y = mx + b$. We'll try the second, easier way first, and then go through the formula for good measure. To put the equation into $y = mx + b$ form, what must you do? Well, clearly the y needs to be isolated.

Subtract 5 from both sides.

$$y + 5 - 5 = x - 5$$

This gives you $y = x - 5$. You now have the equation in $y = mx + b$ form. The coefficient for x is 1, so the slope of the line is 1, choice A.

How do we go about putting this equation into the slope formula? Well, the formula needs two coordinate pairs.

The line's equation is $y + 5 = x$; if $y = 0$ then $x = 5$, and if $y = 1$ then $x = 6$. The slope formula is the difference in y-coordinates over the difference in x-coordinates. You get $\dfrac{1-0}{6-5}$, also known as 1. Pretty slick, no?

Slippery Slopes

When is a hill not a hill? When it's flat. A flat, or horizontal, line is a line whose y-coordinate is constant. All horizontal lines have the same slope: 0. That's because there is no change in y, so you have a fraction with the numerator 0, which is always equal to 0.

Vertical lines, on the other hand, have an x-coordinate which is constant. This means that they form fractions with 0 denominators, which are undefined; this means that *the slope of a vertical line is undefined.*

From Chapter 11, you know that a positive slope indicates a line that rises to the right, and a negative slope indicates a line that falls to the right.

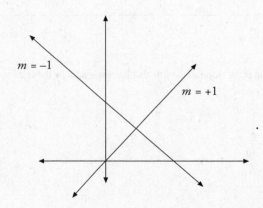

The numerical value of the slope—which is the absolute value if the slope is negative—represents the steepness of a slope and the angle that the slope makes with the *x*-axis. Thus, a line of slope $\frac{1}{2}$ is less steep than a line of slope 1, which in turn is less steep than a line of slope 2.

Parallel lines must have equal slopes. So if you come across two distinct lines with the same slope, they must be parallel. Perpendicular lines, on the other hand, must have slopes that multiply together to equal −1. If you see two algebraic lines—linear equations—$y = 2x + 3$ and $y = -\frac{1}{2}x + 2$, you now know a geometric fact about them: They're perpendicular, because when you multiply their slopes $\left(-\frac{1}{2} \text{ and } 2\right)$, the result is −1.

SUMMARY

- Familiarize yourself with these types of visual representations of data: table, bar chart, line chart or line graph, pie chart, box-and-whisker plot, and stem-and-leaf plot.

- Do not be intimidated by problems that involve a chart or figure—just zero in on the information you need and crunch the necessary numbers. Be aware of partial answer choices that will try to entice you.

- The formula for percent change is $\dfrac{\text{difference}}{\text{original amount}}$.

- A linear equation is an algebraic equation in which each term is either a constant or the product of a constant and (the first power of) a single variable.

- The slope-intercept form for two variables x and y is $y = mx + b$. In this formula, m is the the slope and b is the y-intercept.

- Slope is the measure of the steepness of a line. Shorthand for slope is $\dfrac{\text{rise}}{\text{run}}$.

- The slope of a horizontal line is 0. The slope of a vertical line is undefined.

KEY TERMS

table
bar chart
line chart (line graph)
pie chart
box-and-whisker plot
stem-and-leaf plot
PQRST wave
percent change
linear equation
slope-intercept form
slope

Chapter 13
English Verbal
Mechanics

COMMUNICATION IN NURSING

Proper Communication

Communication is a process by which information is conveyed from one person or group of persons to another. There are myriad forms of communication in the world today, but let's discuss communication that you, as a future nurse, will recognize and use in your day-to-day duties. For example, if you are running late to start your shift and you see a colleague in the hall, you may exchange the perfunctory "Hello. How are you? So nice to see you," while you continue your decaffeinated sprint to the elevator that is about to close. Whether that colleague returned the pleasantries or not, you just participated in **verbal communication.**

Communication is Key

To effectively communicate as a nurse, you must have a solid command of the English language and strong writing skills. Speak concisely and write legibly. Proper history taking and documenting can save a patient's life and your career. Doctors often rely heavily on what the nurses write in their initial notes. In the future, you may even be called to testify in court based on information you documented in a chart several years prior.

Other types of communication include **written communication** (a doctor's order: Give 2 mg Epinephrine IV now), **signed communication** (sign language), and **electronic communication** (email or text messages).

Many Types of Communication

Communication can be verbal (a word), nonverbal (a look with eyes that are welling up with tears), passive aggressive ("Don't give me more food," while ladling heaps of potatoes on to the plate), direct ("Give me the syringe"), or indirect (walking by a group and saying "Hey").

You may someday have a patient who is wincing in pain and is curled up into a ball on a bed. He appears to be in pain, although when asked, he may deny (verbally) having pain. His body movements are a form of **nonverbal communication.** The everyday verbal chit-chat that is audible between people on the buses, trains, cell phones, and busy streets is surpassed only by the silent, nonverbal facial expressions that one shows when he or she is suffering as a patient. Reading people's facial expressions and picking up on subtle eyebrow furrows and frowns come with time and understanding. In time, you may learn that for a patient who suffered a stroke and is unable to speak, he or she still has the ability to think, know, and feel. He or she may not be able to express the thought into a word, a condition called **expressive aphasia**. Most often these patients are taught how to communicate by nodding to "yes" or "no" questions, but a **communication board** or picture board is sometimes utilized.

A communication board is a large, lightweight board or poster with preprinted samples, words, and icons. Patients who are unable to speak can simply point to the symbol for hunger, thirst, anger, or pain, or to a picture of the body to indicate the exact location of their discomfort. Or patients can point to the phrase "thank you" to express gratitude to the assisting nurse, family, and friends.

For now, let's discuss the written word and spoken word. Effective communication is key to your success in the nursing profession and to the health of the patients (their families and significant others) entrusted to your care. You do not need to assume a leadership role or dictate business strategies at a meeting to be a good communicator. The basis of **effective communication** is to process a message, say it clearly, do it, write it down, make it happen, and then follow it up. *Remember:* In the nursing field, if something wasn't written down or documented, it was never done. A medication not charted means it was not administered.

Improper Communication

The opposite of effective communication is **inappropriate communication,** which includes grunting, screaming, hitting, immodest dressing, inappropriate and unwelcomed physical contact, yelling, talking down to people, using a condescending tone, using curse words or derogatory words, making slanderous statements, intimidating people, or making the inappropriate request to view the chart of a patient that you are not caring for.

Electronic Communication

Please note that cell phones, laptops, and smart phone wireless devices that are not issued by a hospital are not HIPAA compliant. All information exchanged on these noncompliant devices is a violation of a patient's right to privacy. Do not use your personal cell device at work, while training as a nurse, or as a nurse.

Illegal Communication

As discussed in Chapter 2, it is against the law and inappropriate to view or disclose any information regarding any patient.

If you are a nurse and a coworker is admitted to the hospital where you work, you cannot look at his or her chart or ask a resident how surgery went. If you hear coworkers discussing a patient who is not under their care, or discussing another coworker's private medical information, walk away. Anonymously report the incident. Nurses who assume leadership roles have an obligation to investigate all patient complaints against HIPAA violators. Please make sure that you read your hospital code of conduct manual to be certain your rights are protected as a patient and as a professional representing the hospital.

VERBAL MECHANICS

To do well on the English/Verbal section of the TEAS or NLN PAX-RN, you need to know basic grammar, sentence structure, spelling, punctuation, and mechanics. For the NET, the primary focus of that exam is mathematics, so review this content but don't worry too much about it. English is the standard language in the field of health care, though, so verbal review is useful for all. Let's review.

You will need to be familiar with the following grammar concepts and parts of speech: sentence structure, nouns, pronouns, verbs, adverbs, adjectives, prepositions, conjunctions, interjections, and interrogatives. Yes, this content is a flashback to younger years, but it is a good refresher and it will enhance your writing skills.

Sentences

A **sentence** is a group of words that expresses a complete thought. It has a subject and one or more verbs. Don't forget the period, and always avoid run-on sentences. The following are examples of sentences:

> The cow jumped over the moon.
> I am delayed seeing patients.
> The weather was beautiful today.
> The nurse administered the antibiotic using the proper sterile technique.
> After miles of bumper-to-bumper traffic, the Cooper family arrived safely at the zoo before it closed.

A **phrase** is a part of a sentence that does not have a subject or a verb and can't stand on its own. Here are some examples of phrases:

> in the operating room
> across the street
> on the nightstand
> down the hallway

A **fragment** is a group of words that lacks either a subject or a verb. Here are some examples:

> After multiple failed biopsies
> Pain, suffering, and humiliation
> In the state-of-the-art NICU

A **clause** is part of a sentence that contains both a subject and a verb. Clauses are either **dependent** or **independent**. Here's an example of a dependent clause:

> Whenever the back door opened

This clause has a subject (door) and a verb (opened), but it does not express a complete thought. It depends upon something else—that is, the dependent clause can't stand on its own.

An independent clause makes a complete thought and therefore can stand alone. The following is an example of an independent clause:

> The farmer ate homemade bread every day for many years.

A **run-on sentence** consists of at least two independent clauses incorrectly connected. A run-on sentence may be lengthy, but its problem is one of structure, not length. Here are two examples:

- Run-on sentence: It's hot today drink plenty of water.

  Correct sentence: It's hot today; drink plenty of water.

- Run-on sentence: The NET has 60 math questions, be sure to review basic arithmetic and algebra before you take the exam.

  Correct sentence: The NET has 60 math questions. Be sure to review basic arithmetic and algebra before you take the exam.

Nouns

A **noun** names or identifies a person, place, thing, idea, or creature. The **articles** *the*, *a*, and *an* often appear before nouns in a sentence. Some examples of nouns are *woman, baby, temperature, Texas, climate, religion, doctor, nurse, office, German Shepherd, bus, book, bottle, diploma, degree, temperature,* and *soda*.

An **abstract noun** identifies something that people can't experience through their senses. It indicates something intangible such as *sadness, peace, injustice, guilt, shame, fear, anger,* and *disappointment.* A **concrete noun** identifies something that people can experience through their senses. Some examples of concrete nouns are *book, flower, school, automobile,* and *dog*.

A **singular noun** refers to one thing. Examples are *girl, boat, desk, basket,* and *nurse*.

A **plural noun** refers to more than one thing. Examples are *girls, boats, desks, baskets,* and *nurses*. However, not all nouns are made plural by adding an -s or -es. Consider these examples:

Singular	Plural
nucleus	nuclei
child	children
crisis	crises
fungus	fungi
syllabus	syllabi
phenomenon	phenomena

Common nouns refer to general items; **proper nouns** refer to specific items. Proper nouns are always capitalized. To understand the difference between the two types of nouns, study the following list:

Common Noun	Proper Noun
actor	John Wayne
author	Jane Austen
president	Abraham Lincoln
state	Pennsylvania
building	Empire State Building
school	Cleveland Elementary
nurse	Clara Barton

Pronouns

A **pronoun** takes the place of a noun whose identity is made clear earlier in the text. Pronouns must agree in number with the nouns they refer to, and they must be free from ambiguity. Consider this example of bad use of a pronoun:

> Phil was so angry that he took the chess pieces and threw it across the room.

The term *chess pieces* is plural, but the pronoun *it* is singular. The sentence should read as follows:

> Phil was so angry that he took the chess pieces and threw *them* across the room.

Four common types of pronouns are **personal pronouns** (I, we, you, he, she, they), **possessive pronouns** (mine, your, his, hers, its, our, their), **relative pronouns** (that which, who, whom, whose, whoever, whomever), and **interrogative pronouns** (who, what, when, where, why, how, whom, whose, which).

Verbs

Verbs denote action or state of being. A verb tells the reader what the subject of the sentence is doing or how the subject is being acted upon. Verbs must agree in number with the subject of the sentence. The **verb tense** indicates when the action of the verb occurs. Make sure you're familiar with the common verb tenses. Let's look at some examples that illustrate different verb tenses.

Present tense: I am, you are, he/she is, we are, they are, I am running, you are leaving, she is fleeing

Past tense: I was, you were, he/she went, we expected, they ran

Future tense: I will attend, she will visit, we will laugh, you will decide

Past perfect tense: I had cried, she had run, we had become

Present perfect tense: My neighbor has moved, we have learned, you have seen

Future perfect tense: The attorney will have served the papers, we will have finished, they will have lived

The **infinitive** of a verb is the unconjugated form of the verb. Examples of infinities are *to go, to run, to eat,* and *to study.* Consider the following sentence:

He loved to dance.

That sentence has the verb *to love* conjugated in the past tense (he loved) and the infinitive *to dance.*

Adverbs

Adverbs modify verbs by denoting quality, manner, and degree of the action. They can modify more than just verbs, though. They can also modify adjectives, clauses, sentences, and other adverbs. The following examples illustrate the use of adverbs:

He approached her *gingerly.* (The adverb *gingerly* modifies the verb *approached.*)
We fought *well.* (The adverb *well* modifies the verb *fought.*)
Carla did *unexpectedly well* on her nursing school entrance exam. (The adverb *unexpectedly* modifies the adverb *well.*)
The *extremely* large box was delivered this morning. (The adverb *extremely* modifies the adjective *box.*)
Finally, we made the playoffs, but we lost in the championship game. (The adverb *finally* modifies the clause *we made the playoffs.*)
Surely, he will be on time today. (The adverb *surely* modifies the entire sentence.)

Adjectives

Adjectives modify the nouns in the sentence by providing descriptions, limits, or specific qualities. Here are some examples of adjectives: a *creepy* man, a *tiny* baby, an *angry* defendant, a *happy* father, a *disgruntled* retiree, a *bitter* spouse, a *trusting* patient, a *blue* bonnet, an *exhausted* marathoner, an *animated* film, *English* literature, an *intrusive* coworker, an *evasive* boyfriend, and a *judgmental* attorney.

This review might seem quite elementary, but a review in which we get down to brass tacks can be useful if you encounter vocabulary words that are unfamiliar. You would be wise to use context clues or parts of speech to point you in the right direction. Let's look at a question like one you might see on the NLN PAX-RN.

1. The Battle Hymn of the Republic" is a well-known _____ song.

   A. disruptive
   B. orderly
   C. organized
   D. martial

Here's How to Crack It

The question provides four adjectives that can complete the sentence. Perhaps you already know that martial means "of, relating to, or suited for war or a warrior," so choice D is correct. Choices B and C don't make sense, as songs cannot be orderly or organized, so cross off those two. "The Battle Hymn of the Republic" could perhaps be played at a loud volume in certain instances, and might be seen as disruptive in that situation, but it's not inherently disruptive. So even if you didn't know the meaning of *martial*, you could use POE to reach that answer anyway.

Prepositions

Prepositions are words that show position or place. They are always followed by a noun or a pronoun, which is called the **object of the preposition**. Some examples of prepositions are *above, below, within, under, aside, unlike, through, in, for, behind, among, around, near, beyond, at, on, except, between, to, about, before, beyond, inside, toward, underneath, outside, over,* and *during.* The italicized words in the following sentences are prepositions:

Claire hid *under* the bed *during* the thunderstorm.
Marco played *in* the orchestra *for* many years.
Jessica saw the trespasser *outside* her window.
Above the piano was a beautiful portrait *of* my great aunt.

Conjunctions

A **conjunction** is a word that connects two or more words, phrases, clauses, or sentences. Some examples of conjunctions are *so, and, but, yet, or, both . . . and, either . . . or, if, when,* and *since.* The italicized words in the following sentences are conjunctions:

Aunt Polly ran into the room, *but* Tom was already gone.
Both my sister *and* I were born on August 14.
When the sun goes down, the air at the lake becomes rather cool.

Interjections

An **interjection** is an interruptive expression of sudden feeling. Here are a few examples:

Yay ! You did it.
Bravo ! Your violin recital was beautiful.
Encore ! Do it again.
Yikes ! That wasn't good.

COMMON PUNCTUATION REVIEW

The following is a quick review of the common marks of punctuation:

- A **period** (.) is used to symbolize the end of a sentence. It tells the reader to stop here.
  Example: The patient was discharged from the hospital.

- A **comma** (,) is used to indicate pause. Commas are used between clauses, after an introductory clause or phrase, and to separate listed items—just to name a few uses.
  Examples: Sarla is the nurse, but Cliff is the personal care assistant.
  Despite guidelines in the code of conduct manual, Michelle inappropriately viewed private medical information.
  The hospital course was stormy, complicated, and eventful.

- A **hyphen** (-) joins words and separates syllables.
  Example: She just received some heart-wrenching news.

More Review!

Check out *Word Smart, Word Smart II,* and *Grammar Smart* from The Princeton Review for additional verbal review.

- A **semicolon** (;) separates items in a list that has internal punctuation and links independent clauses.
  Examples: She interviewed three individuals: Joe, the baker; Bob, the builder; and Antonio, the violinist.
  Please come soon; I miss you.

- A **colon** (:) is most often used to introduce something that follows it.
  Example: The committee included the following individuals: a funny stand-up comedian, a financial guru, a mathematician, and a pilates instructor.

- An **em dash** (—) is most often used to show a break in thought or to introduce an appositve.
  Examples: We hate that restaurant—the food tastes so bland.
  The three candidates—Mr. Johnson, Ms. Clapton, and Mr. Ortiz—arrived promptly for the debate.

- An **ellipses** (. . .) shows the intentional omission of a word or the trailing off of a sentence.
  Example: The toddler proudly proclaimed, "I can count to ten—one, two, three . . . nine, ten."
  I started to wonder . . .

- A **question mark** (?) indicates that a sentence asks a question or makes an inquiry.
  Examples: What time did the surgery begin?
  When can we expect the results of the biopsy?

- An **exclamation point** (!) is used after interjections and statements of strong emotion.
  Examples: How dare you!
  Stay away from me!
  Get out!
  Be careful! The floor is still wet.
  Our team won the state championship!

- An **apostrophe** (') shows possession. When the possessor is singular, the apostrophe comes before the s. When the possessor is plural, the apostrophe comes after the s.
  Examples: Manuel's office was destroyed in the flood.
  Eva's prescription won't be ready until tomorrow. (Singular examples)
  The nurses' charts were examined by the supervisor.
  Come to my parents' house. (Plural examples)

- **Quotation marks** ("...") are used to indicate the exact words of a speaker.
  Example: The physician said, "It's very important that my instructions be followed exactly."

- **Parentheses** ( ) are used to set off information that is not closely related to the subject of the sentence.
  Examples: They put out a bid of almost a million dollars (a monetary sum that was less than appropriate) for the work being done.
  You will find the dosage on page 47 (Chapter 4) of your pharmacology book.

Caution

As a nurse, you should prepare your written statements in proper context of person, place, and time—and with a good measure of professionalism. Some people use capital letters to indicate strong emotion. Don't fall into this habit. Overuse of capital letters is interpreted as hostility. Here are some examples of the type of writing you should avoid:

- The resident YELLED at me over the phone.
- The patient screamed, "GET OUT!" The frustrated patient well may have thrown a food tray (with impressive force), cursed at you, and screamed for you to "get out," but a better record of the events would be written as follows: The patient threw his tray table at me and screamed, "Get out." Nursing leadership was notified as well as social worker and patient advocacy services.
- When responding to an email inviting you to attend a non-mandatory meeting, don't write "NO" or "NOT GOING." Instead, you could write, "I am unable to attend due to prior work obligation; however, I would like to discuss the agenda at a later date. Please contact me to discuss future dates to set up a meeting."

MORE KEY VERBAL CONCEPTS

The beginning of Chapter 5: Human Anatomy and Physiology covered a lot of medical terminology. That section offered commonly used prefixes and suffixes that you will use in your nursing profession. Please go back and review that section. It should help with your English section review.

Here are some additional concepts that should help in your nursing exam and in your career:

- **Suffixes** appear after the root of a word and give information about the word. An example is *ese* in Japanese. The suffix *ese* means "a native of" and it is tacked onto the stem Japan.
- **Prefixes** appear before the root of a word and also give information about the word. An example is *post* as in postpartum depression. The prefix *post* indicates that the phrase is about a period of time that comes after partum, or after childbirth.
- **Antonyms** are words that are opposite in meaning. Examples are hot and cold, good and bad, malicious and benevolent, destructive and encouraging, legal and illegal, moral and immoral, ethical and unethical, healthy and unhealthy, and clean and unclean.
- **Synonyms** are words that are similar in meaning. Examples are mean and cruel, heartless and thoughtless, deliberate and intentional, scathed and bitter, kind and compassionate, caring and sympathetic, loving and compassionate, handsome and good-looking, pretty and attractive, intelligent and smart, callow and immature, and struggling and suffering.
- **Contractions** are shortcuts of saying what we want to say. You probably use them every day without even thinking about them. For example, in a conversation, you may say, "We simply *can't* go" instead of saying "We simply *cannot* go." The word *can't* is a contraction of the word *cannot*. The apostrophe in a contraction takes the place of a letter or letters that have been omitted. Here are some common contractions:

Word(s)	Contraction
will not	won't
he is	he's
it is/it has	it's
should not	shouldn't
are not	aren't
that is	that's
we are	we're

Many suffixes and prefixes that can give you information about a word's meaning come from other languages. Let's look at a question that you might see on the NLN PAX-RN.

---

5. Saying that the prisoner is undergoing "enhanced interrogation" merely highlights the _____ flavor of the cruel word *torture*.

   A. aphoristic
   B. archaistic
   C. euphemistic
   D. dysphemistic

Here's How to Crack It

Choice C is correct, as the meaning of the sentence is that certain phrases are softened through different language, which is the meaning of the root word *euphemism*. Choice C, euphemistic, comes from the Greek word *euphemismos*, which is the use of a favorable word in place of an impolite one. If you break down the word, *eu* means good and *pheme* means speak—to speak good, or more polite, words in place of coarse words. Choice D, dysphemistic, has the opposite meaning of euphemistic, so choice D must be incorrect. Choice A is an adjective that means a short saying that describes a general truth, which isn't quite what we need in this question, so cross it off. Perhaps you have heard the word *archaic* before and know that it means retrograde or old-fashioned, so you can cross off choice B, since the meaning of this sentence has nothing to do with outdated vocabulary. Go with choice C.

SOUND ALIKES (HOMOPHONES)

Homophones are words that sound the same but differ in meaning.

Here are some common homophones that often cause problems in usage. Familiarize yourself with the differences in meanings.

> Check out that prefix in action! *Homo* means "same" and *phone* means "sound," so *homophone* means "same sound."

allowed/aloud	lessen/lesson
arc/ark	new/knew
ate/eight	no/know
alter/altar	past/passed
board/bored	peace/piece
break/brake	principal/principle
capital/capitol	rap/wrap
council/counsel	role/roll
dear/deer	sight/site
die/dye	seen/scene
coarse/course	there/their/they're
compliment/complement	to/too/two
its/it's	weather/whether
lead/led	week/weak
	your/you're

USAGE RULES

Sentence Structure

Good sentence structure is about putting words, clauses, and phrases—the essential building blocks of sentences—together in logical ways. Before we talk about the errors of sentence structure, let's spend a moment talking about correct structure. Here's an example:

As he ran across the room, Tom broke the vase.

As you know from our review earlier in the chapter, this sentence consists of two clauses—an independent and a dependent. Each clause has a subject and a verb. The second clause (Tom broke the vase) is the independent clause because it can stand alone, and the first clause (As he ran across the room) is the dependent clause here.

You can easily change a dependent clause into an independent clause and vice versa. Often all it takes is adding or deleting a single word. For example, suppose you remove the word *As* from the dependent clause just mentioned:

He ran across the room.

The result is an independent clause that can stand on its own. On the other hand, notice what happens when you add *As* to the dependent clause.

As Tom broke the vase . . . .

If we stick these two new clauses together now, the meaning of the sentence would be very different.

As Tom broke the vase, he ran across the room.

Could we have kept the meaning more or less the same and still made the first clause independent? Sure. Try this:

Tom ran across the room, breaking the vase.

Now the first half of the sentence contains the main independent clause. We had to change the pronoun *he* to *Tom* so the reader would know who the sentence was talking about. We also had to change the second half of the sentence from a clause into a modifying phrase. While a clause has a subject and a verb, a phrase has neither a subject nor a verb.

Putting the Pieces Together

Proficient writers use a mixture of dependent clauses, independent clauses, and phrases to add variety to their writing and to create emphasis. By combining these building blocks in different ways, writers show their readers which thoughts are most important and at the same time create a rhythm.

Here are the structures used most often:

- Independent clause (period) and new independent clause (period)
  Example: Jane lit the campire. Frank set up the tent.

- Independent clause (comma), conjunction, and second independent clause (period)
  Examples: Jane lit the campfire, and Frank set up the tent.
  Jane lit the campfire, while Frank set up the tent.

- Independent clause (semicolon) and second independent clause (period)
  Example: Jane lit the campfire; Frank set up the tent.

- Dependent clause (comma) and independent clause (period)
  Example: As Jane lit the campfire, Frank set up the tent.

All of the sentences above are correct, and all mean almost the same thing. A writer may choose one over another to emphasize one thought over another. For example, in the last sentence, the writer is choosing to make "setting up the tent" the focus of the sentence. Perhaps the writer is setting the stage for the tent collapsing with Frank inside it.

Here's another example:

- Phrase (comma) and independent clause (period)
  Example: Holding his flashlight in his teeth, Frank set up the tent.

- Independent clause (comma) phrase (period)
  Example: Frank set up the tent, holding his flashlight in his teeth.

Misplaced Modifiers

When constructing a sentence or when spotting sentence errors on your nursing exam, you should be aware of **misplaced modifiers**. A modifying phrase should be near the word or phrase it modifies. If a modifier is too far away, readers may misinterpret the sentence. For example, study the following sentence, which contains a misplaced modifier:

Sweeping up the pieces of glass, the missing key to the jewelry box was found by Aunt Polly.

As it is written, this sentence gives the impression that the missing key was doing the sweeping, which is impossible. When a sentence begins with a modifying phrase (a group of words without a subject), the noun being modified must follow the phrase. Who was sweeping up the pieces of glass? Aunt Polly, of course. The correct version of this sentence would be as follows:

Sweeping up the pieces of glass, Aunt Polly found the missing key to the jewelry box.

The following is a more subtle version of the same type of error:

Happy and excited, Aunt Polly's key opened the jewelry box for the first time in weeks.

At first glance, it looks as if the modifying phrase "happy and excited" is modifying Aunt Polly. However, what is the real subject of this sentence, as written? The key. Aunt Polly's is actually modifying the key. The correct version of this sentence would be as follows:

Happy and excited, Aunt Polly used her key to open the jewelry box for the first time in weeks.

Subject-Verb Agreement

As mentioned earlier in this chapter, the verb of a sentence must always agree with its subject in number. Let's look at an example.

My computer play chess better than I do.

Does that sound right to you? Let's check it out. The subject of this sentence is *computer* (since that is the thing in the sentence doing the action—the computer is playing chess) and *computer* is singular. The verb of the sentence is *play*, which is in the plural form. In this case, the subject and the verb don't agree. Here's a corrected version of the same sentence:

My computer plays chess better than I do.

Not every question will be as simple as that example, though. Sometimes you may not know if a noun or subject is singular or plural, making it tough to determine whether its verb should be singular or plural. Of course you know that subjects like he and cat are singular, but what about *family* and *everybody* ? The following is a list of tricky subjects. These are nouns that typically describe a group of people, but are usually considered singular and thus need a singular verb:

The family is
The jury is
The group is
The team is
The audience is
The congregation is
The United States (or any other country) is

The following pronouns also take singular verbs:

Either is
Neither is
Each is
Anyone is
No one is
Everyone is

SUMMARY

- There are many types of communication, including verbal, nonverbal, passive-aggressive, direct, and indirect.

- Beware of improper communication on the job.

- A sentence is a group of words that explains a complete thought.

- A phrase is part of a sentence that cannot stand on its own. It has neither a subject nor a verb.

- A fragment is a group of words that lacks either a subject or a verb.

- A clause can be dependent or independent. An dependent clause isn't a complete thought—it depends on another clause. An independent clause can stand on its own.

- A run-on sentence is made up of two or more independent clauses incorrectly connected. It is a problem of structure, not necessarily length.

- A noun is a person, place, object, thing, or idea. A noun can be abstract or concrete, singular or plural, common or proper.

- A pronoun is a word that replaces a noun.

- Verbs show action or state of being. They must agree in number with the subject of the sentence.

- Adjectives modify nouns.

- Adverbs modify verbs, adjectives, other adverbs, clauses, and sentences.

- A preposition shows position or place.

- A conjunction is a word that connects two or more words, phrases, clauses, or sentences.

- An interjection is an interruptive expression of sudden feeling.

- Review additional verbal concepts: suffixes, prefixes, antonyms, synonyms, and contractions.

- Beware of homophones; they can lead to error.

- Watch out for misplaced modifiers. A modifying phrase should be near what it modifies.

KEY TERMS

communication
verbal communication
written communication
signed communication
electronic communication
nonverbal communication
expressive aphasia
communication board (picture board)
effective communication
improper communication
sentence
phrase
fragment
clause
dependent clause
independent clause
run-on sentence
noun
articles
abstract noun
concrete noun
singular noun
plural noun
common noun
proper noun
pronoun
personal pronoun
possessive pronoun
relative pronoun
interrogative pronoun
verb
verb tense

present tense
past tense
future tense
past perfect tense
present perfect tense
future perfect tense
infinitive
adverbs
adjectives
preposition
object of the preposition
conjunction
interjection
period
comma
hyphen
semicolon
colon
em dash
ellipses
question mark
exclamation point
apostrophe
quotation marks
parentheses
suffix
prefix
antonym
synonym
contractions
homophones
misplaced modifiers

Chapter 14
Reading
Comprehension

Whether you are planning to take the NET, the TEAS, or the NLN PAX-RN, you will definitely encounter reading comprehension questions. The reason these tests include reading comprehension questions is that you will have to read and write to communicate in your job as a nurse. Therefore, it's important that you have skills to read passages and make deductions, inferences, conclusions, and then decisions.

In a hospital or medical office, written notes detailing events must be coherent, accurate, composed in English, written in black or blue ink, and legible. Your notes and documentation will attest to what you did and what happened during your shift. Records are saved, stored, scanned (sometimes sealed), and soon will be accessible through global computerized systems as more and more medical sites are going paperless. Because records may be subpoenaed and used in a tort malpractice case, nurses are encouraged to read and write coherently and carefully. Imagine if your poor handwriting leads to an incorrect diagnosis or an incorrect dosage of medicine. This chapter introduces a strategic approach for reading comprehension questions in test taking, so that you can ace your exam.

READING COMPREHENSION QUESTIONS

You may have no interest in the reading comprehension passages featured in your exam, but you must be skilled enough to note key information and draw conclusions from that. You must then apply what you read to the questions that you will be asked. The reading comprehension passages might not be about subjects that interest you or about which you have any outside knowledge. You might read about politics, dignitaries, topics in humanities, and other informative passages that explore the journey of the soul, mysticism, health, vitamins, and longevity. Or you might read discussions proving the reincarnation of hedgehogs. The topics don't matter; you're just there to notice the pertinent information you need to answer the questions correctly, and move on.

Reading comprehension exam questions test only what you understood or retained from what you just read. The questions measure how efficiently you can locate specific pieces of information. That is, the questions test your ability to read and comprehend a specific passage. Your answers don't reflect your intelligence or ability to function as a nurse. You may asked to recall events (time-line accuracy), annotate protagonist-antagonist relationships, interpret the author's thoughts, deduce the point of an article, extrapolate inferences from a passage, or find the best solution to a generalized concern concealed in the content of the passage. You may be asked to choose a better meaning for adverbs and adjectives used to modify the nouns and verbs in passages.

The key to reading boring or low-interest vignettes is to skim first, knowing that it will soon be over! Get a general idea first. Read the opening sentences and then the first and last line of each paragraph. Do not personalize what you are reading; there is no room for debate and opinion. You don't have to agree or like what you are reading.

When you are in the process of choosing your answer, don't worry about the need for outside information. If you know outside information about the subject of a passage, that's great, but it's not a requirement. Every question can be answered with just the material in the specific passage that you just read. Even if you are a genius and you know the answer is better found elsewhere, don't be tempted to look elsewhere. You must recall relevant evidence or ideas from the given passage. See if you can pick up on the author's theme, structure, or point of view. Among many passages, you will read different styles of writing, so be flexible. Some authors riddle their passages with sarcasm and wit—you may find yourself chuckling during the exam (but please refrain from rolling on the floor laughing). You may see irony, symbolism, and figurative language, too. If you are a more visual person, close your eyes and see if you can visualize what you read. If you are not visual, tune out all external noises and just read. Imagine that it's just you and the exam proctor in the room.

AN OPEN-BOOK TEST

Answering passage-based reading comprehension questions is like taking an open-book test. All of the information that you may be asked about is sitting right under your nose. You do not need outside knowledge for any of the questions. So, don't worry if you are not familiar with the passage content—the answer is there for you.

THE METHOD

Here's an effective method for approaching reading comprehension questions:

1. **Read the blurb.** Long passages usually begin with a short intro (often italicized), which will give you a little background about the passage. If you see one, read it. If there is no blurb, that's ok. Go to the next step.
2. **Quickly read for the main idea.** Skim the passage to find the main idea. As you're reading, think about what the author is getting at. That is, what's the big idea? Don't get wrapped up in the details at this point—just focus on the big picture.
3. **Choose a question and paraphrase it.** Putting a question into your own words can bolster understanding of both the question and the passage. If a question is easy to understand and paraphrase, then it may be a good question to attack right away.
4. **Read what you need to answer the question.** If the writers of the test found the answer (or the best of all the answers), then you have to find it. It is definitely somewhere within the passage. Go back and find it in your open-book test.
5. **Answer in your own words.** That's right. Before you even pick an answer from the given choices (A through D), first decide for yourself what the correct answer will be. Then choose from the four answer choices that you are given
6. **Use POE** (process of elimination), which you learned about in Chapter 3. Immediately eliminate the two most ridiculous or obviously wrong answers. Then go back to the passage and duke out the answer between the two choices left. Keep in mind that any answer choice that requires you to know outside information is wrong. Everything you need to answer that question in is that passage.

Beware the Buzzwords

Beware of answer choices that contain the following buzz words:

> must
> always
> impossible
> never
> cannot
> each
> every
> everyone
> totally
> all
> solely
> only

This collection of words (and other words that signify extremes) should be a red flag to you. Extreme language is rarely seen on standardized tests, so beware if you see it in an answer choice—chances are, that choice is incorrect.

Beware Exact Phrasing

Some test answers will be verbatim phrases from the reading comprehension passage. These sound familiar and, therefore, test takers are likely to pick these answers. But correct answers to specific questions are usually paraphrases of information in the passage, not direct quotes.

For General Questions, Pay Attention to Scope

Suppose a passage gives a brief overview of the effects of the Industrial Revolution on city growth in England and you are asked for the primary purpose of the passage. In this case, you might find incorrect answers such as "detail the Bessemer process of steel manufacturing" (too specific) or "chart the spread of the Industrial Revolution throughout Europe" (too broad). Often, answers that are too specific are just mentioned once or twice in the passage and answers that are too broad simply cannot be accomplished in the length of a short reading passage.

Which Approach to Take

When it comes to reading passages and their related questions, keep in mind that you are not being tested for reading ability or memory, just for how well you find the information and choose the right answer. There are six major question types that turn up with reading comprehension passages: vocabulary in context, detail, infer/imply/deduce, purpose, tone, main idea. Let's briefly examine each type.

1. **Vocabulary in context questions** ask you for the meaning of a word in the passage. For example, suppose the passage contains the word *floor*. A question may ask "Used this way, *floor* means _____." To answer this question, you must determine how the word *floor* is used in the context of the passage. Your vocabulary review (see Chapter 15) will be helpful with this question type.

2. **Detail questions** are relatively straightforward and essentially ask, "What does the passage say?"

3. **Infer/imply/deduce questions** might seem intimidating, but you're definitely up to the task. They are simply taking what you have read in the passage and going just one step further. They are asking what you can then deduce from the given information, or what is implied by the information, or what conclusion you can now infer. Don't let the test writers trick you into thinking that you need to read between the lines or discover a hidden meaning in the passage. In reality, questions of this type are quite similar to detail questions. In most cases, the answer will simply be a paraphrase of something already stated in the passage.

4. **Purpose questions** are a lot like the questions that you should ask yourself when you are trying to paraphrase the passage. With these questions, the test writers want to see if you know why the author wrote this passage. So, go ahead and ask yourself, "Why did the author write this?" (You don't have to care either.)

5. **Tone questions** ask you to determine the tone of the author. Is the attitude of the author positive, negative, or neutral? Identify the author's attempt to persuade, inform, entertain, or express feelings.

6. **Main idea questions** are straightforward. Such questions ask you to determine the gist of the passage. Don't get caught up in every detail of the passage. Rather, focus on the overall message.

HELPFUL HINTS: BEYOND THE BASICS

In addition to the techniques discussed so far, we have a few final points to round out your repertoire.

Literary Devices

There may be a few questions that ask about the **literary devices** the author uses to make a point. It's probably been a few years since you have seen these. No need to fear. We provided a list of terms for you to review.

Simile

A **simile** is the comparison of two dissimilar things with the use of the words *like* or *as*.

Examples: The smoke uncoiled from the chimney like a snake charmed out of its basket.
She sobbed like a baby.
David is sharp as a tack.

Metaphor

A **metaphor** is also a comparison of two dissimilar things, though without the use of *like* or *as*.

Examples: In a crisis, Kristen is a rock.
A blanket of snow covered the earth.

Extended Metaphor

An **extended metaphor** is like a metaphor turned up to 11. In an extended metaphor, a symbol is used to represent something else throughout a long passage or entire work. The poem "O Captain! My Captain!" by Walt Whitman is a classic example: On the surface, the poem is about a captain who has successfully navigated his ship through a storm, but dies just before reaching port. However, the poem is actually an extended metaphor: The captain represents Abraham Lincoln, the ship is America, the storm is the Civil War, and his sudden death is . . . well, his sudden death.

Personification

Personification is the assigning of human qualities to nonhumans: animals, plants, inanimate objects, and the like.

Examples: The wind whispered in the night.
Every time Janet dove into the pile, the leaves leaped and danced in the air.
The Heavens rejoiced the day you were born.

Alliteration

Alliteration is the repetition of initial consonant sounds.

Examples: Little Lucy loves lavender and lilacs.
Zach zigged and zagged around the zoo.

Hyperbole

Hyperbole is the use of exaggeration to make a point. Hyperboles can sometimes be confused with similes because they often use *like* or *as*.

Examples: I ate my weight in chocolate.
It is four hundred thousand degrees outside today.
To Charlie, his father seemed as tall as a skyscraper.

Imagery

The tendency may be to assume that **imagery** is limited to the use of visual images, but in actuality, imagery is the language that appeals to all of the senses.

> Examples: I stroked the papery skin of her hands.
> As she sang, Hillary's high, clear voice wafted through the hall.

Tone

Tone may also be referred to as **mood**. It's the overall attitude of a piece of writing. Look for words or phrases that evoke emotion.

> Examples: Chris trudged out into the bleak, grey dawn.
> The puppy bounded eagerly into Lindsey's open arms.

Onamatopoeia

Onomatopoeia refers to words that represent sounds. Pretty much every animal sound is included in this group, as well as words such as *slap, crack, swish, click,* and *murmur.*

Verbal Irony

Verbal irony occurs when a discrepancy takes place between what someone says and what the situation indicates the speaker means.

> Examples: Your patient deliberately wrestled you down to the ground and didn't stop kicking until her shoes came off? *Good times!*
> You left your laptop in the taxi? *Smart!*

Sarcasm is the most common type of verbal irony. In real life, however, be mindful not to use it to hurt someone's feelings. People enjoy a good laugh and light humor, but nobody likes a sarcastic person or a sharp, caustic tongue.

Situational Irony

Situational irony occurs when people plan for events to turn out one way, but they actually turn out another way. Here's one funny example of situational irony: A group of nurses takes a vacation in Mexico. To play it safe, one of the nurses deliberately avoids fresh veggies, ice, and water. She's careful to use bottled water when brushing her teeth. Who got Montezuma's revenge? The one who maintained aseptic technique or the ones who enjoyed the fruits of the land? Yup, you guessed it. Ms. Clean. That's situational irony.

Dramatic Irony

Dramatic irony is similar to situational irony, but the audience or reader is given more information than the characters have. The short story "The Gift of the Magi" is a great example of dramatic irony. In this story, a beautiful wife can't afford a Christmas gift for her husband and she wants to buy him a chain for his pocket watch. At the same time, her equally impoverished husband wants to buy his wife a pretty comb for her long, flowing hair. The wife decides to cut off her hair and sell it to make money so that she can purchase the chain for her husband. Meanwhile, the husband sells his watch to get money for the hair comb. Imagine the dramatic irony on Christmas Eve when they exchanged gifts.

Satire

Satire uses sarcasm, humor, exaggeration, absurdity, and/or irony to ridicule human behavior or societal weakness, often with the intent of shedding light on a situation. For great political and human behavioral satire, watch some reruns of *Saturday Night Live* (hilarious political debates).

Soliloquy

A **soliloquy** is a form of a monologue in which the character in the passage expresses feelings and thoughts aloud, but does not intend for other characters to hear these thoughts. (Think of it as a solo—talking to yourself.) Many playwrights love using soliloquies. For example, in Shakespeare's *Hamlet*, all exit the stage but Hamlet. In a short soliloquy, Hamlet reflects that he will be cruel to his mother, showing her the extent of her crime in marrying Claudius, but he determines that he will not actually hurt her.

Foreshadowing

Foreshadowing occurs when the writer of a passage reveals details (hints, clues, suggestions) that will become significant later as the story or plot unfolds. Foreshadowing can be subtle (like mentioning ominous storm clouds gathering), or it can be as concrete and direct as a train wreck that seems random and unimportant at the start of the story, but later becomes an indicator of tragedies to come.

Allusions

An **allusion** is a literary device by which an author refers to a historical event or uses a Biblical, literary, or mythological reference with which the reader is expected to be familiar.

> Examples: The teenage girls chatted into the night about their turncoat friend. "She's such a Judas!" Tiffany seethed.
> Bob couldn't get a job because he had no experience, but he couldn't get experience because no one would hire him for a job. A frustrating catch-22.

Infer

To **infer** is to derive or judge by reasoning. An inference isn't information that is simply given at face value—there is an implied judgment or conclusion with an inference.

> Examples: We can infer from her state of panic, tears, and quick breathing that Deb is clearly upset and afraid.
> Based on your hatred of all things chocolate, it's safe to infer that you won't be buying my chocolate chip cookies at the bake sale.

Imply

To **imply** means to suggest or hint. You might see a question about the author's implied message or the implied meaning of a passage.

> Examples: She didn't outright reject Dean's request for a kiss, but her awkward laugh and head movement implied that she wanted nothing to do with him.
> The company outing isn't mandatory, but the implication is that all staff had better make it their business to attend.

Deduce

To **deduce** means to determine by deduction or conclude based on evidence.

> Examples: Based on the mess that they left in the kitchen, I deduced that the family must have been in a huge hurry to leave the house that morning.
> From the height of the Sun, Chrissy deduced that it was around noontime.

Paradox

A **paradox** is a statement that looks like a contradiction, yet is actually true in a sense.

> Examples: Less is more.
> Freedom is slavery.

GOT ALL THAT?

Now that you have read through a good method for reading comprehension, noted buzzwords to beware of, perused an approach for the reading comprehension passages and questions, and reviewed literary devices, let's tackle a few passages and questions.

Here are some questions like those you might see on the NET.

Impact of Mobile Phones on Human Health

[1] Mobile phones or cellular phones, which have become *sine qua non* in our lives, are extremely handy, but they can cause harm to human health. Mobile phones discharge radio waves, which can lead to potential risks associated with health. The World Health Organization (WHO) has distinguished mobile phone emission as possibly carcinogenic. This means that there could be hazards related to carcinogenicity, or the ability to produce cancer.

[2] One of the effects of mobile phone radiation is dielectric heating, in which the living tissue is heated due to the rotations undertaken by polar molecules, which are catalyzed by the electromagnetic field. The heating effect will occur at the surface of the brain, affecting a temperature increase by a fraction of a degree. Some studies assert that radiofrequency radiation (RFR) released by the cell phones can impact the cognitive functions of humans. Apparently, the response time to a spatial working memory task is longer or slower, and prolonged exposure to RFR may increase the effects on performance. Some users of mobile

phones have alleged feeling burning sensations in the skin, fatigue, sleep disturbance, dizziness, and other symptoms. However, the connection between these symptoms and radiation is yet to be proved.

1. Which of the following conclusions can be **definitely** drawn from the passage?

   A. Excessive use of mobile phones leads to cancer.
   B. Use of mobile phones impacts mental health of humans.
   C. Mobile phones are useful though harmful to human health.
   D. Hands-free usage of phones is the best precautionary measure.

Here's How to Crack It

As we know from this chapter, extreme language is rarely seen on standardized tests. Choice A is wrong because it's an extreme stance and the question asks for a definite conclusion, which is not what the last sentence of the first paragraph gives us. That last sentence says "there could be hazards related to carcinogenicity," but does not definitely conclude that cell phones cause cancer. Eliminate choice A. The effects of prolonged exposure to RFR (listed at the end of the passage) include burning sensations in the skin, fatigue, sleep disturbance, and dizziness, but none of those symptoms concern mental health, so cross off choice B. While hands-free usage of phones is a good precaution against cell phone-related car accidents, this isn't covered in the passage, and the question will ask you only about content in the passage (remember— it's an open-book test), so eliminate choice D. That leaves choice C, which is paraphrased in the first sentence of the passage, so that is the correct answer.

2. What is the meaning of the term *sine qua non* in the first paragraph of the passage above?

   A. Useless
   B. Essential
   C. Demand
   D. Condition

Here's How to Crack It

Sine qua non might look like Greek to you, but the next clause in that first sentence provides a clue about the phrase's meaning: handy. What choice is closest to the meaning of handy? Choice B, essential. Choice A (useless) wouldn't make sense in that first sentence, since something cannot be both handy and useless. Choices C and D (demand and condition) wouldn't make sense in meaning or syntax of this sentence—cross those out. Choice B is the correct answer.

SUMMARY

- Use these steps to answer reading comprehension questions:

  Read the blurb.

  Quickly read the passage for the main idea.

  Choose a question and paraphrase it.

  Read what you need to answer the question.

  Answer in your own words.

  Use POE.

- Beware of buzzwords, extreme language, and exact phrasing.

- Questions that accompany reading comprehension passages will most likely be of the following types: vocabulary in context, detail, infer/imply/deduce, purpose, tone, main idea.

- Review literary devices.

KEY TERMS

literary devices
simile
metaphor
extended metaphor
personification
alliteration
hyperbole
imagery
tone (mood)
onomatopoeia
verbal irony
sarcasm
situational irony
dramatic irony
satire
soliloquy
foreshadowing
allusion
infer
imply
deduce
paradox

Chapter 15
Vocabulary

WILL I NEED A STRONG VOCABULARY FOR MY EXAM?

Having a strong vocabulary is useful in life and in the test-taking world. Vocabulary will be important in your exam, whether you are taking the NLN PAX-RN, the NET, or the TEAS. The NLN PAX-RN tests word knowledge (among other things) in the Verbal section, and the TEAS tests vocabulary in context in the English/Language Usage section. Knowing a large assortment of vocabulary will be beneficial for those of you who are going to take the NET as well, since you might see new words in the reading comprehension passages. So any way you slice it, vocabulary review is useful.

HOW TO LEARN VOCABULARY

The vocabulary list that follows looks daunting, we know. Add the 200 words in this chapter to the Key Terms that you have seen at the close of the content review chapters, and that's a whole lot of words to memorize. Therefore, we recommend that you take things day by day. That is, each day, select a section of words that you will tackle and review them multiple times during the day. A great way to push yourself to look at words throughout the day is by making flash cards. Flash cards are useful, but be sure to write down not only the word and its definition, but also an example sentence in which you use that word. For each word in the list in this chapter, we have provided a sample sentence for you, but feel free to create your own to reinforce memorization. Carry these cards with you everywhere—to the bank, when running errands, to work, to school—everywhere. Anytime that you have a few moments of down time, pull out your flash cards and review. You'll be surprised—all those short review sessions make a difference.

Here is a list of words that you are likely to see on your exam. For every word, we have provided the part of speech of the word, its definition, and a sample sentence that contains it. Enjoy!

abstruse   **(adjective)**
hard to understand

> The assigned text was so abstruse that I have no idea how I'll pass the test.

acquiesce   **(verb)**
to submit without protest

> Jeff rarely stands up to his demanding wife; he pathetically acquiesces to her every whim.

adroit   **(adjective)**
expert, skilled, or nimble

> Timothy is a talented violinist; he makes all of us sound like beginners.

advocate (verb)

to speak or write in favor of

A group of nurses joined together to advocate patient privacy rights on the local and national levels.

affluence (noun)

abundance of wealth

The suspect's affluence disallowed the myriad excuses for gross negligence and passivity.

allude (verb)

to refer to casually or indirectly

Let's not allude to their inappropriate choices and poor judgment of character last year.

anachronism (noun)

something out of place in historical time

If a movie character living in the 1950s were listening to an mp3 player, that would be an anachronism.

antagonistic (adjective)

acting in opposition to another

Shane has an antagonistic streak; he's always picking on someone.

apprehensive (adjective)

uneasy or fearful

Ned always feels apprehensive before a big test.

appropriated (verb)

to take possession of

The detective appropriated my car to chase the criminals down the freeway.

assertion (noun)

a statement or declaration, often without reasoning or support

"I knew that already," was Ted's most common assertion during trivia games.

assuage   **(verb)**

to make milder or less severe

To assuage his guilt about forgetting her birthday, Bob bought his girlfriend a lot of flowers.

astute   **(adjective)**

having practical intelligence

The detective's astute observations helped solve the crime.

atypical   **(adjective)**

not typical; not conforming to type

Joe's love of reading is atypical of the children in his family.

banal   **(adjective)**

lacking originality

Watching scary movies on Halloween is too banal; let's hang out at the graveyard.

belabor   **(verb)**

to explain or work at something beyond what is necessary

We all heard her say not to drink grape juice on the couch, but she belabored the point for an hour.

belittle   **(verb)**

to speak of someone as less impressive or less important

Ian belittles his younger brother, calling him names and teasing him constantly.

bleak   **(adjective)**

bare and desolate

The bleak landscape was depressing, so we closed the curtains.

cacophony   **(noun)**

harsh, loud, discordant sounds

For several months, the hospital administration fed the trusting employee a cacophony of lies.

cantankerous   (adjective)

disagreeable to deal with

Grandma's cantankerous outbursts make it difficult for us to have a peaceful visit.

capricious   (adjective)

subject to or led by whim

Candy's capricious behavior keeps even her best friends guessing.

captivate   (verb)

to attract or hold the interest of

Acrobats captivate even the most reluctant crowds.

cavalier   (adjective)

showing arrogant disregard

Lisa's cavalier attitude about the group project frustrated her classmates.

coerce   (verb)

use of force or intimidation to get results

The class bully coerced Dan into writing his research paper for him again.

coherent   (adjective)

logically connected or consistent

Mike's speech wasn't all that coherent; we think he was too nervous to speak clearly.

cohesive   (adjective)

united, integrated, or unified

After we worked out our differences, we were once again a cohesive group.

complacent   (adjective)

pleased with oneself

After testifying against the defendents, Natasha coiffed her hair and gave herself a complacent smile.

comprehensive (adjective)

of large scope

The course offers a comprehensive study of the history of rock and roll.

compromised (verb)

to make vulnerable

The security of private medical information was compromised when the violator inappropriately accessed the file.

concede (verb)

to acknowledge as true or proper

Behind the scenes, the office conceded that Vanessa was the best provider in their medical group.

connoisseur (noun)

a person with expert knowledge or taste

Debra fancies herself a connoisseur of French wines and brags about her exquisite taste.

conscientious (adjective)

careful; painstaking

Kim's conscientious habits earn her top grades in every class.

consecration (noun)

dedication to the service or worship of a god

The clergy recited a consecration prayer on the feast of the Sacred Heart.

contentious (adjective)

tending to argument or conflict

The contentious brothers were constantly arguing and fighting.

contrite (adjective)

showing sincere remorse

His contrite attitude did not persuade the judge to reduce his punishment.

convoluted   (adjective)

intricately involved

Maria's convoluted explanation of inaccurate facts left the court even more confused.

credible   (adjective)

worthy of belief or confidence

Dave's story about aliens stealing his cell phone isn't exactly credible.

credulous   (adjective)

willing to believe or trust too readily

Joseph is so credulous; he believes everything he reads on the Internet.

culpable   (adjective)

deserving blame

The man culpable of the robbery was never caught or charged.

cultivate   (verb)

to develop through education or training

Lucy cultivated her singing ability through years of intense training.

cynical   (adjective)

distrusting the motives of others

Janet is cynical about Internet dating after her last disastrous relationship.

dearth   (adjective)

an inadequate supply

There's a dearth of water in the desert.

debilitating   (adjective)

to make weak or feeble

George suffered a debilitating injury that ended his dancing career.

deferential (adjective)

showing deference or respect

The office often gave deferential treatment to wealthy patients and neglected the poor.

deficient (adjective)

lacking in some characteristic or trait

The offending client was deficient in honesty and conscience.

deleterious (adjective)

harmful or injurious

Working in a hostile environment can have deleterious effects on employees.

demeanor (noun)

conduct; behavior

Owen's calm demeanor puts everyone at ease.

denuded (verb)

to make naked or bare

Since our state's water shortage has essentially denuded our yard, we're putting in a rock garden instead.

deplore (verb)

to regret deeply or strongly

Patrick deplores reality television, but I secretly like it.

deprecate (verb)

to express disapproval of

Emily's self-deprecating jokes were more sad than funny.

despondent (adjective)

profoundly hopeless

Elizabeth was despondent over dropping her engagement ring in the sewer.

diatribe (noun)

a bitter attack or criticism

After reading our essays, our teacher went on a diatribe about verb tense.

didactic (adjective)

inclined to teach or lecture too much

The professor's didactic speaking style put the class to sleep.

differentiate (verb)

to perceive the difference between

It's sometimes difficult to differentiate between pepperoni and salami.

diffident (adjective)

lacking self-confidence

Pam's diffident demeanor is characterized by her shuffling walk and lack of eye contact.

diligent (adjective)

attentive and persistent

Chelsea's diligent record keeping always helps when she's ready to prepare her tax return.

discern (verb)

to perceive or recognize

I couldn't discern the point of the book, even after reading it twice.

discord (noun)

lack of harmony

Conversations between Maria and her staff often turn from peace to discord without warning.

disdain (noun)

a feeling of contempt or scorn

Four-year-old Annie shows her disdain for vegetables by tossing them off her plate.

disparage (verb)

to belittle; to bring reproach or discredit upon

The athlete disparaged his entire sport with his blatant abuse of performance-enhancing drugs.

dispassionate (adjective)

devoid of feeling or bias

The dispassionate judge heard the case without becoming emotional.

dispel (verb)

to drive off; to eliminate

Michael's changed appearance made it impossible for him to dispel the rumors of plastic surgery.

disseminate (verb)

to scatter or spread widely

The news of the tragedy was immediately disseminated by every major news network.

distinguish (verb)

to mark as different

I can't distinguish between my black and brown shoes and sometimes wear one of each.

divergent (adjective)

moving apart from a common point

There were three divergent paths, so we each followed one to see where they went.

dogmatic (adjective)

asserting opinions in an arrogant manner

Eva's dogmatic political speeches turned some supporters against her.

dormant (adjective)

inactive, as if asleep

The dormant volcano hasn't erupted in more than a century.

ebullient (adjective)

overflowing with excitement

The ebullient crowd went crazy when Manuel took the stage.

elaborate (verb)

to develop thoroughly

Ronnie's boss asked him to elaborate on the reason he hated his job.

elicit (verb)

to draw out or bring forth

The cheerleaders had a hard time eliciting cheers from the bored audience.

eminent (adjective)

high in station or rank

Airports and streets close with the arrival of eminent politicians.

empirical (adjective)

provable from experiment or experience

Without empirical evidence, no one believed there was a UFO.

entrenched (adjective)

firmly established or set

Entrenched in his work, Aaron didn't even notice it was time to go home.

enumerate (verb)

to number or list

I'll enumerate the reasons I love you.

equivocal (adjective)

doubtful; uncertain

Victor gave an equivocal answer when asked if he liked Betsy's new dress.

evoke (verb)

to call up or produce

Disco music evokes memories of polyester leisure suits.

excoriate (verb)

to criticize or berate severely

The fraternity's hazing actions were excoriated in local and national news.

exonerate (verb)

to clear from guilt or blame

Peter was exonerated after he proved someone else stole the cookies.

exorbitant (adjective)

highly excessive

We spent an exorbitant amount of money on plane fare to Fiji.

extravagant (adjective)

spending more than is wise or necessary

Celebrities' extravagant lifestyles are the subject of much MTV programming.

facetious (adjective)

not meant seriously or literally

I was being facetious when I said I liked your acid-wash jeans.

fallacy (noun)

a deceptive or false notion

It's a fallacy that butter heals a burn.

flamboyant (adjective)

strikingly bold or brilliant

Elvis's flamboyant jumpsuits are as famous as his music.

flippant (adjective)

frivolously disrespectful

Sandy's flippant comments covered up her disappointment.

frank (adjective)

direct in speech

People love to hate Howard and the frank opinions he shares on the radio.

gaffe (noun)

a social blunder

Anita made the embarrassing gaffe of publicly mispronouncing the director's name.

gullible (adjective)

easily deceived or cheated

Jack is so gullible that we were able to convince him he could fly if he jumped off the roof.

hypothesis (noun)

an explanation for the occurrence of a process or event

The chemistry final required us to prove or disprove a given hypothesis.

idiosyncratic (adjective)

belonging to one's particular character

Ursula's idiosyncratic movements got her kicked off the drill team.

impartial (adjective)

not biased

None of the judges of the talent show were impartial; each had a clear favorite.

imperturbable (adjective)

incapable of being upset or agitated

Regardless of how much noise we make, my dad is imperturbable when he's reading.

implacable (adjective)

not to be appeased or pacified

An implacable opponent, Bobby was aggressive even after the match.

improvise (verb)

to compose, recite, or play on the spur of the moment

Keith was cut from jazz band because he couldn't improvise his solos.

impudent (adjective)

having or showing offensive boldness

Ralph's impudent comments got him sent to his room without dinner.

impugn (verb)

to challenge as false

In order to win the popularity contest, Lisa had to impugn her opponent's charitable deeds.

incongruous (adjective)

out of place, unbecoming, or inappropriate

Amy's charming smile is incongruous with the anger she is feeling.

inconsequential (adjective)

of little or no importance

Since Kate doesn't have a curfew, it's inconsequential if she stays out late.

indignant (adjective)

expressing strong displeasure at something offensive

Maggie was indignant when her boss accused her of stealing.

indulgent (adjective)

giving in to a desire in an excessive manner

My aunt is indulgent, letting me break all of Mom's rules when I visit.

inevitable (adjective)

unable to be avoided

Slipping on banana peels is inevitable if you're in a cartoon.

inherent   (adjective)

existing as an inseparable quality or element

The delicious taste of chocolate is inherent to its appeal.

innocuous   (adjective)

harmless or inoffensive in effect

Most spider bites are itchy, but otherwise innocuous.

intransigent   (adjective)

refusing to agree or compromise

Joe was intransigent, refusing to share any of his fries with us.

intuition   (noun)

insight not depending on reason

Janet's intuition told her to look under the rug for her missing earrings.

inured   (verb)

accustomed to something, especially a hardship or difficulty

Lauren was inured to the freezing weather and just bundled up before going for a run.

itinerant   (adjective)

traveling from place to place

The itinerant preacher wandered from town to town.

jocular   (adjective)

joking or facetious

Hal is always so jocular; it's strange when he's serious.

languid   (adjective)

lacking energy or vitality

Carrie's languid spirit concerned her friends.

laud   (verb)

to praise

Fans laud great athletes by carrying them around on their shoulders.

licentious **(adjective)**

unrestrained by law or morality

The licentious sheriff chased women and broke all of his own laws.

loquacious **(adjective)**

tending to talk too freely or too much

Loquacious Lucy purchased a big cell phone plan.

mediocrity **(noun)**

the state of being average or unremarkable

Impatient with mediocrity, the coach pushed his team to be champions.

mercenary **(adjective)**

motivated purely by money

The mercenary corporation bought rival businesses and fired all the employees.

metaphor **(noun)**

a direct comparison between two dissimilar things

When he tells you that you are his sunshine, he's using a metaphor.

meticulous **(adjective)**

showing extreme care about small details

Danielle is a very meticulous person; nothing in her room is ever out of place.

mollify **(verb)**

to soften in feeling or temper

In order to mollify her, Karen's mom baked a pie for her.

mundane **(adjective)**

uninteresting; common

Tired of the same mundane chores every week, I offered to rake leaves.

munificent (adjective)

great generosity in giving

The munificent CEO gave raises to all of his employees.

muted (adjective)

of low intensity or volume

The painting's muted colors conveyed a peaceful feeling.

nebulous (adjective)

hazy, vague, or indistinct

The decision lay in that nebulous area between wrong and right.

negligible (adjective)

not important; of little consequence; trifling

The money I spend on gum is negligible and not worth including in the budget.

nihilism (noun)

total rejection of laws or institutions

Mich's philosophy of nihilism keeps her from caring about rules and laws.

nonchalant (adjective)

coolly unconcerned

Melanie tried to be nonchalant about winning the scholarship, but we knew she was excited.

novelty (noun)

state of being new or unique

Oscar loves his toys until their novelty wears off.

obfuscate (verb)

to confuse, bewilder, or stupefy

The message was obfuscated by his use of mixed metaphors.

obliterate (verb)

to destroy completely

A week of sunny days can obliterate all traces of snow.

obscure (adjective)

unclear; hard to perceive or understand

Karen is always making obscure references to *Star Trek* episodes.

obstinate (adjective)

adhering to one's opinion or course

Kendra can be obstinate, refusing to follow rules she doesn't like.

onerous (adjective)

causing hardship

Lance's onerous debt caused him and his family continual stress.

ostentatious (adjective)

intended to attract notice

The wedding decorations were so ostentatious that we almost overlooked the bride.

overt (adjective)

open to view; not concealed

In an overt attempt to cheat, Sarah wrote the answers on the back of her hand.

paragon (noun)

a model or pattern of excellence

Though Selden is a nice guy, Lily doesn't see him as a paragon of virtue.

parody (noun)

a humorous imitation of something serious

The comedian's parody of the president was so realistic that it was eerie.

partisan (adjective)

influenced or controlled by a certain group

The journalist's partisan politics kept him from reporting the election results objectively.

patronizing (adjective)

in an offensively condescending manner

The way my grandmother still pinches my cheek is so patronizing.

pensive (adjective)

dreamily thoughtful

Feeling pensive, Andrea spent the afternoon writing in her journal.

perfidy (noun)

deliberate breach of trust

Jason's perfidy was obvious when he was caught driving his father's car without permission.

perfunctory (adjective)

performed merely as a routine

A perfunctory kiss accompanied the deliverence of his diploma at the commencement exersises.

perusal (noun)

a survey or reading

After a quick perusal of the magazine, Cary decided to buy a subscription.

pious (adjective)

having a spirit of reverence for God

Because of his pious nature, Bob prayed before every meal, every test, and every game.

placid (adjective)

pleasantly calm or peaceful

The placid lake was perfect for waterskiing.

plasticity (noun)

capacity for being molded or shaped

Silly Putty's most important quality is its plasticity.

plausible (adjective)

appearing truthful or reasonable

Her excuse for being late didn't sound plausible.

polemical (adjective)

involving dispute or controversy

The polemical discussion about adopting school uniforms went on for hours.

pompous (adjective)

arrogant; exhibiting self-importance

Ever since she was voted prom queen, Janie has had a pompous attitude.

portend (verb)

to indicate in advance

Dark clouds portend bad weather.

potentate (noun)

a person who possesses great power; a ruler

The queen, a gentle potentate, called for an end to the beheadings.

presumption (noun)

an assumption or supposition

Juries should have a presumption of innocence regarding the accused.

pretension (noun)

an attitude of dignity or importance

The family's air of pretension is so false it's ridiculous.

prevalent (adjective)

widespread

Mosquitoes are prevalent in swampy areas.

prodigious   (adjective)

extraordinary in size, amount, or degree

Nate's prodigious backpack rose well over his head when he put it on.

prolific   (adjective)

producing abundantly

Don is a prolific author, publishing a book a year.

prophetic   (adjective)

having the abilities of a prophet to predict what will happen

I had a prophetic dream that I'd one day become a nurse.

prosaic   (adjective)

commonplace or dull

Dolores uses prosaic passwords, so it's easy to hack into her email accounts.

provident   (adjective)

providing carefully for the future

A provident homeowner, Jessica stores extra food and water in case of emergencies.

provincial   (adjective)

belonging to a particular area

The provincial newspaper rarely discussed events beyond the neighborhood.

provoke   (verb)

to anger or enrage

Allison tries to provoke her brother by flicking him in the forehead.

querulous   (adjective)

full of complaints

The querulous group of ladies made it hard for us to enjoy the concert.

quiescence (noun)

the quality of being at rest

The quiescence of the morning was shattered by the arrival of a freight train.

reciprocity (noun)

a mutual exchange

In an act of reciprocity, Jen gave me a book after I gave her a CD.

reclusive (adjective)

living apart from society

Many famous writers are reclusive and wary of personal publicity.

recrimination (noun)

a retaliatory accusation; a charge made in retaliation for an accusation

Accusations and recriminations passed back and forth between the divorcing couple.

refute (verb)

to prove wrong

The senator tried to refute the accusation that he took bribes.

regimen (noun)

a strict plan for living, usually designed to improve the health of an individual

After his heart attack, Brett's doctor gave him a strict diet and exercise regimen.

remonstrate (verb)

to say or plead in protest or disapproval

The student body remonstrated against the proposed shortened lunch hour.

renowned (adjective)

celebrated; famous

The renowned playwright had a nationwide reputation for arrogance.

reserved (adjective)

formal or self-restrained

Karen is always reserved around new people until she gets to know them.

resilient (adjective)

springing back; recovering readily

Always resilient, Mabel makes lemonade when life gives her lemons.

resolute (adjective)

firmly determined

Bill is resolute in his decision never to marry.

respite (noun)

a delay or temporary rest

The movie provided a respite from our long day of studying.

reticent (adjective)

reserved or reluctant

Though she's outgoing at home, Tanya is reticent about talking in class.

retribution (noun)

something given as repayment, often punishment

The criminal sought retribution against the informant who turned him in.

reverent (adjective)

having or showing respect

The pastor always spoke in a reverent tone of voice.

sagacious (adjective)

having keen practical sense

The sagacious attorney built a strong case to defend her client.

salutary (adjective)

promoting health or some beneficial purpose

The health spa boasted a nutritious and salutary cuisine.

satire (noun)

the use of ridicule to point out weaknesses

The candidate was a frequent object of satire on late-night comedy shows.

scathing (adjective)

bitterly severe

The mean girls shouted scathing insults at each other.

sensationalistic (adjective)

meant to produce startling or thrilling impressions

Sensationalistic stories about aliens and UFOs are popular in tabloids.

serene (adjective)

calm or peaceful

Louise feels most serene after a hot bath and a cup of chamomile tea.

servile (adjective)

slavishly submissive

Erica's servile boyfriend follows her everywhere, hoping she'll drop something so he can pick it up.

somber (adjective)

gloomily dark

It's traditional to wear somber colors at a funeral.

spurious (adjective)

not genuine, authentic, or true

Joe's spurious remark did not fool the police officer.

squander   (verb)

to spend or use wastefully

Because Danny squanders every penny he earns, he has no retirement savings.

stringent   (adjective)

extremely strict or severe

The stringent rules were difficult for the rowdy children to follow.

superfluous   (adjective)

more than is sufficient or required

The streamers were superfluous to the overly decorated party room.

supplant   (verb)

to replace one thing with another

The Republican nominee wants to supplant the incumbent Democrat.

suppress   (verb)

to keep in or repress

Nick doesn't even try to suppress the urge to yell at other drivers.

tedious   (adjective)

long and tiresome

Ms. Bart's lectures were so tedious that I would start to nod off halfway through.

tenacious   (adjective)

holding fast; stubborn

The team was tenacious, finally defeating its opponent in double overtime.

torpor   (noun)

sluggish inactivity or indifference

After he ate three helpings of turkey, Wendell's torpor was understandable.

tractable (adjective)

easily managed or controlled

The tractable group of teens was talked into staying out after curfew.

uniformity (noun)

the state of being the same or homogenous

School dress codes are meant to encourage uniformity.

veiled (adjective)

covered or concealed as if by a veil

Andrea asked to borrow my phone in a veiled attempt to get Seth's number.

venerable (adjective)

demanding respect due to dignity or age

Many cultures see the elderly as wise and venerable.

versatility (noun)

the state or quality of adapting easily

A sofa bed's best feature is its versatility, not its comfort.

vignette (noun)

a small, pleasing sketch or view

Selena took a few moments to write a vignette about Paris in the spring.

vociferous (adjective)

crying out noisily

Martha shouted vociferously for her friend to meet her across the street.

volatile (adjective)

threatening to break out into violence

Howie's volatile temper makes others uncomfortable.

wary (adjective)

on guard against danger

I'm wary of sales pitches that sound too good to be true.

Chapter 16
Helpful Advice

BE POSITIVE AND SMART

If you made it to this page, you have probably completed most, or perhaps all, of your review. Bravo! Well done! Now, let's talk about the experience of actually taking the test. Be gentle with yourself. No pressure. No drama. There will be plenty of drama once you begin your career. You've taken exams before. Think of this exam as a cross between high school and college courses. The exams are made to test your abilities to answer their questions. Your score on the exam is a reflection only of how well you take that exam. It's not a measure of your intelligence. Sure, a successful nurse must know a lot about a lot of things (science, math, reading comprehension), but most important, a fantastic nurse must have brain and heart. A good nurse must have that balance of head and heart to show real compassion to a patient, not to mention the people skills required to intervene in a crisis and be a patient advocate. We all have different gifts. For some people, things come easily, without challenge and with very little effort. Others may have to study a bit more, but that's okay.

This test is no reflection of the kind of nurse you will become. That comes with inspiration, courage, conviction, further education, skills, practice, clinicals, and time. You can't make bread from scratch without first mixing the ingredients, allowing it to rise, punching it down, and allowing it to rise again before greasing the pan and placing it in the oven to bake. Otherwise you will be lucky to get a cracker or flatbread instead of a nice fluffy loaf. The same goes for nursing prep. There are necessary next steps.

BE CONSISTENT

Don't do anything differently the week before your exam. If you never played basketball, don't start now. If you don't eat meat, don't agree to eat a burger for the first time ever. No new vitamins, colonic cleanses, facials, exercise regimens, mystery foods, or diet fads. Pulling all-nighters is also not advisable either. Do not pack on pounds or sleep the days away to ensure extra sleep. The week before your exam, try to eat three healthy, balanced meals and healthy snacks each day. Preparing for a test isn't like marathon preparation when you stack and pack the carbs! Drink plenty of water, not excess iced teas, coffees, and sodas, as they have unwanted calories, sugar, and sodium. You don't want to be on a sugar high, with caffiene jitters and stomach rumbles on test day. Restroom passes may be frowned upon at the testing site, so don't do any smooth moves to offset your tummy. Stay away from over-the-counter medications and beverages that contain any amount of alcohol. Both are central nervous system depressants.

SLEEP EASY AND DISCONNECT

Everyone needs adequate sleep, regardless of test-taking appointments. Unfortunately, many people do not get enough sleep. Try to make yourself go to bed at least eight hours before you want to get up on test day, and get into that sleep pattern by observing it every night for at least one week before the test. Also during that week, break up with your friends for a short while—they'll be there when you finish your exam. Refrain from excessive chatting on the phone, wasting time on the internet, and outings and events with friends for just one week. Just one week.

EMERGENCY EXITS AND BULK HEAD

A few days before the exam, get together a bag of items you want to take to the exam. Be sure to wear a comfortable, breathable outfit on test day, and pack layers in case the test site is chilly. Exam day is not a fashion show or interview—you don't have to dress to impress. Instead, dress as if you were taking a long flight and you're not sure of the temperature on the airplane. Dress in layers. Avoid perfume or cologne in case you're seated near someone who might be allergic or sensitive to scents.

BE FOCUSED

For computerized exams, throwing the computer chair through a window at the testing facility is never a good idea, no matter how frustrated or stressed you might become. Breathing exercises and counting to ten will help you get through moments of frustration and eliminate harmful thoughts. If you find yourself stumped by a question and if your test permits, just take a breath and move on to the next question. If you have time, you can come back to the question later. Pack your sharpened and used (not brand new) No. 2 pencils and take plenty to spare. Recall the information that you have studied as best you can. Don't let yourself get paranoid about hidden agendas in test answers, and don't waste precious time hovering over a difficult question. Remember—these are multiple-choice questions and the answers ARE there. Cross out (mentally or physically) the wrong choices (distractors) immediately, and narrow down your choices, as discussed in Chapter 3.

When moving from section to section, focus only on the section that you are in at that moment, and then move along. For example, once you complete the Math section, think about it no more and focus on the next subject matter.

Also, pay attention to yourself. It's easy to get distracted when it seems as if others are plugging away and cranking out answers left and right and moving at a fast clip. Pay attention to where you are, your time, your focus, and your test—not to a neighbor or friend in your exam. Getting caught up in someone else's game can cost you points, time, and peace of mind.

EAT, DRINK, AND POTTY

Have a meal a few hours before your exam. In other words, don't go to a drive-thru on your way to the test site. At the same time, don't take the test on an empty stomach. You don't want to feel faint and sluggish, and you certainly don't want to become hypoglycemic. Instead, you want to feel nourished, refreshed, well-rested, confident, and content on test day. Some test takers enjoy foods that have low glycemic indices. Eating such foods helps maintain your blood sugar level, rather than causing your blood sugar to rapidly increase, peak, and then drop below normal, leaving you sluggish and potentially agitated. To avoid this crash, stay away from sweet foods like pancakes with heavy syrup, for instance. You might consider fruit, almonds, egg whites (as long as you have no allergy to nuts and are not a strict vegan), whole wheat toast with peanut butter and light jam, scones, oatmeal, and even cereal (but nothing too sugary). Acceptable foods include any food that you have had and tolerated before and any food that will not affect your blood sugar dramatically. Also, be sure to use the restroom facilities immediately before the exam.

NO WRINKLES IN TIME

The clock is ticking on exam day and there's no stopping it. It's there and it's moving—forward. You should be moving forward, too. Move carefully and thoughtfully through your exam, selecting answers, skipping around if necessary (and if it's allowed), and racking up points. Be present. Be in the moment. Be in the question. Be in the answer. Then move to the next. The clock does not care where you are or what your needs are. The clock will not applaud if you have eight minutes to spare or scold you if you are filling in the bubbles down to the very last tick of the clock. Be mindful of your time and pace yourself. That's why it's a very good idea to practice ahead of time with a timer so you can feel more confident on exam day.

AVOID WHAT-IFS

One the test is over, reward yourself with a nice meal, a beverage, a treat, or just the enjoyment of your pre-test prep mania routine. It's easy to fall into the "rush home and look up answers" trap, but that serves no point at all. Many test takers agonize and rehash the "shoulda coulda wouldas" with friends and peers, regarding the answer choices that they picked. By that time, the test is over and out of your hands, so it's best not to let anxiety get the best of you. Just go back to your normal routine. Once you receive communication that you achieved the score that you were shooting for, sure go ahead and celebrate. Then get ready for the necessary next steps. If, after receiving your score, your reality is that you now find yourself preparing for the NLN PAX-RN, NET, or TEAS exam again, that's okay too.

Keep in mind that the test does not take into consideration what life brought you on that particular test day, nor how well you prepared, how you felt, how anxious you were, the possibility of illness, sadness, stress, trauma, drama, or any other external variables. Once you've gone through the experience of taking an actual exam, some test anxiety should be alleviated because at least you know exactly what to expect.

DO YOUR BEST

Give it your all, knowing that you studied, reviewed, and practiced. Thank your family, friends and loved ones for their undying support and understanding. Now do your best and keep moving forward.

Best wishes and good luck!

About the Author

Kristen Marie Haight is a Certified Pediatric Nurse Practitioner, lecturer, and published author. Devoted to the "caring and healing profession" for nearly twenty years, her area of clinical expertise includes, but is not limited to, pediatric primary care, neurosurgery, neurology, emergency, pediatric, and neonatal critical care. As adjunct faculty, she has taught adult med-surg as well as pediatrics in the clinical and classroom settings. She earned her BSN from the College of Mount Saint Vincent, Riverdale, NY, in 1992 and her Master of Science degree from Columbia University, New York, NY, in 1997.

She began writing in 2001, added a strong medical flare in 2004, and a juvenile fiction genre in 2006. She brought forth and meshed her writing career with an already impressive advanced practice health care arena: fourteen years of primary care and nine years of a unique neurosurgical (both critical and non-acute) background. In addition to continuing her medical and non-medical writing, she has consistently maintained professional positions in both the hospital and private practice settings in Manhattan, where she served as a licensed health care provider (Registered Nurse and Nurse Practitioner), clinical expert, educator and mentor, counselor, volunteer and also having held leadership roles in a variety of settings. Her interests have always been in the ethics and sciences related to medicine and nursing care, but Ms. Haight's heart is with the preemies.

In her spare time, she has been deployed as an American Red Cross Nurse, Disaster Relief Services Volunteer, both locally and nationally as well as has served medical relief missions in Haiti (pre-earthquake). In her other spare time, she happily took on the invitation to write for The Princeton Review/Random House, early 2011, in hopes to share her extensive knowledge base and clinical skills in writing. Kristen is currently in the final stages of completing another medical manuscript and continues to advocate patient privacy rights, cancers awareness, and heart health. She knows that illness and life issues certainly do not spare health care providers or their loved ones, which keeps everyone connected and the demand for dedicated doctors and nurses high.

NOTES

NOTES

NOTES

NOTES

NOTES

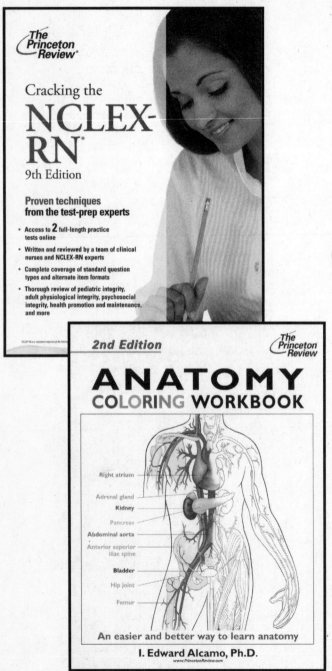
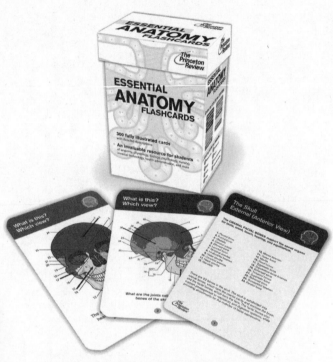
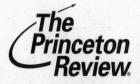